Handbook of Experimental Pharmacology

Volume 259

The *Handbook of Experimental Pharmacology* is one of the most authoritative and influential book series in pharmacology. It provides critical and comprehensive discussions of the most significant areas of pharmacological research, written by leading international authorities. Each volume in the series represents the most informative and contemporary account of its subject available, making it an unrivalled reference source.

HEP is indexed in PubMed and Scopus.

More information about this series at http://www.springer.com/series/164

Julian Gomez-Cambronero •
Michael A. Frohman
Editors

Lipid Signaling in Human Diseases

Springer

Editors
Julian Gomez-Cambronero
Department of Biochemistry
and Molecular Biology
Wright State University
Dayton, OH, USA

Michael A. Frohman
Department of Pharmacological Sciences
Stony Brook University
Stony Brook, NY, USA

ISSN 0171-2004 ISSN 1865-0325 (electronic)
Handbook of Experimental Pharmacology
ISBN 978-3-030-33667-7 ISBN 978-3-030-33668-4 (eBook)
https://doi.org/10.1007/978-3-030-33668-4

This Springer imprint is published by the registered company Springer Nature Switzerland AG.
The registered company address is: Gewerbestrasse 11, 6330 Cham, Switzerland

In memory of Dr. Julian Gomez-Cambronero

Preface

Lipid signaling, of the type covered in this HEP volume, has been a topic of investigation for upwards of three-quarters of a century, starting with early observations that acetylcholine stimulation of pancreatic slices in the presence of ^{32}P led to most of the radioactivity being incorporated into phosphatidic acid (PA) and phosphoinositides (PI), followed by the eventual discovery that elevation of intracellular calcium was triggered by PI bisphosphate hydrolysis. Many different types of lipids, lipid signals, mechanisms of coupling to receptors, and interaction with downstream effectors were subsequently uncovered, along with the families of genes responsible for signaling-activated lipid metabolism.

In this HEP volume, authors from across the field review their respective fields of expertise for what has become an enormous expanse of cell biology with profound impacts on normal and pathophysiology. Finally, under some circumstances, inhibition of some forms of lipid signaling is beneficial in the treatment of selected diseases; also discussed here is the status of small molecule therapeutics as modulators of cancer, thrombosis, autoimmunity, and neurological disease.

We start with sphingolipids, with a chapter from Dr. Sarah Spiegel in the Department of Biochemistry and Molecular Biology at Virginia Commonwealth University on the lipid sphingosine-1-phosphate (S1P) and its precursors, sphingosine and ceramide, and how their balance functions as a cellular rheostat that determines whether a cell survives or dies. S1P plays important roles in cancer (cell growth, inhibition of apoptosis, angiogenesis, and metastasis), the immune system (asthma, anaphylaxis, autoimmunity, sepsis, tissue rejection, and atherosclerosis), and development (fertility, vascular maturation, cardiac, and ear and brain development). S1P is formed inside cells by two sphingosine kinases, SphK1 and SphK2, which her lab cloned and characterized, and can be exported out by specific transporters to activate S1P's receptors in autocrine and/or paracrine manners. S1P also has intracellular targets when produced by nuclear SphK2, binding to histone deacetylases and inhibiting their activity, thus linking S1P and sphingolipid metabolism in the nucleus to gene expression and epigenetic regulation. S1P is important in cytokine signaling and NF-κB activation in inflammatory, anti-apoptotic, and immune processes.

Complementing this is a discussion by Dr. Yusuf Hannun, Director of the Stony Brook Cancer Center and Professor of Biochemistry and Cell Biology. Dr. Hannun discovered many of the bioactive sphingolipids and studied sphingolipid metabolism, structure, mechanisms, and roles in cell function. Neutral sphingomyelinase deficiency results in Niemann–Pick disease and is also involved in the regulation of cell migration and survival. His chapter delineates specific functions of individual pathways of sphingolipid metabolism, with a specific focus on sphingomyelinases and cancer biology and therapeutics. Finally, Professor Nigel Pyne at the Strathclyde Institute of Pharmacy and Biomedical Sciences in the UK reviews sphingosine kinases and isoform diversity, with special attention to inhibitors that are currently in preclinical studies for colon cancer.

Phospholipase D (PLD) lipid signaling through the production of PA first became of interest in the context of alternate ways of generating diacylglycerol kinase (DAG) via DAG kinases, as a means of activating protein kinase C. Subsequent observation of high levels of agonist-stimulated PLD activity in secretory cells and the identification of ARF-family GTPases as direct activators of PLD created excitement concerning the potential role of PLD in membrane vesicle trafficking and regulated exocytosis. Dr. Michael Frohman's research group at Stony Brook University cloned the mammalian PLD genes and was involved in the first studies of "knockout" PLD mice and PLD-specific inhibitors. He reviews here the use of PLD inhibitors to treat thrombotic disease and cancer progression, linking long-standing cell biological findings to human therapeutic opportunities. Another approach to PLD function is presented by Dr. Julian Gomez-Cambronero, the Brage Golding Distinguished Professor of Research and Professor of Biochemistry and Molecular Biology at Wright State University, on the roles of PLD in cell migration as related to cardiovascular repair after injury and cancer metastasis and the potential for use of PLD inhibitors in the clinic. Finally, Dr. Nicholas Vitale, at the Institute of Cellular and Integrative Neurosciences in Strasbourg, summarizes two decades of investigation into the role of PLD in regulated exocytosis in the central and peripheral nervous system in connection to neurodegenerative diseases and some forms of intellectual disability.

Complementary to the actions of the phospholipases, lipid kinases are also key in signaling pathways. Here, Dr. Isabel Mérida, Group Leader in the Department of Immunology and Oncology, Centro Nacional de Biotecnología (CNB-CSIC), Madrid, describes the contribution of DAG kinase-regulated mechanisms to T cell activation and oncogenic transformation, with focus on inhibitors and their potential therapeutic use. Paralleling this topic, Dr. Ana Carrera, a Group Leader at the same institution, covers class I phosphoinositide 3-kinases (PI3K) at the interface of immunology and cancer.

Turning to secreted signaling lipids, Dr. Jeffrey Travers, Professor and Chair of Pharmacology and Toxicology at Wright State University, reviews the biochemistry and pharmacology of the lipid mediator platelet-activating factor (PAF), which in combination with the related oxidized glycerophosphocholines (Ox-GPCs) is produced in response to numerous pro-oxidative environmental stimuli from UV radiation to chemotherapy and cigarette smoke exposure.

Therapeutics in this field are focused on inhibitors of the PAF receptor as anti-inflammatory therapeutics. Another important category of secreted signaling lipids are the lysophospholipids, as reviewed by Dr. Andrew Morris, Professor of Pharmacology at the University of Kentucky and the co-discoverer of the mammalian phospholipase D gene family with Dr. Frohman. Synthesis and inactivation of bioactive lysophospholipids is important in the setting of cardiovascular disease. Dr. Morris discusses their contributions to CVD genetics/functional genomics, with special attention to the lipid phosphate phosphatase genes in determining cardiovascular disease risk.

Dr. Miriam Greenberg, Professor at Wayne State University, reviews genetic, molecular, and cell biological tools of the yeast system and relevant mammalian cell cultures to elucidate the essential functions of inositol phospholipids and metabolites and the cellular consequences of inositol-depleting drugs, with implications for understanding the pathology underlying cardiovascular disorders and the therapeutic mechanisms of action of drugs used in the treatment of psychiatric disorders. In a newer and fascinating field, Dr. Vanina Zaremberg, Associate Professor of Biochemistry at the University of Calgary, reviews the first and rate-limiting step in the synthesis of all glycerolipids as catalyzed by glycerol 3-phosphate acyltransferase (GPAT) and the mode of action of the lipid analog, edelfosine, a prototypical member of the alkylphosphocholine class of cancer chemotherapeutic drugs. Although edelfosine and its analogs show promise for the treatment of cancers, it has been difficult to further optimize their efficacy, as the cellular target of this class of drugs has yet to be identified. Based on the results of unbiased yeast genetic screens, new hypotheses are being tested involving studies on lipid microdomains, sterol traffic, and phosphatidic acid signaling in yeast.

The last two chapters address the nuclear trafficking of lipids, from Dr. Lucio Cocco, Professor of Biomedical and Neuromotor Sciences at the University of Bologna, and Dr. Pascal Zimmerman, Director of Research at the Cancer Research Center of Marseille. Dr. Cocco discovered nuclear signaling via inositol lipid cycling and signaling activity of polyphosphoinositides during myogenic differentiation, giving new insight to mechanisms underlying some myotonic dystrophies. He has also studied nuclear PLC and phosphoinositide signaling during hemopoietic differentiation in health and disease, particularly myelodysplastic syndrome (MDS). Dr. Zimmerman studies spatiotemporal regulation of cell signaling, with emphasis on phosphoinositides in the context of cell signaling and cell–cell communication as it affects cancer pathways, and with a new focus on exosomes and lipid signaling in exosome biogenesis (particularly in connection to PLD and PA) in cancer propagation and drugs that can affect these processes.

Taken together, the chapters offered here present a broad field of current areas of investigation in the field of lipid signaling and offer windows into the areas of active research and therapeutics that are or will be under clinical investigation in the coming years.

Dayton, OH, USA — Julian Gomez-Cambronero
Stony Brook, NY, USA — Michael A. Frohman

Julian Gomez-Cambronero Passing

Of great sadness, Julian Gomez-Cambronero became afflicted with a serious illness during the preparation of this volume and passed away on November 12, 2018. Almost all of the senior authors in this volume knew him well, some for many decades, and felt his loss acutely. Julian is survived by his loving and always supportive wife Teresa Madrid and his two children, Julia and David (Melissa), who illuminated his life and for whom he cared for deeply. I never met Julian's family, but felt a connection to them nonetheless through the holiday photographs Julian sent each year, with his pride and love for them demonstrative in the accompanying text.

Julian was the Brage Golding Distinguished Professor of Research in the Department of Biochemistry and Molecular Biology at Wright State University, where he had been a faculty member for 23 years. Julian had come to the USA from Spain, his native country, where he earned his PhD in Biochemistry and Immunology at the Complutense University of Madrid in 1986, following which he undertook postdoctoral studies at the University of Connecticut.

Despite his long sojourn in the USA, Julian maintained a connection to his homeland, and in particular, his hometown, Manzanares, which bestowed upon him the Professional Achievement "Sembrador" Award in 2004, named him as the city's "Hijo Predilecto" (Favorite Son) in a grand ceremony in 2014 and celebrated him as Keynote Speaker in the 2016 Patron Saint festivities. Julian even constructed a scale model of the solar system in one of the city's public parks in remembrance of the time he had spent with his daughter Julia on her science homework and initiated the formation of a science museum for children there based on his passion for supporting early childhood education as a means to create the researchers of the future.

Speaking from my own experience, Julian was an outrageously charismatic, energetic, and optimistic individual. He had an unquenchable enthusiasm for science, for the mentoring and advancement of his trainees, and for collaboratively engaging with his colleagues. Over our 20+ years of professional interaction, which involved two co-publications and many meetings in person at conferences, there were numerous moments of stimulated discussion and humor.

Julian was the first person I thought of to be editor for this HEP topic. He had so many friends in the field and had such enthusiasm for it that he immediately came up with dozens of potential authors targeted to create a "Best of" list for lipid signaling. Julian will be missed by all of us.

Stony Brook, NY, USA Michael A. Frohman

Contents

Part I

New Roles for Sphingolipid Signaling and Cell Function

Role of Sphingosine Kinase 1 and Sphingosine-1-Phosphate Axis in Hepatocellular Carcinoma

Michael Maceyka, Timothy Rohrbach, Sheldon Milstien, and Sarah Spiegel

Contents

Abstract

Hepatocellular carcinoma (HCC) is primarily diagnosed in the latter stages of disease progression and is the third leading cause of cancer deaths worldwide. Thus, there is a need to find biomarkers of early HCC as well as the development of more effective treatments for the disease. Sphingosine-1-phosphate (S1P) is a pleiotropic lipid signaling molecule produced by two isoforms of sphingosine kinase (SphK1 and SphK2) that is involved in regulation of many aspects of mammalian physiology and pathophysiology, including inflammation, epithelial and endothelial barrier function, cancer, and metastasis, among many others. Abundant evidence indicates that SphK1 and S1P promote cancer progression and metastasis in multiple types of cancers. However, the role of SphK/S1P in HCC is less well studied. Here, we review the current state of knowledge of SphKs and S1P in HCC, including evidence for the correlation of SphK1 expression and S1P levels with progression of HCC and negative outcomes,

M. Maceyka · T. Rohrbach · S. Milstien · S. Spiegel (✉)
Department of Biochemistry and Molecular Biology, Massey Cancer Center, Virginia Commonwealth University School of Medicine, Richmond, VA, USA
e-mail: sarah.spiegel@vcuhealth.org

J. Gomez-Cambronero, M. A. Frohman (eds.), *Lipid Signaling in Human Diseases*, Handbook of Experimental Pharmacology 259, https://doi.org/10.1007/164_2019_217

and discuss how this information could lead to the design of more effective diagnostic and treatment modalities for HCC.

Keywords
Hepatocellular carcinoma · S1P receptors · Sphingosine kinase · Sphingosine-1-phosphate (S1P)

Abbreviations

HCC	Hepatocellular carcinoma
NAFLD	Nonalcoholic fatty liver disease
NASH	Nonalcoholic steatohepatitis
S1P	Sphingosine-1-phosphate
S1PR	S1P receptor
SphK	Sphingosine kinase
Spns2	Spinster 2

1 Introduction

Hepatocellular carcinoma (HCC) is cancer of the liver arising from malignant hepatocytes and accounts for nearly 90% of all primary liver cancers. HCC has a high level of morbidity, being the third leading cause of cancer deaths (El-Serag 2011). Due in part to both delayed diagnosis of HCC as well as its general aggressiveness, the median 5-year survival rate is less than 7%. Major risk factors for HCC include hepatitis virus B and C infections, overconsumption of alcohol, and nonalcoholic fatty liver disease (NAFLD), particularly when it progresses to nonalcoholic steatohepatitis (NASH). NAFLD/NASH are often associated with obesity and type 2 diabetes, and the rapid increase in the occurrence of these two disorders may contribute to the rise in non-viral associated HCC observed in the industrialized countries (Satapathy and Sanyal 2015). The hallmarks of NAFLD progression including insulin resistance, oxidative stress, and inflammation are all factors that also promote cancer initiation and progression (Cohen et al. 2011).

Sphingolipids, including sphingomyelin and glycosphingolipids, are essential lipid components of mammalian membranes. Sphingolipids consist of various head groups attached to ceramide, which is structurally analogous to the glycerolipid backbone diacylglycerol and, like diacylglycerol, is a second messenger involved in signaling pathways, typically promoting apoptosis and suppressing cell growth (Newton et al. 2015; Coant et al. 2017; Ogretmen 2018). Deacylation of ceramide yields sphingosine that has also been implicated in cell signaling. Sphingosine can be reacylated back to ceramide by a salvage pathway or phosphorylated by one of two sphingosine kinases (SphK1 and SphK2) forming sphingosine-1-phosphate (S1P). There are two fates for S1P: irreversible degradation by S1P lyase or dephosphorylation back to sphingosine. The metabolism of S1P is critical because S1P is a potent pleiotropic signaling molecule that regulates many physiological and pathological processes that are important for cancer including cell growth, proliferation, and cell motility, immune cell recruitment, epithelial and endothelial barrier function, and angiogenesis and lymphangiogenesis, among many others (Ogretmen 2018; Pyne and Pyne 2010; Kunkel et al. 2013; Maceyka and Spiegel 2014). Multiple stimuli, including growth factors, cytokines, and hormones, stimulate phosphorylation and activation of cytosolic SphK1 leading to its translocation to the plasma membrane where its substrate sphingosine resides and/or is generated (Maceyka and Spiegel 2014). S1P can be transported out of the cell, either by a specific S1P transporter called spinster 2 (Spns2), a member of the major facilitator superfamily of transporters, or via a subset of ATP-binding cassette (ABC) transporters, including ABCC1 and ABCG2 (Takabe and Spiegel 2014). This S1P can activate a family of five, S1P-specific G protein-coupled receptors (S1PR1–5) that mediate many of its known actions in an autocrine or paracrine manner, termed "inside-out signaling by S1P" (Takabe et al. 2008). These receptors are differentially expressed and couple to a wide array of heterotrimeric G proteins, leading to a diverse, and at times opposing, range of cellular and physiological responses (Pyne and Pyne 2010; Maceyka and Spiegel 2014). S1P produced inside cells also has intracellular actions; however, only a handful of intracellular targets and pathways have been identified so far. For example, S1P produced by activation of SphK1 binds to and activates proteins such as TNF receptor-associated factor 2 (TRAF2) (Alvarez et al. 2010; Park et al. 2015, 2016; Liu et al. 2017), a key adaptor molecule in TNFR signaling complexes that promotes downstream signaling cascades leading to activation of the master transcription factor NF-κB (Alvarez et al. 2010; Park et al. 2015). S1P can also activate NF-κB through formation of a signaling complex, consisting of S1P, TRAF2, and RIP1 that further associates with heat shock proteins GRP94 and HSP90α and IRE1α (Park et al. 2016). S1P produced in the nucleus by SphK2 is an endogenous histone deacetylase inhibitor (Hait et al. 2009, 2014; Nguyen-Tran et al. 2014; Nagahashi et al. 2015; Gardner et al. 2016) and also binds to hTERT and increases telomerase activity and enhances cancer cell growth (Panneer Selvam et al. 2015).

S1P is present at high levels in the blood and lymph, and the functions of S1P and its receptors as well as Spns2 in the regulation of immune cell trafficking have recently been implicated in tumor immunology and metastasis (Fang et al. 2017; van der Weyden et al. 2017). Moreover, numerous studies have also shown that expression of SphK1 and S1P promotes progression and metastasis of many types of cancers and correlates with poor prognosis (Ogretmen 2018; Pyne and Pyne 2010; Maceyka and Spiegel 2014). However, while the SphK1/S1P/S1PR signaling axis has been associated with initiation, progression, and chemoresistance of a variety of cancers, much less is known about its role in HCC. SphK1 and S1P expression have been correlated with initiation and progression of NAFLD, which is a risk factor for HCC, and thus, it is not surprising that they would also play a role in HCC. Here we discuss current evidence indicating that SphK1 and S1P are upregulated in human HCC patients and that they may serve as valuable biomarkers for early stage disease detection. We also examine the molecular mechanisms in HCC leading to SphK1/S1P upregulation, evidence that their upregulation promotes epithelial-mesenchymal transition and HCC progression, and the participation of downstream effectors of SphK1/S1P in HCC progression.

2 SphK1 and S1P Are Upregulated in HCC

Several studies have suggested that the SphK1/S1P axis could play a role in the promotion of HCC based on the observations that SphK1 is overexpressed in HCC cell lines and in patient samples and that S1P is increased in both patient serum and HCC tumors (Shi et al. 2015; Cai et al. 2017). For example, using immunohistochemistry techniques, both SphK1 and S1P levels were observed to be upregulated in HCC (Reynolds et al. 2017). Moreover, expression of SphK1 in HCC tumors was higher than in normal adjacent tissues, and SphK1 expression positively correlated with tumor size, tumor stage, and histological differentiation and negatively correlated with overall survival (Cai et al. 2017). Similarly, it was shown that SphK1 levels correlated with increased recurrence and decreased survival of patients with portal vein tumor thrombosis after primary tumor resection (Shi et al. 2015). However, in one study, though HCC tissues had elevated levels of SphKs, they had reduced levels of S1P compared to normal adjacent tissues (Uranbileg et al. 2016), findings that were linked to the elevated expression of the S1P-degrading enzyme, S1P lyase. These results highlight the importance of localized coupling of S1P synthesis, release, and S1PR activation that may not correlate with bulk S1P levels but are still sufficient to promote S1P signaling and HCC progression. Importantly, however, several studies have shown by mass spectrometry that serum levels of S1P are elevated in HCC compared to patients with cirrhosis (Ressom et al. 2012) and significantly elevated compared to normal controls (Grammatikos et al. 2016; Zeng et al. 2016). These results suggest that serum S1P may be a useful diagnostic marker for patients with liver disease that has progressed to HCC, particularly for patients at risk for liver cancer given its typically late stage of diagnosis.

3 Inflammation and Fibrosis

Many studies have linked SphK1 and S1P to the promotion of inflammatory responses, and it is well known that inflammation can promote the initiation and progression of cancer (Kunkel et al. 2013; Pyne et al. 2016). Indeed, several studies have also linked SphK1/S1P signaling to liver inflammation, fibrosis, and NAFLD/NASH (Rohrbach et al. 2017). For example, SphK1 is elevated in NAFLD patients and in obese mice that have many of the hallmarks of the disease, including NF-κB activation, elevated cytokine production, and immune cell infiltration (Geng et al. 2015) (Fig. 1). SphK1 null mice are resistant to these obesity-driven effects, and

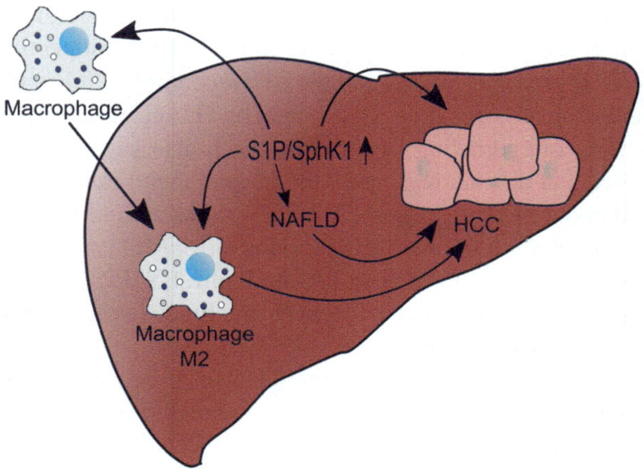

Fig. 1 Role of S1P in promotion of liver cancer. SphK1 and S1P have been shown to promote NAFLD, which is a risk factor for HCC development. Moreover, increased SphK1 and S1P production by the liver can enhance recruitment of macrophages that migrate to the tumor site, remain there, and aid in angiogenesis, termed tumor-associated macrophages (TAMs), and are thought to express an M2 phenotype

inflammatory mediator production in hepatocytes is reduced when S1PR1 is knocked down. Similarly, liver fibrosis in humans and in CCl4-induced fibrosis in mice have been correlated with increased levels of S1P, which stimulate fibrotic angiogenesis through activation of S1PR1 and S1PR3 (Yang et al. 2013).

Myeloid cells, particularly tumor-associated macrophages (TAMS), are frequently increased in the HCC microenvironment and are associated with worse prognosis (Wan et al. 2015). Although the role of the SphK/S1P axis in recruitment and function of TAMS has not been investigated in HCC, in many other cancers, S1P secreted by the tumor due to elevation of SphK1 plays a key role in the recruitment and phenotypic shift of the tumor macrophages from pro-inflammatory (M1) to anti-inflammatory (M2) that promotes tumorigenesis and angiogenesis (Rodriguez et al. 2016; Mrad et al. 2016) (Fig. 1).

4 Regulation of the S1P Signaling Axis in HCC

The observations that SphK1 and S1P are elevated in HCC tumor samples suggest that the tumors have mechanisms for increasing S1P signaling. One group has shown that the HCC cell line HepG2 secretes S1P and that inhibition of this secretion blocks cell proliferation that can be rescued by exogenous S1P, indicative of an autocrine S1P signaling loop (Jin et al. 2016). They linked the secretion of S1P to AKR1B10, a protein involved in lipid metabolism that is elevated in HCC, as siRNA against AKR1B10 reduced S1P levels and cell growth. They further showed that high expression of AKR1B10 correlated with both more negative outcomes and higher levels of S1P in tumor but not peripheral liver tissue. This study utilized an ELISA method to measure S1P that is not as sensitive as mass spectrometry methods and did not detect any changes in S1P synthesis or degradation that could affect S1P levels, although other studies have implicated pathways that control SphK1 expression in HCC. For example, similar to many other growth factors, hepatocyte growth factor

(HGF) stimulates SphK activity, S1P production, and motility in HCC cells that can be blocked by downregulating SphK1. HGF induced translocation of SphK1, the S1P transporter Spns2, and the S1P receptor S1PR1 to the lamellipodia at the leading edge of moving lung vascular cells (Fu et al. 2016). This not only reaffirms the inside-out signaling hypothesis, but it also suggests that the pro-motility signaling occurs at distinct regions of the plasma membrane to promote directed motility up a chemoattractant gradient. Similarly, motility and invasion of several HCC cell lines were dependent on overexpression of SphK1 and signaling via S1PR1 (Bao et al. 2012), supporting a role for the SphK1/S1P/S1PR1 axis in liver metastasis and suggesting that this axis might be an attractive therapeutic target for the development of new anti-HCC drugs.

Expression of highly upregulated in liver cancer (HULC), which was originally identified as a very highly overexpressed long noncoding RNA in HCC, was suggested to correlate with both SphK1 mRNA and ELISA-measured S1P levels in patient samples (Lu et al. 2016). Functionally, HULC-induced angiogenesis in situ and in HCC xenografts depended on SphK1 expression. Mechanistically, HULC sequestered miR-107, increasing the transcription of E2F1, which activated the transcription of SphK1. Together, these results suggest that HULC promotes tumor angiogenesis in liver cancer in part by upregulation of SphK1 (Lu et al. 2016). Another miR, miR-506, was also claimed to downregulate SphK1 mRNA and protein, to reduce secreted S1P in vitro, and to negatively correlate with mRNA levels of SphK1 in clinical HCC samples (Lu et al. 2015). Thus, it was proposed that miR-506 depresses angiogenesis of liver cancer by targeting the 3′UTR of SphK1 mRNA. Interestingly, a second group has found a similar downregulation of miR-506 in pancreatic cancer that correlated with the upregulation of SphK1/AKT/NF-κB signaling (Li et al. 2016). Further studies are needed to support the significance of these miRs in HCC and conclusively demonstrate their specific targets.

5 Downstream Effectors/Pathways of SphK1/S1P that Promote HCC

5.1 S1PRs

The most obvious and druggable proximal targets of the S1P signaling axis are the cell surface S1P receptors, which have been linked to progression of many cancers (Ogretmen 2018; Pyne and Pyne 2010; Maceyka and Spiegel 2014; Patmanathan et al. 2017). Indeed, several studies have correlated expression of S1PR1 to HCC progression and poor prognoses. Consistent with previous studies suggesting that SphK1 produced S1P promotes tumor cell migration and invasion by activating S1PR1 (Bao et al. 2012), in diethylnitrosamine-induced HCC in mice, SphK1, SphK2, S1PR1, and S1PR3 were upregulated, while the S1P-degrading enzyme

S1P lyase was downregulated (Sanchez et al. 2018). Other studies also suggested that S1P-S1PR1 signaling is involved in the progression of HCC in patients. miR-148a dysregulation discriminated overall survival and recurrence-free survival rates of HCC. In human HCC samples, both ubiquitin-specific protease 4 (USP4) and S1PR1 were identified as targets of miR-148a. USP4 and S1PR1 were upregulated in mesenchymal-type liver tumor cells with miR-148a dysregulation, facilitating migration and proliferation of tumor cells, though a significant negative correlation was not found between miR148a and S1PR1 in three heterotopic patient-derived HCC xenografts (Heo et al. 2014). Another putative tumor-suppressing microRNA, miR-363, decreased S1PR1 expression by binding its 3′UTR and also inhibited the proliferation of HCC cells (Zhou et al. 2014).

5.2 The S1P Signaling Axis Promotes EMT in HCC

The epithelial-mesenchymal transition (EMT), a process by which epithelial cells dedifferentiate to multipotent mesenchymal stem cells, is a hallmark of cancer initiation (Kalluri and Weinberg 2009). Cells that undergo EMT lose the expression of epithelial markers, polarity, and become more motile. Several studies suggest that the S1P signaling axis promotes EMT in HCC. For example, inhibition of SphK activity with N,N-dimethylsphingosine in HCC cells was originally shown to upregulate liver-specific markers of differentiation, including albumin and alpha-fetoprotein (AFP) (Osawa et al. 2001). Intriguingly, in a set of 77 HCC patient samples, not only did expression of SphK1 and SphK2 correlate with decreased differentiation so did expression of S1P lyase. However, in this sample set, there was no correlation between SphK1/2 expression and S1P levels in the tumor (Uranbileg et al. 2016). Once again, these results suggest that localized S1P production rather than absolute levels may be critical to its function in promoting HCC.

It was recently shown that SphK1 induces the EMT in HepG2 cells by accelerating lysosomal degradation of the cell-cell adhesion molecule E-cadherin (CDH1), thus facilitating their invasion and metastasis (Liu et al. 2017). Of note, in HepG2 cells, SphK1-produced S1P bound to TRAF2 and stimulated lysine 63-linked ubiquitination and activation of beclin1 that in turn stimulated autophagic degradation of E-cadherin (Liu et al. 2017). These intriguing findings define a novel mechanism for the regulation of the EMT via SphK1-TRAF2-beclin1-E-cadherin signaling cascade in HCC cells. Moreover, this study suggests that inhibition of SphK1 to attenuate autophagy may be a promising strategy for treatment of HCC. In agreement, a non-isozyme-specific SphK inhibitor promoted the Wnt5a-dependent degradation of the tumor-promoter β-catenin and inhibited HepG2 cell proliferation (Liu et al. 2016). Another group put forward a different mechanism to explain how S1P induces the EMT in HCC showing that signaling through S1PR1 stimulated the MMP7-dependent shedding of syndecan-1, leading to the activation of the TGF-β signaling pathway and the promotion of the EMT phenotype (Zeng et al. 2016) (Fig. 2). Although there is strong evidence for EMT in HCC patients, so far, data are missing that demonstrate that the process of EMT is reversible after intrahepatic or

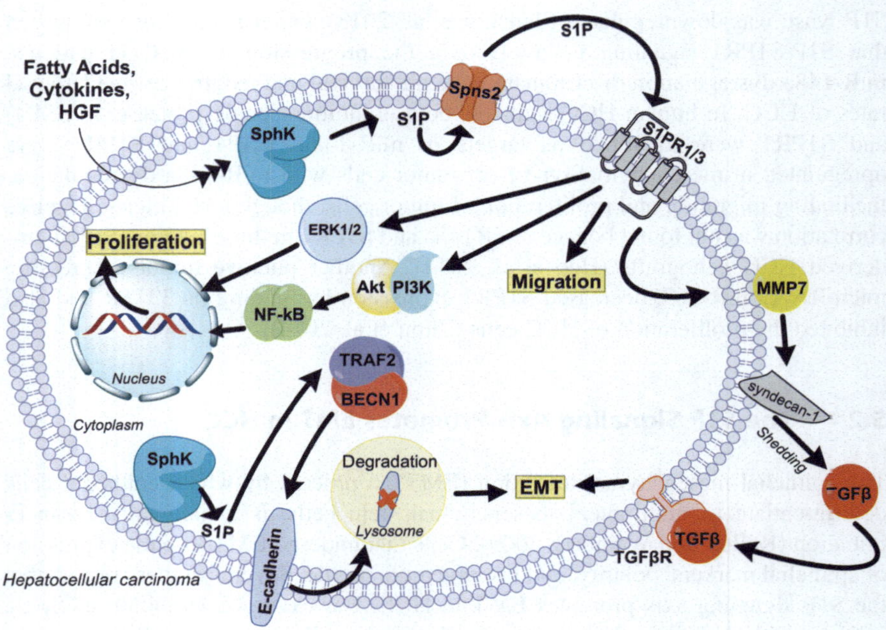

Fig. 2 S1P signaling in HCC progression. S1P can regulate signaling and physiological processes in several pathways to promote HCC. As indicated in the text, these include increasing cell motility and proliferation through S1PR1/3 activation, S1PR1/3-mediated activation of ERK and AKT, degradation of E-cadherin to promote EMT, and proteolysis of syndecan-1 to induce HGF signaling. The EMT can be regulated by a unique pathway involving the SphK1-TRAF2-beclin1-E-cadherin signaling cascade in HCC cells

even distal metastatic colonization. Future studies are needed to clarify whether targeting the SphK/S1P axis and inhibition of EMT could lead to development of effective therapies against HCC.

6 Inhibition of the S1P Signaling Axis as Treatment for HCC

The studies discussed clearly demonstrate that SphK1 and S1P signaling axis are associated with and likely promote the initiation and progression of HCC. Therefore, it has been suggested that inhibiting SphK1 might be a useful approach for treatment of HCC. Preclinical studies have suggested that effects of drugs that reduce HCC tumor cell growth, such as melatonin (Sanchez et al. 2018) or the natural prenylflavonoid icaritin (Lu et al. 2017), might be due to inhibition of SphK1 and decreased activation of S1PRs. Several groups have investigated the efficacy of inhibiting S1P signaling more directly in vitro and for treatment of tumor-bearing mice. It has been shown that the dual SphK1/2 inhibitor SKI-II acts synergistically with 5-fluorouracil (5-FU), a common drug used for the treatment of advanced HCC, to both promote HCC cell death and inhibit migration of HCC cells through downstream inhibition of FAK, ERK, and NF-κB (Grbcic et al. 2017). Similar effects were obtained when SKI-II was used in combination with the MEK1/2 inhibitor U0126 (Zhang et al. 2013) (Table 1). It has also been shown that SKI-II, alone or in combination with the ROS-generating drug selenite, is effective at killing Huh7 HCC cells, but not non-tumorigenic hepatocyte cells (Chatzakos et al. 2012). Interestingly, ABC294640, which was developed as a SphK2 inhibitor and decreases serum S1P levels, was found to be effective in two HCC xenograft models when used in combination with sorafenib, a multikinase inhibitor and emerging drug for treatment HCC (Beljanski et al. 2011). It was further shown that ABC294640 decreased the level of S1P in the xenograft tumors themselves (Table 1). Furthermore, ABC294640 is currently in a phase II clinical trial for the treatment of patients with sorafenib-resistant HCC (https://clinicaltrials.gov/ct2/show/NCT02939807).

Several studies examined the potential of FTY720 as a therapeutic option for HCC. FTY720 is a prodrug that is phosphorylated by SphK2 to the S1P analog FTY720-phosphate, which acts a functional antagonist for S1PR1 (Brinkmann et al. 2010) and is also a class I HDAC inhibitor (Hait et al. 2015). FTY720 is orally available, generally well tolerated, and already widely used for treatment of multiple sclerosis. As such, it is an attractive drug for cancer chemotherapy, and it has been found to effectively inhibit proliferation of many types of cancer cells. In HCC xenograft models, FTY720 administration inhibited tumor growth, tumor microvessel density, and metastases (Ho et al. 2005), effects that were linked to inhibition of AKT activation (Lee et al. 2004). In an orthotopic rat model, FTY720 was shown to reduce both intrahepatic and lung metastases as well as reducing tumor angiogenesis, likely through its function as a S1PR1 modulator (Li et al. 2012) (Table 1). Consistent with these results, FTY720 also decreased circulating endothelial progenitor cells. In this model, FTY720 suppressed tumor proliferation index, as well as activation of AKT and FAK (Ng et al. 2007). FTY720 also effectively downregulated S1PR1, decreased cell migration and ERK activation, and markedly extended life span in rats whose cancerous liver was transplanted with a non-cancerous one (Ushitora et al. 2009). This result is important as liver transplantation after cancer resection can provide long-term survival if recurrence can be avoided. While the clinical translation of FTY720 for cancer treatment is currently limited due to its immune suppression effects, future studies aimed at more complete understanding of the mechanism of action of FTY720, developing approaches for its specific delivery, and reducing effective concentrations and its immunosuppressive effects by using it in synergistic combinations with other drugs could enhance its rapid acceptance as an important anti-HCC drug.

Table 1 Compounds that target the S1P axis in liver fibrosis and in preclinical HCC animal models

Compound	Target(s)	Mechanism	Effects	References
N,N-dimethylsphingosine	SphK1/SphK2	SphK1 (Ki = 5 μM) and PKC inhibitor	Blocked bone marrow-derived mesenchymal stem cell differentiation to myofibroblasts during liver injury	Yang et al. (2012)
PF-543	SphK1	SphK1-specific inhibitor (Ki = 3.6 nM)	Reduced liver fibrosis	Gonzalez-Fernandez et al. (2017)
SEW2871	S1PR1	Agonist (EC50 = 14–140 nM)	Reduced hepatic parenchymal damage and fibrosis	Ding et al. (2016)
VPC23019	S1PR1/3	Antagonist (pKi = 7.9/5.9 for S1PR1/3)	Reduced liver fibrosis	Yang et al. (2013)
W146	S1PR1	Antagonist (Ki = 10–20 nM)	Reduced liver fibrosis	Yang et al. (2012)
JTE-013	S1PR2	Antagonist (Ki = 17 nM)	Reduced hepatic inflammation and fibrosis in mice with BDL ligation	Yang et al. (2015)
			Reduced bile acid-induced cholangiocyte proliferation	Wang et al. (2017)
SKI-II	SphK1/SphK2	SphK inhibitor (IC50 = 16 μM for SphK1; 8 μM for SphK2)	Reduced survival and migration of HCC cells	Lu et al. (2017) and Zhang et al. (2013)
			Reduced liver injury	Yang et al. (2013)
FTY720/FTY720-P	S1PR1,3,4,5	S1PR1 agonist/functional antagonist of S1PR1, 3, 4, 5 HDAC inhibitor	Reduced intrahepatic and lung metastases in orthotopic rat model	Li et al. (2012)
			Extended life span of tumor-bearing rats	Ushitora et al. (2009)
ABC294640	SphK2	SphK2 inhibitor	Reduced HCC xenograft in mice	Beljanski et al. (2011)
ABC294640	SphK2	SphK2 inhibitor	Phase II clinical trial for sorafenib-resistant HCC patients	https://clinicaltrials.gov/ct2/show/NCT02939807

7 Future Perspectives

That multiple mechanisms that promote HCC converge on the activation of the S1P signaling axis suggests that targeting this axis may prove therapeutically useful. S1P is elevated in patient tumors, as is the enzyme that produces it, SphK1, indicating it may be a node for HCC progression and thus a promising drug target. Tumor profiling and published preclinical studies with the functional S1PR1 antagonist FTY720 suggest that S1PR1 may also be a target for HCC treatment. The results discussed here indicate the need for further studies of inhibition of the SphK/S1P/S1PR signaling axis as one arm of a combination therapy for the treatment of this deadly disease.

Acknowledgments This work was supported by National Institutes of Health Grant R01 GM043880 to S.S. T.R. was supported by T32 training grant in Digestive Disease and Liver Disease 5T32DK007150-39.

Conflict of Interest Statement The authors declare that they have no conflicts of interest with the contents of this article.

References

Alvarez SE, Harikumar KB, Hait NC, Allegood J, Strub GM, Kim EY, Maceyka M, Jiang H, Luo C, Kordula T, Milstien S, Spiegel S (2010) Sphingosine-1-phosphate is a missing cofactor for the E3 ubiquitin ligase TRAF2. Nature 465:1084–1088

Bao M, Chen Z, Xu Y, Zhao Y, Zha R, Huang S, Liu L, Chen T, Li J, Tu H, He X (2012) Sphingosine kinase 1 promotes tumour cell migration and invasion via the S1P/EDG1 axis in hepatocellular carcinoma. Liver Int 32:331–338

Beljanski V, Lewis CS, Smith CD (2011) Antitumor activity of sphingosine kinase 2 inhibitor ABC294640 and sorafenib in hepatocellular carcinoma xenografts. Cancer Biol Ther 11:524–534

Brinkmann V, Billich A, Baumruker T, Heining P, Schmouder R, Francis G, Aradhye S, Burtin P (2010) Fingolimod (FTY720): discovery and development of an oral drug to treat multiple sclerosis. Nat Rev Drug Discov 9:883–897

Cai H, Xie X, Ji L, Ruan X, Zheng Z (2017) Sphingosine kinase 1: a novel independent prognosis biomarker in hepatocellular carcinoma. Oncol Lett 13:2316–2322

Chatzakos V, Rundlof AK, Ahmed D, de Verdier PJ, Flygare J (2012) Inhibition of sphingosine kinase 1 enhances cytotoxicity, ceramide levels and ROS formation in liver cancer cells treated with selenite. Biochem Pharmacol 84:712–721

Coant N, Sakamoto W, Mao C, Hannun YA (2017) Ceramidases, roles in sphingolipid metabolism and in health and disease. Adv Biol Regul 63:122–131

Cohen JC, Horton JD, Hobbs HH (2011) Human fatty liver disease: old questions and new insights. Science 332:1519–1523

Ding BS, Liu CH, Sun Y, Chen Y, Swendeman SL, Jung B, Chavez D, Cao Z, Christoffersen C, Nielsen LB, Schwab SR, Rafii S, Hla T (2016) HDL activation of endothelial sphingosine-1-phosphate receptor-1 (S1P1) promotes regeneration and suppresses fibrosis in the liver. JCI Insight 1:e87058

El-Serag HB (2011) Hepatocellular carcinoma. N Engl J Med 365:1118–1127
Fang V, Chaluvadi VS, Ramos-Perez WD, Mendoza A, Baeyens A, Rivera R, Chun J, Cammer M, Schwab SR (2017) Gradients of the signaling lipid S1P in lymph nodes position natural killer cells and regulate their interferon-gamma response. Nat Immunol 18:15–25
Fu P, Ebenezer DL, Berdyshev EV, Bronova IA, Shaaya M, Harijith A, Natarajan V (2016) Role of sphingosine kinase 1 and S1P transporter Spns2 in HGF-mediated lamellipodia formation in lung endothelium. J Biol Chem 291:27187–27203
Gardner NM, Riley RT, Showker JL, Voss KA, Sachs AJ, Maddox JR, Gelineau-van Waes JB (2016) Elevated nuclear and cytoplasmic FTY720-phosphate in mouse embryonic fibroblasts suggests the potential for multiple mechanisms in FTY720-induced neural tube defects. Toxicol Sci 150:161–168
Geng T, Sutter A, Harland MD, Law BA, Ross JS, Lewin D, Palanisamy A, Russo SB, Chavin KD, Cowart LA (2015) SphK1 mediates hepatic inflammation in a mouse model of NASH induced by high saturated fat feeding and initiates proinflammatory signaling in hepatocytes. J Lipid Res 56:2359–2371
Gonzalez-Fernandez B, Sanchez DI, Crespo I, San-Miguel B, Alvarez M, Tunon MJ, Gonzalez-Gallego J (2017) Inhibition of the SphK1/S1P signaling pathway by melatonin in mice with liver fibrosis and human hepatic stellate cells. Biofactors 43:272–282
Grammatikos G, Dietz J, Ferreiros N, Koch A, Dultz G, Bon D, Karakasiliotis I, Lutz T, Knecht G, Gute P, Herrmann E, Zeuzem S, Mavromara P, Sarrazin C, Pfeilschifter J (2016) Persistence of HCV in acutely-infected patients depletes C24-ceramide and upregulates sphingosine and sphinganine serum levels. Int J Mol Sci 17:18095–18105
Grbcic P, Tomljanovic I, Klobucar M, Kraljevic Pavelic S, Lucin K, Sedic M (2017) Dual sphingosine kinase inhibitor SKI-II enhances sensitivity to 5-fluorouracil in hepatocellular carcinoma cells via suppression of osteopontin and FAK/IGF-1R signalling. Biochem Biophys Res Commun 487:782–788
Hait NC, Allegood J, Maceyka M, Strub GM, Harikumar KB, Singh SK, Luo C, Marmorstein R, Kordula T, Milstien S, Spiegel S (2009) Regulation of histone acetylation in the nucleus by sphingosine-1-phosphate. Science 325:1254–1257
Hait NC, Wise LE, Allegood JC, O'Brien M, Avni D, Reeves TM, Knapp PE, Lu J, Luo C, Miles MF, Milstien S, Lichtman AH, Spiegel S (2014) Active, phosphorylated fingolimod inhibits histone deacetylases and facilitates fear extinction memory. Nat Neurosci 17:971–980
Hait NC, Avni D, Yamada A, Nagahashi M, Aoyagi T, Aoki H, Dumur CI, Zelenko Z, Gallagher EJ, Leroith D, Milstien S, Takabe K, Spiegel S (2015) The phosphorylated prodrug FTY720 is a histone deacetylase inhibitor that reactivates ERalpha expression and enhances hormonal therapy for breast cancer. Oncogenesis 4:e156
Heo MJ, Kim YM, Koo JH, Yang YM, An J, Lee SK, Lee SJ, Kim KM, Park JW, Kim SG (2014) microRNA-148a dysregulation discriminates poor prognosis of hepatocellular carcinoma in association with USP4 overexpression. Oncotarget 5:2792–2806
Ho JW, Man K, Sun CK, Lee TK, Poon RT, Fan ST (2005) Effects of a novel immunomodulating agent, FTY720, on tumor growth and angiogenesis in hepatocellular carcinoma. Mol Cancer Ther 4:1430–1438
Jin J, Liao W, Yao W, Zhu R, Li Y, He S (2016) Aldo-keto reductase family 1 member B 10 mediates liver cancer cell proliferation through sphingosine-1-phosphate. Sci Rep 6:22746
Kalluri R, Weinberg RA (2009) The basics of epithelial-mesenchymal transition. J Clin Invest 119:1420–1428
Kunkel GT, Maceyka M, Milstien S, Spiegel S (2013) Targeting the sphingosine-1-phosphate axis in cancer, inflammation and beyond. Nat Rev Drug Discov 12:688–702
Lee TK, Man K, Ho JW, Sun CK, Ng KT, Wang XH, Wong YC, Ng IO, Xu R, Fan ST (2004) FTY720 induces apoptosis of human hepatoma cell lines through PI3-K-mediated Akt dephosphorylation. Carcinogenesis 25:2397–2405

Li CX, Shao Y, Ng KT, Liu XB, Ling CC, Ma YY, Geng W, Fan ST, Lo CM, Man K (2012) FTY720 suppresses liver tumor metastasis by reducing the population of circulating endothelial progenitor cells. PLoS One 7:e32380

Li J, Wu H, Li W, Yin L, Guo S, Xu X, Ouyang Y, Zhao Z, Liu S, Tian Y, Tian Z, Ju J, Ni B, Wang H (2016) Downregulated miR-506 expression facilitates pancreatic cancer progression and chemoresistance via SPHK1/Akt/NF-κB signaling. Oncogene 35:5501–5514

Lu Z, Zhang W, Gao S, Jiang Q, Xiao Z, Ye L, Zhang X (2015) MiR-506 suppresses liver cancer angiogenesis through targeting sphingosine kinase 1 (SPHK1) mRNA. Biochem Biophys Res Commun 468:8–13

Lu Z, Xiao Z, Liu F, Cui M, Li W, Yang Z, Li J, Ye L, Zhang X (2016) Long non-coding RNA HULC promotes tumor angiogenesis in liver cancer by up-regulating sphingosine kinase 1 (SPHK1). Oncotarget 7:241–254

Liu H, Zhang CX, Ma Y, He HW, Wang JP, Shao RG (2016) SphK1 inhibitor SKI II inhibits the proliferation of human hepatoma HepG2 cells via the Wnt5A/beta-catenin signaling pathway. Life Sci 151:23–29

Liu H, Ma Y, He HW, Zhao WL, Shao RG (2017) SPHK1 (sphingosine kinase 1) induces epithelial-mesenchymal transition by promoting the autophagy-linked lysosomal degradation of CDH1/E-cadherin in hepatoma cells. Autophagy 13:900–913

Lu PH, Chen MB, Liu YY, Wu MH, Li WT, Wei MX, Liu CY, Qin SK (2017) Identification of sphingosine kinase 1 (SphK1) as a primary target of icaritin in hepatocellular carcinoma cells. Oncotarget 8:22800–22810

Maceyka M, Spiegel S (2014) Sphingolipid metabolites in inflammatory disease. Nature 510:58–67

Mrad M, Imbert C, Garcia V, Rambow F, Therville N, Carpentier S, Segui B, Levade T, Azar R, Marine JC, Diab-Assaf M, Colacios C, Andrieu-Abadie N (2016) Downregulation of sphingosine kinase-1 induces protective tumor immunity by promoting M1 macrophage response in melanoma. Oncotarget 7:71873–71886

Nagahashi M, Takabe K, Liu R, Peng K, Wang X, Wang Y, Hait NC, Allegood JC, Yamada A, Aoyagi T, Liang J, Pandak WM, Spiegel S, Hylemon PB, Zhou H (2015) Conjugated bile acid activated S1P receptor 2 is a key regulator of sphingosine kinase 2 and hepatic gene expression. Hepatology 61:1216–1226

Newton J, Lima S, Maceyka M, Spiegel S (2015) Revisiting the sphingolipid rheostat: evolving concepts in cancer therapy. Exp Cell Res 333:195–200

Ng KT, Man K, Ho JW, Sun CK, Lee TK, Zhao Y, Lo CM, Poon RT, Fan ST (2007) Marked suppression of tumor growth by FTY720 in a rat liver tumor model: the significance of down-regulation of cell survival Akt pathway. Int J Oncol 30:375–380

Nguyen-Tran DH, Hait NC, Sperber H, Qi J, Fischer K, Ieronimakis N, Pantoja M, Hays A, Allegood J, Reyes M, Spiegel S, Ruohola-Baker H (2014) Molecular mechanism of sphingosine-1-phosphate action in Duchenne muscular dystrophy. Dis Model Mech 7:41–54

Ogretmen B (2018) Sphingolipid metabolism in cancer signalling and therapy. Nat Rev Cancer 18:33–50

Osawa Y, Nagaki M, Banno Y, Nozawa Y, Moriwaki H, Nakashima S (2001) Sphingosine kinase regulates hepatoma cell differentiation: roles of hepatocyte nuclear factor and retinoid receptor. Biochem Biophys Res Commun 286(4):673–677

Panneer Selvam S, De Palma RM, Oaks JJ, Oleinik N, Peterson YK, Stahelin RV, Skordalakes E, Ponnusamy S, Garrett-Mayer E, Smith CD, Ogretmen B (2015) Binding of the sphingolipid S1P to hTERT stabilizes telomerase at the nuclear periphery by allosterically mimicking protein phosphorylation. Sci Signal 8:ra58

Park ES, Choi S, Shin B, Yu J, Hwang JM, Yun H, Chung YH, Choi JS, Choi Y, Rho J (2015) Tumor necrosis factor (TNF) receptor-associated factor (TRAF)-interacting protein (TRIP) negatively regulates the TRAF2 ubiquitin-dependent pathway by suppressing the TRAF2-sphingosine 1-phosphate (S1P) interaction. J Biol Chem 290:9660–9673

Park K, Ikushiro H, Seo HS, Shin KO, Kim YI, Kim JY, Lee YM, Yano T, Holleran WM, Elias P, Uchida Y (2016) ER stress stimulates production of the key antimicrobial peptide,

cathelicidin, by forming a previously unidentified intracellular S1P signaling complex. Proc Natl Acad Sci U S A 113:E1334–E1342
Patmanathan SN, Wang W, Yap LF, Herr DR, Paterson IC (2017) Mechanisms of sphingosine 1-phosphate receptor signalling in cancer. Cell Signal 34:66–75
Pyne NJ, Pyne S (2010) Sphingosine 1-phosphate and cancer. Nat Rev Cancer 10:489–503
Pyne NJ, McNaughton M, Boomkamp S, MacRitchie N, Evangelisti C, Martelli AM, Jiang HR, Ubhi S, Pyne S (2016) Role of sphingosine 1-phosphate receptors, sphingosine kinases and sphingosine in cancer and inflammation. Adv Biol Regul 60:151–159
Ressom HW, Xiao JF, Tuli L, Varghese RS, Zhou B, Tsai TH, Ranjbar MR, Zhao Y, Wang J, Di Poto C, Cheema AK, Tadesse MG, Goldman R, Shetty K (2012) Utilization of metabolomics to identify serum biomarkers for hepatocellular carcinoma in patients with liver cirrhosis. Anal Chim Acta 743:90–100
Reynolds GM, Visentin B, Sabbadini R (2017) Immunohistochemical detection of sphingosine-1-phosphate and sphingosine kinase-1 in human tissue samples and cell lines. Methods Mol Biol 1697:43–56
Rodriguez YI, Campos LE, Castro MG, Aladhami A, Oskeritzian CA, Alvarez SE (2016) Sphingosine-1 phosphate: a new modulator of immune plasticity in the tumor microenvironment. Front Oncol 6:218
Rohrbach T, Maceyka M, Spiegel S (2017) Sphingosine kinase and sphingosine-1-phosphate in liver pathobiology. Crit Rev Biochem Mol Biol 52:543–553
Sanchez DI, Gonzalez-Fernandez B, San-Miguel B, de Urbina JO, Crespo I, Gonzalez-Gallego J, Tunon MJ (2018) Melatonin prevents deregulation of the sphingosine kinase/sphingosine 1-phosphate signaling pathway in a mouse model of diethylnitrosamine-induced hepatocellular carcinoma. J Pineal Res 62:12369
Satapathy SK, Sanyal AJ (2015) Epidemiology and natural history of nonalcoholic fatty liver disease. Semin Liver Dis 35:221–235
Shi J, He YY, Sun JX, Guo WX, Li N, Xue J, Cheng SQ (2015) The impact of sphingosine kinase 1 on the prognosis of hepatocellular carcinoma patients with portal vein tumor thrombus. Ann Hepatol 14:198–206
Takabe K, Spiegel S (2014) Export of sphingosine-1-phosphate and cancer progression. J Lipid Res 9:1839–1846
Takabe K, Paugh SW, Milstien S, Spiegel S (2008) "Inside-out" signaling of sphingosine-1-phosphate: therapeutic targets. Pharmacol Rev 60:181–195
Uranbileg B, Ikeda H, Kurano M, Enooku K, Sato M, Saigusa D, Aoki J, Ishizawa T, Hasegawa K, Kokudo N, Yatomi Y (2016) Increased mRNA levels of sphingosine kinases and s1p lyase and reduced levels of s1p were observed in hepatocellular carcinoma in association with poorer differentiation and earlier recurrence. PLoS One 11:e0149462
Ushitora Y, Tashiro H, Ogawa T, Tanimoto Y, Kuroda S, Kobayashi T, Miyata Y, Itamoto T, Asahara T, Ohdan H (2009) Suppression of hepatocellular carcinoma recurrence after rat liver transplantation by FTY720, a sphingosine-1-phosphate analog. Transplantation 88:980–986
van der Weyden L, Arends MJ, Campbell AD, Bald T, Wardle-Jones H, Griggs N, Velasco-Herrera MD, Tuting T, Sansom OJ, Karp NA, Clare S, Gleeson D, Ryder E, Galli A, Tuck E, Cambridge EL, Voet T, Macaulay IC, Wong K, Sanger Mouse Genetics P, Spiegel S, Speak AO, Adams DJ (2017) Genome-wide in vivo screen identifies novel host regulators of metastatic colonization. Nature 541:233–236
Wan S, Kuo N, Kryczek I, Zou W, Welling TH (2015) Myeloid cells in hepatocellular carcinoma. Hepatology 62:1304–1312
Wang Y, Aoki H, Yang J, Peng K, Liu R, Li X, Qiang X, Sun L, Gurley EC, Lai G, Zhang L, Liang G, Nagahashi M, Takabe K, Pandak WM, Hylemon PB, Zhou H (2017) The role of sphingosine 1-phosphate receptor 2 in bile-acid-induced cholangiocyte proliferation and cholestasis-induced liver injury in mice. Hepatology 65:2005–2018
Yang L, Chang N, Liu X, Han Z, Zhu T, Li C, Yang L, Li L (2012) Bone marrow-derived mesenchymal stem cells differentiate to hepatic myofibroblasts by transforming growth

factor-beta1 via sphingosine kinase/sphingosine 1-phosphate (S1P)/S1P receptor axis. Am J Pathol 181:85–97

Yang L, Yue S, Yang L, Liu X, Han Z, Zhang Y, Li L (2013) Sphingosine kinase/sphingosine 1-phosphate (S1P)/S1P receptor axis is involved in liver fibrosis-associated angiogenesis. J Hepatol 59:114–123

Yang L, Han Z, Tian L, Mai P, Zhang Y, Wang L, Li L (2015) Sphingosine 1-phosphate receptor 2 and 3 mediate bone marrow-derived monocyte/macrophage motility in cholestatic liver injury in mice. Sci Rep 5:13423

Zeng Y, Yao X, Chen L, Yan Z, Liu J, Zhang Y, Feng T, Wu J, Liu X (2016) Sphingosine-1-phosphate induced epithelial-mesenchymal transition of hepatocellular carcinoma via an MMP-7/syndecan-1/TGF-beta autocrine loop. Oncotarget 7:63324–63337

Zhang C, He H, Zhang H, Yu D, Zhao W, Chen Y, Shao R (2013) The blockage of Ras/ERK pathway augments the sensitivity of SphK1 inhibitor SKI II in human hepatoma HepG2 cells. Biochem Biophys Res Commun 434:35–41

Zhou P, Huang G, Zhao Y, Zhong D, Xu Z, Zeng Y, Zhang Y, Li S, He F (2014) MicroRNA-363-mediated downregulation of S1PR1 suppresses the proliferation of hepatocellular carcinoma cells. Cell Signal 26:1347–1354

Exploring the Therapeutic Landscape of Sphingomyelinases

Prajna Shanbhogue and Yusuf A. Hannun

Contents

P. Shanbhogue
Biochemistry and Cell Biology, Stony Brook University, Stony Brook, NY, USA

Y. A. Hannun (✉)
Biochemistry and Cell Biology, Stony Brook University, Stony Brook, NY, USA

Stony Brook University Cancer Center, Stony Brook, NY, USA

Department of Medicine, Stony Brook University, Stony Brook, NY, USA
e-mail: yusuf.hannun@stonybrookmedicine.edu

J. Gomez-Cambronero, M. A. Frohman (eds.), *Lipid Signaling in Human Diseases*,
Handbook of Experimental Pharmacology 259, https://doi.org/10.1007/164_2018_179

Abstract

Sphingosine, ceramide, sphingosine-1-phosphate, and other related sphingolipids have emerged as important bioactive molecules involved in a variety of key cellular processes such as cell growth, differentiation, apoptosis, exosome release, and inter- and intracellular cell communication, making the pathways of sphingolipid metabolism a key domain in maintaining cell homeostasis (Hannun and Obeid, Trends Biochem Sci 20:73–77, 1995; Hannun and Obeid, Nat Rev Mol Cell Biol 9:139–150, 2008; Kosaka et al., J Biol Chem 288:10849–10859, 2013). Various studies have determined that these pathways play a central role in regulating intracellular production of ceramide and the other bioactive sphingolipids and hence are an important component of signaling in various diseases such as cancer, diabetes, and neurodegenerative and cardiovascular diseases (Chaube et al., Biochim Biophys Acta 1821:313–323, 2012; Clarke et al., Adv Enzyme Regul 51:51–58, 2011b; Horres and Hannun, Neurochem Res 37:1137–1149, 2012). In this chapter, we discuss one of the major enzyme classes in producing ceramide, sphingomyelinases (SMases), from a biochemical and structural perspective with an emphasis on their applicability as therapeutic targets.

Keywords

Cancer · Ceramide · Niemann-Pick disease · Sphingomyelinase

Abbreviations

alk-SMase	Alkaline sphingomyelinase
APL	Anionic phospholipid
aSMase	Acid sphingomyelinase
BMP	Bis(monoacylglycero)phosphate
CDase	Ceramidase
CerK	Ceramide kinase
CerS	Ceramide synthase
$cPLA_2$	Phospholipase A_2
DES	Dihydroceramide desaturase
DSS	Dextran sodium sulfate
ENPP	Ectonucleotide pyrophosphate phosphodiesterase
ER	Endoplasmic reticulum
ERCP	Endoscopic retrograde cholangiopancreatography
GBA	Acid glucocerebrosidase
GCS	Glucosylceramide synthase
GSH	Glutathione
HDL	High-density lipoprotein
IL-1	Interleukin 1
IL-6	Interleukin 6
IPC	Inositol phosphorylceramide

ISC1	Inositol phosphosphingolipid phospholipase C1
MA-nSMase	Mitochondria-associated neutral sphingomyelinase
MAPK	Mitogen-activated protein kinase
MIPC	Mannosylinositol phosphorylceramide
NMDA	*N*-methyl D-aspartate
NPD	Niemann-Pick disease
nSMase	Neutral sphingomyelinase
PA	Phosphatidic acid
POPG	1-Palmitoyl-2-oleoyl-*sn*-glycero-3-phospho-(1′-*rac*-glycerol)
PS	Phosphatidylserine
S1P	Sphingosine-1-phosphate
SAR	Structure-activity relationship
SK	Sphingosine kinase
SM	Sphingomyelin
SMase	Sphingomyelinase
SMPD	Sphingomyelin phosphodiesterase
SMS	Sphingomyelin synthase
SPP	Sphingosine-1-phosphate phosphatase
SPT	Serine palmitoyltransferase
TNF	Tumor necrosis factor
WT	Wild-type

1 Introduction

Ceramide is produced via three major pathways in cells – a de novo synthesis pathway catalyzed by ceramide synthases; a relatively faster direct hydrolytic mechanism by metabolizing sphingomyelin (SM), in a pathway catalyzed by SMases (Bartke and Hannun 2009; Milhas et al. 2010); and the salvage pathway which recycles sphingoid bases, formed from hydrolysis of sphingomyelin and glycolipids, into ceramide (Fig. 1).

Sphingomyelin phosphodiesterases or SMases are hydrolases involved in breaking sphingomyelin down to ceramide and phosphocholine. These have emerged as critical enzymes in regulating the levels of ceramide as well as downstream metabolites. SMases have been found to play important roles in inflammation (Aslan et al. 2014; Becker et al. 2010; Duan and Nilsson 2009), cancer (Chen et al. 2015; Ito et al. 2012; Petersen et al. 2013; Saftig and Sandhoff 2013; Shamseddine et al. 2015b), atherosclerosis, and Alzheimer's disease (Horres and Hannun 2012; Jana and Pahan 2010; Lee et al. 2014). Although these studies emphasize the role of the family of SMases as important therapeutic targets, no clinical SMase inhibitors are currently under use as therapeutics.

Early studies of SMases were performed in the 1960s as a result of work on Niemann-Pick disease (NPD – types A and B) which identified unusual accumulation of SM in organs such as the spleen. This line of investigation attributed a drastic

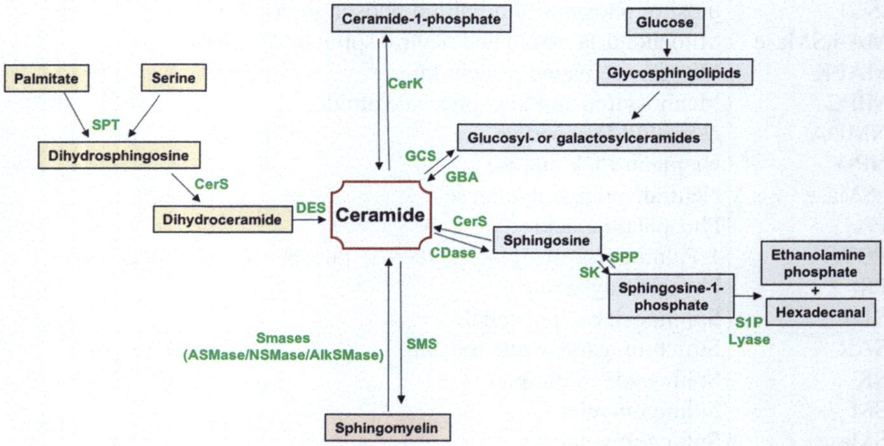

Fig. 1 Ceramide generation pathway. Flowchart of the various ceramide generation pathways – de novo, hydrolytic, and salvage. Yellow boxes indicate the de novo ceramide synthesis pathway, orange and grey boxes indicate the many hydrolytic and recycling pathways. *SPT* serine palmitoyltransferase, *CerS* ceramide synthase, *DES* dihydroceramide desaturase, *SMS* sphingomyelin synthase, *CDase* ceramidase, *GCS* glucosylceramide synthase, *GBA* acid glucocerebrosidase, *CerK* ceramide kinase, *SK* sphingosine kinase, *SPP* sphingosine-1-phosphate phosphatase, *S1P* sphingosine-1-phosphate. Adapted from (Hannun and Obeid 2011)

loss of activity of a SMase in NPD and thus culminated in the identification and description of acid SMase (aSMases) (Brady et al. 1966; Kanfer et al. 1966).

SMases are classified based on their pH optimum and subcellular localization, which direct their substrate and organelle specificity. ASMases have a pH optima between pH 4.0 and 5.0 and are further subclassified based on their cellular location into lysosomal aSMase and secretory aSMase (Kornhuber et al. 2015). The second class of SMases is neutral sphingomyelinases (nSMases) that have a pH optimum around pH 7.0 and can be subclassified into anionic phospholipid (APL)-independent nSMase1 and APL-dependent nSMase2, a third class identified from *Bovine* brain called nSMase3 and a fourth class called the mitochondria-associated SMase (MA-nSMase or nSMase4). These enzymes are found in the inner plasma membrane (Tani and Hannun 2007b), endoplasmic reticulum, trans-Golgi network, mitochondria, exosomes, and nucleus (Airola et al. 2017; Chaube et al. 2012; Shamseddine et al. 2015b). The third class of SMases, the alkaline sphingomyelinases (alk-SMases), have an alkaline pH optimum at around pH 10.0 and are found in microvillar membranes in human colon cells.

Although the three classes of isoenzymes all function as sphingomyelin phosphodiesterases, they do not share the same protein fold or use the same catalytic mechanism (Lim et al. 2015). Thus, aSMases belong to the calcineurin-like phosphodiesterase family, while nSMases 1, 2, and 4 belong to the DNase-I-like superfamily, and alk-SMases encode the type 1 nucleotide phosphodiesterase family fold. There are, however, common threads in the operation of the three classes of isoenzymes as they all have a membrane-associated domain that appears to play a role in positioning the catalytic portion of the enzyme in the correct orientation and provides an additional layer of regulation by adding spatiotemporal specificity to enzyme activation. The availability of high-resolution structures over the last 5 years has tremendously impacted our understanding of how these enzymes function, how they are regulated, and how they can be inhibited or activated using small molecules.

2 Acid Sphingomyelinases

2.1 Roles and Functions

ASMase was the first sphingomyelinase to be identified and characterized, and extensive research in studying this enzyme has revealed its role in a variety of pathophysiologies (Bai and Guo 2017; Brodowicz et al. 2017; Perrotta et al. 2015; Schuchman and Desnick 2017).

ASMase is primarily involved in neurovisceral disease, in particular NPD-A, and the visceral disease NPD-B but also possibly in Alzheimer's disease and depression. NPD-A involves a complete loss of aSMase activity leading to rapid neurodegeneration and is typically lethal in early childhood. NPD-B involves reduction of aSMase activity, has a later onset, and involves neurological and visceral organ abnormalities (Schuchman 2007). In NPD-A and B, there is generalized dysfunction of lysosomes due to the accumulation of SM (Kuemmel et al. 1997a, b; Schram et al. 1984; Schuchman and Desnick 2017; Volk et al. 1972). In addition, there is secondary accumulation of cholesterol in lysosomes and late endosomes due to the accumulation of SM, which prevents cholesterol egress from the lysosomes. This alteration of cholesterol homeostasis in cells has been shown to trigger cell death by autophagy (Kuzu et al. 2017; Perrotta et al. 2015).

In a study of major depressive disorder, it was noted that alternative splicing of aSMase occasionally occurred, resulting in increased amounts of enzymatically active aSMase (Rhein et al. 2017). ASMase is also involved in regulation of neuronal stem cell proliferation in the hippocampus (Gulbins et al. 2016). Further, in a study probing sphingolipid changes in Alzheimer's disease, aSMase was found to be increased in fibroblasts, brain and plasma in patients, as well as in a mouse model of the disease, leading to defective autophagy. Genetic inhibition of aSMase in this mouse model restored lysosomal biogenesis, leading to reduction of amyloid-ß deposition and improved memory (Lee et al. 2014).

ASMase has been implicated in various cancer pathologies. Interaction between melanoma cells and platelets results in activation and secretion of aSMase leading to the stimulation of P-selectin, which further activates the p38 MAPK pathway. Intravenous injection of melanoma cells into WT mice caused multiple lung metastases, while in P-selectin-deficient mice, a significant reduction in lung metastasis was observed. This suggests a novel pathway for metastasis occurring through aSMase activation (Becker et al. 2017). A study on cancer invasiveness and inflammation suggested that aSMase is involved in the regulation of IL-6 through transcriptional mechanisms and also in p38 phosphorylation pathways, thus revealing aSMase as a key player in the aggressiveness of breast carcinoma cells (Perry et al. 2014). In keeping with the theme of cancer metastases, several other groups have also shown evidence for the role of aSMase in these pathways (Carpinteiro et al. 2015; Ellegaard et al. 2013; Zeidan et al. 2008). A study in aSMase-deficient mice highlighted the role of aSMase as a negative regulator of regulatory T cells (Zhou et al. 2016a), and it also has roles in $CD4^{+}$ T cell activation, as reviewed in Bai and Guo (2017).

ASMase has additionally been implicated in regulating uptake and responses to pathogens (viruses and bacteria) (Falcone et al. 2004; Heinz et al. 2015; Kramer et al. 2015; Miller et al. 2012; Yu et al. 2009).

The potential of aSMase inhibitors has long been proposed for a variety of disease pathologies, yet there is a paucity of development of specific inhibitors for it. This can be attributed to a lack of mechanistic information about the enzyme. However, with increasing research in the last decade, and very recent availability of high-resolution structures and elucidation of the catalytic mechanism of aSMases, there is now increased promise for therapeutic development.

2.2 Protein Architecture and Biochemical Properties

Acid SMase (the product of the SMPD1 gene) is translated as a 75 kDa proenzyme, which then undergoes differential posttranslational modifications into either the secretory or the lysosomal forms. Secretory aSMase is possibly regulated via the phosphorylation of S508, whereas the lysosomal fraction is targeted to lysosomes via the mannose-6-phosphate pathway (Jenkins et al. 2010). It is then further processed by lysosomal proteases at both termini to a 70 kDa protein that is N-glycosylated at six sites. The basic layout of human aSMases consists of an N-terminal saposin domain, a proline-rich linker region, and the C-terminal catalytic domain (Xiong et al. 2016; Zhou et al. 2016b). A unique characteristic of this enzyme as compared to other lysosomal hydrolases or even its paralogs sphingomyelin phosphodiesterase acid-like-3A (SMPDL3A) and sphingomyelin phosphodiesterase acid-like-3B (SMPDL3B) is the presence of an appended saposin domain (Gorelik et al. 2016a; Xiong et al. 2016). Saposins are lysosomal proteins that typically bind to and extract lipids from the membrane for subsequent breakdown by various sphingolipid acid hydrolases (Olmeda et al. 2013) and thus function as "accessory" proteins for these hydrolases. The presence of the saposin domain in aSMase renders the enzyme independent of external saposin activity. The saposin domain consists of four alpha helices stabilized by three disulfide bonds arranged as a V-shaped lid over a concave inner hydrophobic surface. The residues that make contacts between the saposin domain and the concave catalytic surface and linker regions are evolutionarily conserved, suggesting that the orientation of this lid-like domain with respect to the catalytic core is important in orienting the substrate SM in the active pocket of the enzyme. The angle of the "V shape" determines whether or not the concave core is able to interact with hydrophobic molecules (open state) or not (closed state) and also determines whether or not aSMase exists as a monomer or a dimer (Acuna et al. 2016; Xiong et al. 2016; Zhou et al. 2016b). Deletion of the saposin domain and its connecting linker completely eliminates enzyme activity for murine aSMase, indicating that the positioning of the enzyme as well as delivery of substrate to the active site is extremely important for its activity (Gorelik et al. 2016b) (Fig. 2).

The saposin domain and the catalytic domain are connected via a proline-rich linker region which makes important contacts with the saposin domain as well as the catalytic domain through a series of polar and nonpolar interactions. The C-terminus of the molecule is the catalytic domain that has a characteristic calcineurin-like phosphodiesterase fold, with six beta sheets in the core surrounded by alpha helices, forming a bowl-like active pocket. The glycosylation sites along the bowl-like catalytic domain likely help stabilize the protein, as a 15°C destabilization was observed in the related de-glycosylated SMPDL3A protein (Lim et al. 2015). The center of the pocket coordinates two zinc ions that are required for aSMase activity. The active site is also proposed to coordinate the oxygen atoms of the substrate head group as well as a water molecule. The residues involved in these coordinated structures are highly conserved, and mutations in these residues have been found in NPD1 and NPD2 patients. The catalytic domain also has a cysteine-rich loop region that seems to be important in aSMase activation, possibly by contributing to a stable active site conformation since multiple known NPD mutations are present here (Xiong et al. 2016; Zhou et al. 2016b).

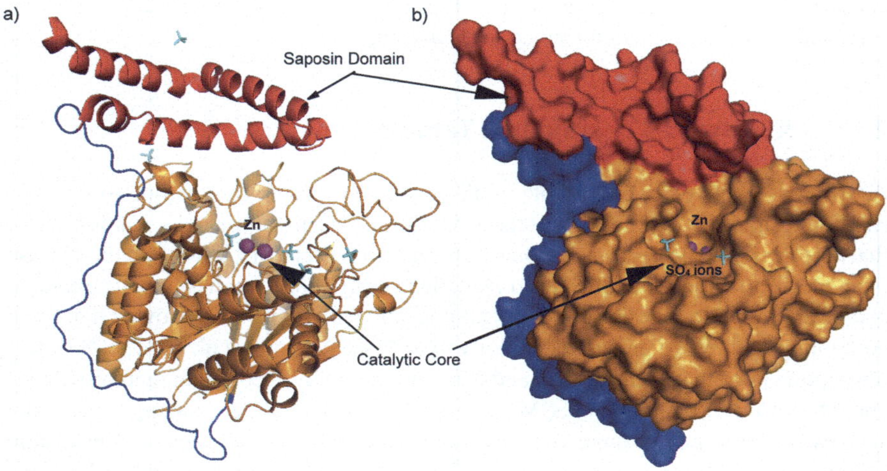

Fig. 2 Open structure of acid sphingomyelinase. (**a**) Cartoon representation of open conformation of human acid sphingomyelinase (Structure obtained from PDB ID: 5JG8). Red helices represent saposin domain in the open conformation. Orange represents the catalytic domain, at the center of which are two zinc ions in magenta. Blue color represents the proline-rich linker domain. Original structure information from Xiong et al. (2016). (**b**) Surface representation of active structure of human acid sphingomyelinase. Red color represents the saposin domain in open conformation. Orange color represents the catalytic domain. The core contains two zinc ions in magenta and two sulfate ions in cyan. Blue region represents the proline-rich linker domain

2.3 Mechanism of Action

The requirements for aSMase activation are an acidic pH, zinc ions, and anionic lipids, mostly bis(monoacylglycero)phosphate (BMP), which is particularly enriched in late endosomes and lysosomes. Interaction of aSMase with a POPG bilayer studied using a coarse-grained simulation model showed that the saposin domain binds to the membrane, placing the catalytic domain facing the lipid head groups of the membrane. Two types of associations are observed – one involving a partial insertion of the saposin domain into the head group region of the bilayer and the other where the saposin domain is in the "open" position, presenting all four helices deeper in the bilayer. This movement of the saposin domain when bound to BMP from a closed to an open state causes a disruption in the bilayer and places the hydrophobic cleft of the catalytic domain facing the substrate molecules in the membrane (Xiong et al. 2016).

At the catalytic core, aSMase catalyzes its substrate through an associative acid-base type reaction. The two zinc ions are coordinated stringently by D206, D278, N318, and a water molecule. The phosphate atom from the substrate SM is positioned at this di-zinc center for attack by the zinc-activated nucleophile generated from the water molecule. The structure of the aSMase analog SMPDL3A with AMP shows the formation of a cation-π box with stacking of the phosphate group with amino acid side chains (Gorelik et al. 2016c). H319 seems to be the energy-favored hydrogen donor in the reaction, allowing for quick exchange of protons. Other conserved polar residues in the active site such as H282, N325, and D251 may be involved in substrate recognition and positioning.

2.4 ASMases as Therapeutic Targets

As discussed above, given the role of aSMase in various disease pathologies, it is a candidate target for a variety of diseases. Unlike classical pharmacological inhibitors that act directly on proteins, functional inhibitors of aSMase (FIASMs) act on aSMase in an indirect fashion to reduce its enzymatic activity. Early studies with imipramine and desipramine in fibroblast, neuroblastoma, and C6 glioma cells showed that these compounds decreased enzymatic activity of aSMase (Albouz et al. 1981, 1983). It is now appreciated that amitriptyline and desipramine act by accumulating in lysosomes and interfering with binding of aSMase to lysosomal membranes, making the enzyme susceptible to intralysosomal proteases and leading to its subsequent degradation (Albouz et al. 1981; Hurwitz et al. 1994; Kolzer et al. 2004). However, it is to be noted that chlorpromazine and tricyclics such as desipramine also cause loss of acid ceramidase and lead to a pronounced downregulation of sphingosine compared to ceramide, suggesting their role in acid ceramidase inhibition as well (Elojeimy et al. 2006; Zeidan et al. 2008). Nevertheless, these compounds are increasingly being studied as an avenue to develop better antidepressants and in treatment of neurodegenerative conditions such as Alzheimer's disease, with some studies even indicating induction of neurogenesis. This comes from various studies connecting the functional effects of tricyclic antidepressants such as fluoxetine, desipramine, imipramine, and amitriptyline to their effects on aSMase activity (Albouz et al. 1981; Beckmann et al. 2014; Gulbins et al. 2013; Hoehn et al. 2016; Hurwitz et al. 1994; Kornhuber et al. 2010).

Studies of various anti-cancer drugs have suggested that many of them function via aSMase. For example, gemcitabine has been shown to function selectively via aSMase in proliferating bovine aortic endothelial cells (BAEC). In this study, the authors showed that baseline aSMase is increased and secreted only in proliferating BAEC as opposed to growth-arrested confluent cells. Additionally, only proliferative BAEC are sensitive to gemcitabine-induced apoptosis, and this effect is blocked by use of an aSMase-specific inhibitor, imipramine, or by using surface anti-ceramide antibody. Growth-arrested confluent cells could also be re-sensitized to gemcitabine by application of exogenous bacterial SMase to these cells (van Hell et al. 2017). In one study, compounds SU11652 and sunitinib (tyrosine kinase inhibitors) were also shown to act as lysosomal destabilizers in drug-resistant Du145 prostate cancer cells as effectively as drug-sensitive parental cells by inducing membrane permeabilization, increasing lysosomal pH, and inhibiting aSMase activity, thus reverting the multidrug resistance (Ellegaard et al. 2013). In single-dose radiation therapy (SDRT), the ionizing radiation-induced damage to tumor endothelium is initiated by ceramide produced by aSMase. Angiogenic factors such as VEGF prevent aSMase-mediated ceramide formation, subsequently reducing endothelial dysfunction in tumors. Pretreatment with axitinib (a VEGF/tyrosine kinase inhibitor) in mice bearing radiosensitive sarcoma or radio-resistant B16F1 melanoma flank tumors was shown to radiosensitize cells to single-dose radiation therapy (Rao et al. 2014). This may permit dose de-escalation and expand the range of SDRT.

ASMase has also been implicated as mediator of cell death in response to several stimuli, and its potential as a target for cancer therapy has been addressed in detail in several studies (Canals and Hannun 2013; Groth-Pedersen and Jaattela 2013; Perrotta et al. 2015; Savic and Schuchman 2013; Smith and Schuchman 2008). This highlights the role of this enzyme in various cancer pathologies, thus providing an alternate mechanism for cancer treatment.

ASMase has been implicated as a target in fibrotic and inflammatory conditions. A study in Caco2 cells and IEC6 intestinal cells showed the effectiveness of a type of pentacyclic triterpenoid, ursolic acid, specifically against aSMase, making it useful in intestinal inflammatory conditions. ASMase was also shown to be involved in bleomycin-induced pulmonary fibrosis as well as in pulmonary edema induced by platelet-activating factor in acute lung injury (Dhami et al. 2010; Goggel et al. 2004). The role of aSMase in hepatic fibrosis has been established. In a recent study of mechanisms of liver fibrosis, aSMase was demonstrated to be linked to acute phase of sepsis as well as fibrogenesis in murine liver. Partial genetic deficiency of aSMase ($smpd1^{+/-}$) had a beneficial effect on liver function. Interestingly, similar to the partial deficiency, using desipramine also significantly improved liver function and survival (Chung et al. 2017). Tricyclic antidepressants were also shown to be promising as a therapeutic strategy to reverse liver fibrosis in a study that screened several compounds in hepatic stellate cells (HSCs). Here, nortriptyline induced an antifibrotic phenotype through inhibition of acid ceramidase as well as aSMase leading to reduced collagen formation in HSCs (Chen et al. 2017). In a study using amitriptyline, it was shown that aSMase inhibition protected mice from *Staphylococcus aureus* sepsis and consequent lung edema, thus making aSMase inhibitors useful in a combinatorial treatment strategy alongside antibiotics (Peng et al. 2015).

Another practical application of aSMase inhibitors is in long-term blood storage for transfusion purposes. Typically, during long-term storage, erythrocyte-derived microparticles form that subsequently promote transfusion-associated lung inflammation. This phenomenon was recently attributed to aSMase formation of ceramide leading to release of microparticles, since it could be attenuated with the use of a functional inhibitors of aSMase, amitriptyline (Hoehn et al. 2017).

Several efforts on development and optimization of inhibitors for acid SMase have relied on designing uncleavable substrate analogs or analogs of endogenous inhibitory molecules such as bisphosphonates and phosphoinositides (Roth et al. 2009). L-Carnitine and L-acylcarnitine have been reported to moderately inhibit aSMase (Arenz 2010; Di Marzio et al. 1997). Thiourea and difluoromethylene analogs of SM have also been mildly effective (Yokomatsu et al. 2001). Detailed SAR studies on geminal bisphosphonates led to the development of the potent inhibitor ARC39, an aminobisphosphonate, with an IC50 of 20 nM, which suppressed dexamethasone-induced cell death in HEK293 cells. A study on secretory aSMase using plasma showed that the enzyme can be activated by oxidation and inhibited by reductants such as glutathione and dithiothreitol. Further, it was shown that the catechin, (−)-epicatechin 3-O-gallate, inhibited aSMase at an $IC_{50}=25.7\ \mu M$. As well, a synthetic catechin, (−)-3′-O-methyepigallocatechin 3-O-gallate, inhibited aSMase at $IC_{50}=1.7\ \mu M$ (Kobayashi et al. 2016).

Thus far, we have discussed the therapeutic advantages of using aSMase inhibitors. However, for diseases in which loss of function needs to be countered (such as NPD), a possible treatment strategy is to use olipudase alfa, the recombinant version of aSMase, which is currently in phase 2 pediatric trials and phase 3 for adults as an enzyme replacement therapy for non-neurological manifestations of NPD (McGovern et al. 2016). Another strategy for treatment of NPD is enzyme enhancement therapy or active site-specific chaperone (ASSC) therapy wherein low concentrations of potent enzyme inhibitors or chemical chaperones are used to enhance folding and activity of mutant proteins. This has been under development to treat Fabry's disease and Gaucher's disease. Use of ceramide, SM, or phosphonucleotide analogs as NPD ASSCs along with aSMase gene therapy or with enzyme replacement therapy has been discussed in a patent by Schuchman and Desnick (2010). Activators of aSMase may help NPD-B patients with mutational defects in protein rather than genetic defects (pertaining to lack of expression of aSMase) to a certain extent as well.

3 Neutral Sphingomyelinases

3.1 Roles and Functions

NSMases have been characterized thoroughly, elucidating their roles in several cellular and pathological processes. One of the major fields of extensive study for role of nSMases is in apoptotic pathways, making it particularly important in cancer progression. Approximately 5% of acute myeloid and acute lymphoid leukemia samples have mutations in nSMase2 (Kim et al. 2008). In hepatocarcinoma, nSMase2 was identified as a tumor suppressor gene, shown to be regulated by epigenetic mechanisms, and confirmed to play a role in cell invasion and migration after being knocked down with siRNA (Revill et al. 2013). NSMase2 has also been shown to play a role in exosome release, thus promoting cancer metastasis (Kong et al. 2015; Singh et al. 2014).

NSMases were first identified in high quantities in the brain; thus dysregulation in nSMase activity would be expected to lead to neurological disorders. In relation to this, several groups have concluded that nSMase2 plays an important role in disease pathologies of the nervous system. Neuronal cell death caused by aggregated Aß1-42, which is a key player in Alzheimer's disease, was shown to be mediated by activation of nSMase as a consequence of cPLA2-A (Sagy-Bross et al. 2013). In a study using Alzheimer's disease model mice (fro; 5XFAD), decreased secretion of exosomes, ceramide levels, glial activation, total $Aß_{42}$, and plaque burden were observed in nSMase2-deficient mice as compared to wild-type 5XFAD. This reduction of exosome release improved pathology and cognition. A study in astrocytes demonstrated a role for nSMase2 in attenuating inflammatory responses and neuronal damage after cerebral ischemia (Gu et al. 2013). Further, age-related accumulation of ceramide may impair cognition through nSMase2, as this enzyme was shown to be upregulated by TNF-α, thus modulating synaptic plasticity through NMDA receptors (Wheeler et al. 2009).

Cardiovascular roles of nSMases have also been studied, with nSMase2 activation being associated with a vasoconstrictor phenotype. For example, nSMase2 overexpression mimics ER stress, which further reduces production of nitrous oxide, a vasodilator (Chaube et al. 2012). In cultured aortic smooth muscle cells, apoC-I and apoC-I-enriched HDL activate the sphingolipid pathway, leading to apoptosis. An nSMase2 inhibitor, GW4869, was shown to inhibit this potential plaque rupture response (Kolmakova et al. 2004). A report on obese type 2 diabetic patients showed increased nSMase activity although ceramide levels were unaffected (Baranowski et al. 2010).

These are just some of the representative literature on the role of nSMases in various disease pathologies (see recent reviews on roles of nSMases (Bienias et al. 2016; Hwang et al. 2015; Shamseddine et al. 2015a; Zhang and Guo 2013)), and as one can appreciate, inhibitors of nSMases have potential therapeutic implications in neurological and cardiovascular conditions, while activators of nSMases have a potential role in cancer therapy. Recent structural and mechanistic data on nSMase function has opened new avenues for nSMases as therapeutic targets.

3.2 Protein Architecture and Biochemical Properties

NSMases belong to the DNase-I superfamily of enzymes and were first structurally characterized from bacteria *Bacillus cereus* and *Staphylococcus aureus* (Ago et al. 2006). They primarily act as toxins in bacteria by aiding in cell membrane disruption, thus causing hemolysis in host cells (Kruse et al. 2011). The yeast homolog of nSMase, inositol phosphosphingolipid phospholipase C (ISC1), hydrolyzes inositol phosphorylceramide (IPC), generating phytoceramide and inositol phosphate. It is also, however, capable of using mannosylinositol phosphorylceramide (MIPC) and mannosyldiinositol phosphorylceramide and SM as substrates (Henry et al. 2011; Sawai et al. 2000).

Mammals have four different classes of nSMases. nSMase1 (product of the SMPD2 gene) is a 47.5 kDa protein with catalytic activity against SM as well as lysophospholipid phosphatase C (lysoPC) in vitro. However, it shows cellular activity preference toward lysoPC and lyso-PAF (platelet-activating factor) as opposed to SM. It has an N-terminal region followed by the catalytic domain and two C-terminal hydrophobic domains. It is dependent on divalent cations such as Mg^{2+} for activity with H136 and H272 playing an important role in enzymatic activity (Rodrigues-Lima et al. 2000). nSMase2 (product of SMPD3) is a 71 kDa Mg^{2+} and APL-dependent phosphodiesterase most abundantly found in the inner plasma membrane. Topology studies have shown that it is characterized by two N-terminal membrane-inserted hydrophobic segments followed by a short linker region and a C-terminal catalytic domain (Tani and Hannun 2007a). The nSMase3 protein (product of SMPD4 gene) has a molecular mass of about 98 kDa and possesses no homology to the other three nSMase classes. It has an N-terminal proline-rich region and a magnesium-binding site followed by the catalytic domain. However, the catalytic domain residues are not the conserved residues found in other members of the nSMase family. The C-terminus has a single transmembrane domain followed by an ER localization motif. It is currently unclear if nSMase3 functions directly on SM. A study on TNF-alpha-mediated activation of SMases indicated an absence of in vivo or in vitro activity of nSMase3 on SM (Clarke et al. 2011a); however, other studies have indicated that it does play a role in regulating sphingolipid levels in cells (Corcoran et al. 2008; Krut et al. 2006; Moylan et al. 2014). Finally, the fourth mammalian SMase termed MA-nSMase is the product of the SMPD5 gene and contains a mitochondrial localization signal followed by a transmembrane domain, a regulatory region, and a cytosolic catalytic domain (Rajagopalan et al. 2015). Similar to nSMase2, it is dependent on Mg2+ or Mn2+ as well as APLs such as phosphatidylserine and cardiolipin for activation. It has a high sequence homology to nSMase2 and has the same catalytic core residues and cation-binding motifs as well as the P-loop-like or the DK switch loop (Wu et al. 2010) (Fig. 3).

The first high-resolution structure of human nSMase2 catalytic domain has recently been determined, providing a detailed mechanism of action. The N-terminal domain is an integral membrane domain consisting of two hydrophobic segments that bind the APLs phosphatidylserine (PS) and phosphatidic acid (PA) that

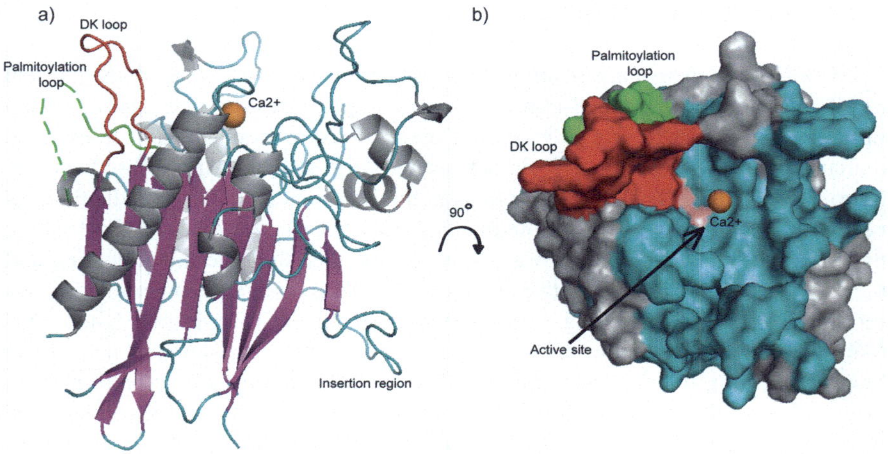

Fig. 3 3-D apo-structure of neutral sphingomyelinase-2. (**a**) This is a cartoon representation of apo-structure of nSMase2. In magenta is the core beta-sandwich structure (Structure obtained from PDB ID: 5UVG). Gray represents the helices surrounding the catalytic core. Red loop is the DK loop in the "closed" position. Green dotted loop represents the palmitoylation loop. Dotted lines indicate the absence of electron density, indicating loop's flexible nature. Teal color represents loops. At the catalytic core is an orange sphere which represents the calcium ion. Original structure information from Airola et al. (2017). (**b**) Surface representation of the catalytic core of nSMase2 showing a clear groove for substrate to dock in. Red region represents the DK loop obstructing the catalytic domain. Teal regions represent loops facing the membrane. Gray region represents the remaining catalytic domain. Orange sphere at the core of the active pocket represents where magnesium would bind during catalysis

are required for full nSMase2 activity (Wu et al. 2011). This domain is followed by a short linker region called the juxtamembrane region that plays a role in nSMase2 activation by acting as an allosteric activator region and enabling domain interaction between the membrane-inserted N-terminus and the C-terminal catalytic domain (Airola et al. 2017). The catalytic domain is cytoplasmic in nature and folds similarly to DNase-I superfamily proteins, with a beta-sandwich core connected by loops of varying lengths. A large 165 amino acid insertion region is present within the catalytic domain and is presumed to add an additional layer of nSMase2 regulation. Indeed, this region contains five conserved serine residues that are known phosphorylation sites aiding in protein stability and can be dephosphorylated by direct binding of calcineurin (also known as protein phosphatase 2B), thereby deactivating nSMase2 (Filosto et al. 2012). The active pocket is a bowl-like cavity that contains divalent cation-binding as well as SM-binding residues, all of them participating in acid-base hydrolysis reaction (Airola et al. 2017). Two clusters of palmitoylation sites (cysteine residues) are present in nSMase2 that direct this protein to the plasma membrane, the first present between the two hydrophobic segments and the second in a loop connecting two beta sheets in the catalytic domain (Tani and Hannun 2007b).

3.3 Mechanism of Action

NSMase2 is fully active at a neutral pH in the presence of Mg^{2+} ions and APLs such as PS and PA. Deleting the N-terminal domain traps the nSMase2 catalytic domain in a low activity state that is enhanced upon co-expression with the N-terminal domain, indicating that this domain acts as allosteric activator of nSMase2 activity (Airola et al. 2017). Two distinct regions in the N-terminal domain are identified as necessary and sufficient for APL binding and subsequently trafficking and activating the enzyme (Wu et al. 2011). It was further shown that the N-terminal domain and the catalytic domain interact with each other via a juxtamembrane linker region, thus transmitting the APL binding signal downstream to the cytoplasmic C-terminus (Airola et al. 2017). In the crystal structure of the catalytic domain, one of the loops connecting the core beta sheets, called the DK switch loop, is present as an extended loop that projects into the hydrophobic groove of the active site, thus possibly blocking SM entry into the catalytic center. Mutating the key residues D430A and K435A led to a dramatic decrease in nSMase2 activity, suggesting that these residues may be involved in SM recognition or binding (Airola et al. 2017). Regulation of nSMase2 activity by this mechanism may provide an advantage to localized production of ceramide.

Once the catalytic domain is in the active conformation, it is proposed to catalyze SM in an acid-base-type hydrolysis reaction. Although the sequence homology between the bacterial and mammalian nSMases is low, the catalytic core and active site residues are all conserved, with the same mode of divalent ion binding across all the structures. Hence, the proposed bacterial mode of SM catalysis can likely be extended to the human nSMase2 as well. In the active site, two Asp, two Asn, one Glu, and one His residues are conserved across species. According to this model, a conserved His residue functions as a nucleophile generated by to the presence of Mg^{2+} ions. The resulting tetrahedral reaction intermediate is now able to deprotonate a nearby water molecule that initiates a nucleophilic attack on the phosphate moiety of SM bound to this cleft, resulting in the formation of ceramide and phosphocholine (PC) (Ago et al. 2006). A major difference between the bacterial SMase structure and the mammalian nSMase structure is the presence of a hydrophobic beta hairpin in the bacterial enzymes that protrudes into the solvent and plays a role in liposome/membrane lipid binding (Ago et al. 2006).

3.4 NSMases as Therapeutic Targets

NSMases are upregulated in inflammatory pathways pertaining to cardiovascular, pulmonary, and neurodegenerative conditions, thus making inhibition of nSMases a potential target for therapeutic development.

Several studies have reported use of the uncompetitive inhibitor GW4869 as a molecular tool to probe the involvement of nSMase2 in pathological settings. GW4869 was identified in a screen for inhibitors of nSMase (Luberto et al. 2002) and offers specificity for nSMase2 over aSMase at an IC_{50} of 1 μM, but does not completely abolish nSMase2 activity. Outcomes with GW4869 suggested roles of nSMase2 in hypoxic pulmonary vasoconstriction, inflammation in liver ischemia-reperfusion injury, and synaptic plasticity (Aslan et al. 2014; Cogolludo et al. 2009; Wheeler et al. 2009). Blocking exosome release from RAW264.7 macrophages by treating them with GW4869 significantly impaired release of pro-inflammatory cytokines, thus also reducing sepsis-induced cardiac inflammation, reducing myocardial depression, and prolonging survival (Essandoh et al. 2015). Stimulation of exosome release by monensin increases the intercellular transmission of prions, and treatment with GW4869 opposes it. This highlights the role for nSMase2 in prion transfer, with potential relevance to Alzheimer's disease progression (Guo et al. 2016).

The fungal compound scyphostatin was discovered as an NSmase2 inhibitor by screening natural compounds. Neurite outgrowth is inhibited in hippocampal neurons cultured with scyphostatin (Brann et al. 2002). Similarly, inflammatory activity triggered by IL-1beta and lipopolysaccharide were shown to be suppressed by treatment with scyphostatin (Rutkute et al. 2007). Another fungal derivative that exhibits anti-nSMase activity is manumycin A, which was shown to have antitumor and anti-inflammatory activities (Bernier et al. 2006; Sonoda et al. 1998). However, although these compounds inhibited nSMase activity, they are not specific to any one subclass of nSMase. Moreover, these compounds also showed inhibition of aSMase activity at higher concentrations. To overcome this issue, irreversible analogs of these compounds have been developed with modifications to the cyclohexane ring and the amide side chain (Arenz et al. 2001a, b; Arenz and Giannis 2000; Pitsinos et al. 2003). Unfortunately, these compounds were discovered to be unstable and hard to dissolve, making them unusable as inhibitors in vivo.

Deprenyl and benzofenone-type congeners of alpha mangostin 1, a xanthone class of natural plant products, have also been used as SMase inhibitors, with loss of the prenyl group improving their efficacy. However, they could not differentiate between aSMase and nSMase activities and worked only after preincubation for at least 30 min, thus making them irreversible and non-specific (Hamada et al. 2003). More recently, a fluorescence-based high-throughput screen yielded another novel, uncompetitive nSMase2 inhibitor called cambinol with a K_i of 7 μM. Unlike its predecessors, which are either against rat, mouse, or bovine forms of nSMases, this was generated against the human recombinant form of the enzyme. SAR studies identified the thiourea and naphthol portions of this compound as essential moieties for inhibition, and it was shown to decrease TNF-alpha- or IL-1beta-related increases of ceramide and cell death in primary neurons (Figuera-Losada et al. 2015).

NSMases have been heavily studied in many pro-apoptotic pathways. Chemotherapeutic agents such as doxorubicin and daunorubicin, as well as the cannabinoid anandamide, were shown to exert their antitumor effects through nSMase2, placing this enzyme at an important juncture in cancer therapy (Di Scala et al. 2017; Shamseddine et al. 2015a, b). As an antitumor strategy, caffeic acid phenethyl ester was used in C6 glioma cells where it induced apoptosis by activation of nSMase2, and pretreatment with the nSMase2 inhibitor GW4869 reduced this effect (Tseng et al. 2014). Interestingly, a natural compound from sea cucumbers called stichoposide C has also been shown to induce apoptosis in leukemia and colorectal cancer cells through aSMase- and nSMase-dependent ceramide generation, and this effect is partially reversible with use of SMase siRNA (Yun et al. 2012). In a series of guanidinium compounds with increasing lipophilicity, the compound C11AG was found to be effective against nSMase2 in vitro (Amtmann et al. 2003; Canals et al. 2011). Other noncompetitive inhibitors of nSMases include glutathione (GSH), ubiquinol, S-methyl glutathione, and glutathione disulfide. GSH was shown to inhibit TNF-alpha-induced ceramide generation in MCF7 cells (Liu et al. 1998). Anticancer studies targeting nSMases have generated two anomeric oleyl glucosamides as anticancer agents wherein the presence of a trifluoroacetyl group close to the center makes them resistant to hydrolysis by hexosaminidases. The alpha anomer however caused death of C6 glioma cells by inducing ER stress via nSMase2. Pretreatment with nSMse2 inhibitor 3-O-methyl SM restored SM levels and prevented ER stress-related cell death in the cancer cells (Romero-Ramirez et al. 2015). Taken together, these studies highlight the importance of nSMase activators as having therapeutic potential in numerous cancer conditions.

4 Alkaline Sphingomyelinase

4.1 Roles and Functions

Alk-SMase is primarily expressed in colon cells and is thought to act on dietary SM. In alk-SMase knockout mice, the intestinal mucosa appears to be thicker as compared to wild-type mice. When azoxymethane/dextran sodium sulfate (DSS) is used as a carcinogen to study formation of aberrant crypt foci in the mucosa, an increased number and size (4.5×) of tumors are observed in the knockout mice as compared to wild-type mice (Chen et al. 2015). In a study in bile from patients undergoing endoscopic retrograde cholangiopancreatography (ERCP), alk-SMase activity is significantly lower in cholangiocarcinoma patients compared to patients who underwent the procedure for gallstones or other benign diseases (Duan et al. 2014). Alk-SMase activity is low in HepG2 liver cancer cells and in human liver biopsy samples supporting its role in liver tumorigenesis (Cheng et al. 2007). These results suggest that Alk-SMase may have a tumor suppressor function.

Expression of alk-SMase can be affected by drugs and dietary factors. It was shown that a diet rich in water-soluble, dietary fiber psyllium increases alk-SMase and caspase-3 activities, driving apoptosis pathways, whereas a high-fat diet had the opposite results, thus attenuating pro-apoptotic effects of psyllium. The opposing effects of high-fiber and high-fat diets on alk-SMase activity hint at an underlying biochemical mechanism of tumorigenesis and inflammation in the gut (Cheng et al. 2004). Alk-SMase purified from *Pichia pastoris* used to treat DSS-induced colitis in a rat model (by delivering alk-SMase intrarectally every week) reduced TNF-alpha expression and inflammation in the treated rats and further protected their colonic epithelium (Andersson et al. 2009). An age-associated decrease of alk-SMase activity has been correlated with premature senescence of colonic mucosal samples of patients with chronic colitis (Sjoqvist et al. 2002).

These studies highlight the role of alk-SMase in various inflammatory and tumorigenic conditions, especially of the GI system, with an emphasis on a loss of alk-SMase function or expression in these models. It would be interesting to study if the effects of alk-SMase activation reduce disease progression. Extensive biochemical and biophysical data are now available to address these questions and aid in the design of alk-SMase agonists as potential therapies.

4.2 Protein Architecture and Biochemical Properties

Alk-SMase (ENPP7), as the name suggests, is active at alkaline pH and in the presence of anionic bile salts such as taurocholate and taurochenodeoxycholate. It has no sequence homology to the nSMase and aSMase families but belongs instead to the nucleotide pyrophosphatase/phosphodiesterase family. Similar to nSMase1, it is also able to use lysoPC as substrate to convert it to monoacylglycerol (Duan et al. 2003).

The basic architecture of this 97.8 kDa enzyme consists of an N-terminal signal peptide followed by a divalent metal-binding site, a catalytic domain, and a C-terminal transmembrane segment and an ER localization motif. The transmembrane segment helps the protein anchor to the luminal side of the intestinal microvillar membrane and can be cleaved off by trypsin (Wu et al. 2004). The high-resolution crystal structure was solved recently (Gorelik et al. 2017). It does not contain the N-terminal signal peptide or C-terminal transmembrane anchor. The overall fold of the enzyme follows that of the alkaline phosphatase family, with a beta-sandwich core flanked by alpha helices on both sides. It also comprises a cap sub-domain packed against one side of the catalytic domain. It is made up of four beta strands at the core connected by various loops and a single helix. Full activity of the enzyme requires *N*-glycosylation of the enzyme at five different residues (Wu et al. 2005) (Fig. 4).

4.3 Mechanism of Action

Alk-SMase is activated by anionic bile salts possibly by directly interacting with alk-SMase aiding in its activation. A cationic patch consisting of residues Arg-271 and Arg-343 and a loop consisting of three solvent-exposed hydrophobic residues, Ile-344, Val-346, and Phe-348, are suggested to be important for alk-SMase activity due to their potential role in taurocholate binding (Gorelik et al. 2017). Upon binding taurocholate, the loop could be inserted into the membrane or alternatively could interact with the acyl chains of the SM molecule, positioning the catalytic domain in a stable conformation (Gorelik et al. 2017).

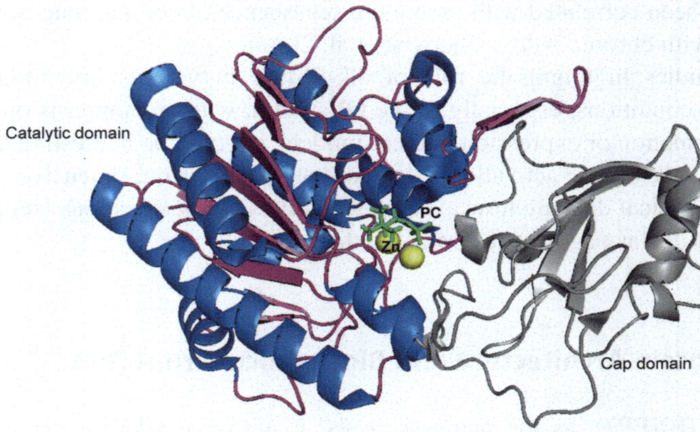

Fig. 4 Active structure of alkaline sphingomyelinase. Cartoon representation of alk-SMase shows the core of N-terminal catalytic domain in pink and the surrounding helices in blue. The C-terminal gray region is the cap domain. In the catalytic core are two zinc ions in yellow and a phosphocholine molecule in green. The interactions made by the phosphocholine molecule with alk-SMase active pocket may represent the binding motif during catalysis (Structure obtained from PDB ID: 5TCD). Original structure information from Gorelik et al. (2017)

The shallow cavity of the catalytic domain, as with aSMase, harbors two zinc ions that participate in hydrolysis of SM and are coordinated by a series of His and Asp residues. The PC-bound structure and biochemical analysis of alk-SMase reveal two Tyr molecules as substrate recognition residues. The choline moiety of the substrate molecule stacks against the aromatic residues, forming a cation- π box (Gorelik et al. 2017). The mechanism of catalysis involves two scissile attacks by nucleophiles generated by each of the two zinc ions. The substrate phosphate makes strong electrostatic interactions with zinc ions and Asn-96 where it undergoes a nucleophilic attack by the side-chain hydroxyl of Thr-75 activated by one of the zinc ions, releasing ceramide (Gorelik et al. 2017). The intermediate phosphocholyl-threonine undergoes a subsequent nucleophilic attack by a water molecule activated by the other zinc ion, thus releasing choline phosphate as the reaction byproduct (Gorelik et al. 2017).

4.4 Alk-SMases as Therapeutic Targets

Since alk-SMase is expressed mostly in the colon and primarily acts on dietary SM, a study on alk-SMase activity in human colorectal cancer was performed. Alk-SMase activity levels were found to be reduced by over 75% of patients with colorectal cancer (Hertervig et al. 1997), suggesting that activators of either alk-SMase transcription pathways or correction of any mutations in alk-SMase by use of enzyme activators could be therapeutic in nature. With regard to this, a study reported the effects of ursodeoxycholate in inhibiting the development of colon carcinoma by unknown mechanisms. It was shown to increase alk-SMase and caspase 3 activities, suggesting a mechanism for its anticarcinogenic effects (Cheng et al. 1999; Liu et al. 2006). Another study of a similar nature used ursolic acid in HT29 cells, where its antiproliferative and apoptotic properties were accompanied by activation of alk-SMase followed by activation of caspases 3, 8, and 9 (Andersson et al. 2003). Ursolic acid is also indicated as a chemoprotective agent, since it reduced the incidence of aberrant crypt foci containing three or more crypts in the initiation phase of colon cancer in azoxymethane-treated rats (Andersson et al. 2008).

Alk-SMase activity is also significantly lowered in models of ulcerative colitis. Two studies tackled this condition using a probiotic, VSL#3, both in a mouse model of colitis and in patients with ulcerative colitis. Treatment with VSL#3 increased alk-SMase activity in both the colon and ileum of mice and in human patients, thus reducing their disease activity index scores (Soo et al. 2008). None of the probiotic-treated mice showed signs of carcinoma, and there was no high-grade dysplasia in the proximal or mid-colon, as compared to roughly 29% in the control mice that did not receive the probiotic (Appleyard et al. 2011). This provides a potential therapeutic use in patients with long-standing colitis, since transition to dysplasia and cancer is potentially delayed due to attenuation of pro-inflammatory pathways.

5 Conclusions

SMases have been shown to play various signaling and regulatory roles in cell proliferation, apoptosis, and exosome release, thus playing a vital role in many disease pathways. Although belonging to the same functional class of enzymes, they have low structural homology, providing an advantage to specifically target each hydrolase with different compounds. With the availability of high-resolution structures of all classes of SMases, a new avenue of therapeutic development is now possible. Specific, more potent, reversible, competitive inhibitors of SMases can now be developed more readily, with focus on building more drug-like compounds, rather than more substrate analogs with poor stability. Insight into how these enzymes are regulated by their various activators such as BMP, PS, and taurocholate also opens up potential to design more antitumor, anti-inflammatory compounds that act as SMase agonists and are competitive with the natural activators of these enzymes.

Acknowledgments We would like to thank Dr. Christopher J. Clarke, Dr. Michael V. Airola, and Dr. Benjamin Newcomb for providing valuable feedback. This work was supported in part by NIH grant R35 GM118128.

References

Acuna M, Castro-Fernandez V, Latorre M, Castro J, Schuchman EH, Guixe V, Gonzalez M, Zanlungo S (2016) Structural and functional analysis of the ASM p.Ala359Asp mutant that causes acid sphingomyelinase deficiency. Biochem Biophys Res Commun 479:496–501. https://doi.org/10.1016/j.bbrc.2016.09.096

Ago H, Oda M, Takahashi M, Tsuge H, Ochi S, Katunuma N, Miyano M, Sakurai J (2006) Structural basis of the sphingomyelin phosphodiesterase activity in neutral sphingomyelinase from Bacillus cereus. J Biol Chem 281:16157–16167. https://doi.org/10.1074/jbc.M601089200

Airola MV, Shanbhogue P, Shamseddine AA, Guja KE, Senkal CE, Maini R, Bartke N, Wu BX, Obeid LM, Garcia-Diaz M, Hannun YA (2017) Structure of human nSMase2 reveals an interdomain allosteric activation mechanism for ceramide generation. Proc Natl Acad Sci U S A 114:E5549–E5558. https://doi.org/10.1073/pnas.1705134114

Albouz S, Hauw JJ, Berwald-Netter Y, Boutry JM, Bourdon R, Baumann N (1981) Tricyclic antidepressants induce sphingomyelinase deficiency in fibroblast and neuroblastoma cell cultures. Biomedicine 35:218–220

Albouz S, Vanier MT, Hauw JJ, Le Saux F, Boutry JM, Baumann N (1983) Effect of tricyclic antidepressants on sphingomyelinase and other sphingolipid hydrolases in C6 cultured glioma cells. Neurosci Lett 36:311–315

Amtmann E, Baader W, Zoller M (2003) Neutral sphingomyelinase inhibitor C11AG prevents lipopolysaccharide-induced macrophage activation. Drugs Exp Clin Res 29:5–13

Andersson D, Liu JJ, Nilsson A, Duan RD (2003) Ursolic acid inhibits proliferation and stimulates apoptosis in HT29 cells following activation of alkaline sphingomyelinase. Anticancer Res 23:3317–3322

Andersson D, Cheng Y, Duan RD (2008) Ursolic acid inhibits the formation of aberrant crypt foci and affects colonic sphingomyelin hydrolyzing enzymes in azoxymethane-treated rats. J Cancer Res Clin Oncol 134:101–107. https://doi.org/10.1007/s00432-007-0255-4

Andersson D, Kotarsky K, Wu J, Agace W, Duan RD (2009) Expression of alkaline sphingomyelinase in yeast cells and anti-inflammatory effects of the expressed enzyme in a rat colitis model. Dig Dis Sci 54:1440–1448. https://doi.org/10.1007/s10620-008-0509-2

Appleyard CB, Cruz ML, Isidro AA, Arthur JC, Jobin C, De Simone C (2011) Pretreatment with the probiotic VSL#3 delays transition from inflammation to dysplasia in a rat model of colitis-associated cancer. Am J Physiol Gastrointest Liver Physiol 301:G1004–G1013. https://doi.org/10.1152/ajpgi.00167.2011

Arenz C (2010) Small molecule inhibitors of acid sphingomyelinase. Cell Physiol Biochem 26:1–8. https://doi.org/10.1159/000315100

Arenz C, Giannis A (2000) Synthesis of the First Selective Irreversible Inhibitor of Neutral Sphingomyelinase This work was supported by grants from the Fonds der Chemischen Industrie. C.A. is grateful to the Land of Baden-Wurttemberg for a scholarship from the Landesgraduiertenforderung. Angew Chem Int Ed Engl 39:1440–1442

Arenz C, Gartner M, Wascholowski V, Giannis A (2001a) Synthesis and biochemical investigation of scyphostatin analogues as inhibitors of neutral sphingomyelinase. Bioorg Med Chem 9:2901–2904

Arenz C, Thutewohl M, Block O, Waldmann H, Altenbach HJ, Giannis A (2001b) Manumycin A and its analogues are irreversible inhibitors of neutral sphingomyelinase. ChemBioChem 2:141–143

Aslan M, Ozcan F, Tuzcu H, Kirac E, Elpek GO (2014) Inhibition of neutral sphingomyelinase decreases arachidonic acid mediated inflammation in liver ischemia-reperfusion injury. Int J Clin Exp Pathol 7:7814–7823

Bai A, Guo Y (2017) Acid sphingomyelinase mediates human CD4+ T-cell signaling: potential roles in T-cell responses and diseases. Cell Death Dis 8:e2963. https://doi.org/10.1038/cddis.2017.360

Baranowski M, Blachnio-Zabielska A, Hirnle T, Harasiuk D, Matlak K, Knapp M, Zabielski P, Gorski J (2010) Myocardium of type 2 diabetic and obese patients is characterized by alterations in sphingolipid metabolic enzymes but not by accumulation of ceramide. J Lipid Res 51:74–80. https://doi.org/10.1194/jlr.M900002-JLR200

Bartke N, Hannun YA (2009) Bioactive sphingolipids: metabolism and function. J Lipid Res 50 (Suppl):S91–S96. https://doi.org/10.1194/jlr.R800080-JLR200

Becker KA, Riethmuller J, Luth A, Doring G, Kleuser B, Gulbins E (2010) Acid sphingomyelinase inhibitors normalize pulmonary ceramide and inflammation in cystic fibrosis. Am J Respir Cell Mol Biol 42:716–724. https://doi.org/10.1165/rcmb.2009-0174OC

Becker KA, Beckmann N, Adams C, Hessler G, Kramer M, Gulbins E, Carpinteiro A (2017) Melanoma cell metastasis via P-selectin-mediated activation of acid sphingomyelinase in platelets. Clin Exp Metastasis 34:25–35. https://doi.org/10.1007/s10585-016-9826-6

Beckmann N, Sharma D, Gulbins E, Becker KA, Edelmann B (2014) Inhibition of acid sphingomyelinase by tricyclic antidepressants and analogons. Front Physiol 5:331. https://doi.org/10.3389/fphys.2014.00331

Bernier M, Kwon YK, Pandey SK, Zhu TN, Zhao RJ, Maciuk A, He HJ, Decabo R, Kole S (2006) Binding of manumycin A inhibits IkappaB kinase beta activity. J Biol Chem 281:2551–2561. https://doi.org/10.1074/jbc.M511878200

Bienias K, Fiedorowicz A, Sadowska A, Prokopiuk S, Car H (2016) Regulation of sphingomyelin metabolism. Pharmacol Rep 68:570–581. https://doi.org/10.1016/j.pharep.2015.12.008

Brady RO, Kanfer JN, Mock MB, Fredrickson DS (1966) The metabolism of sphingomyelin. II. Evidence of an enzymatic deficiency in Niemann-Pick disease. Proc Natl Acad Sci U S A 55:366–369

Brann AB, Tcherpakov M, Williams IM, Futerman AH, Fainzilber M (2002) Nerve growth factor-induced p75-mediated death of cultured hippocampal neurons is age-dependent and transduced through ceramide generated by neutral sphingomyelinase. J Biol Chem 277:9812–9818. https://doi.org/10.1074/jbc.M109862200

Brodowicz J, Przegalinski E, Muller CP, Filip M (2017) Ceramide and its related neurochemical networks as targets for some brain disorder therapies. Neurotox Res. https://doi.org/10.1007/s12640-017-9798-6

Canals D, Hannun YA (2013) Novel chemotherapeutic drugs in sphingolipid cancer research. Handb Exp Pharmacol 211–238. doi: https://doi.org/10.1007/978-3-7091-1368-4_12

Canals D, Perry DM, Jenkins RW, Hannun YA (2011) Drug targeting of sphingolipid metabolism: sphingomyelinases and ceramidases. Br J Pharmacol 163:694–712. https://doi.org/10.1111/j.1476-5381.2011.01279.x

Carpinteiro A, Becker KA, Japtok L, Hessler G, Keitsch S, Pozgajova M, Schmid KW, Adams C, Muller S, Kleuser B, Edwards MJ, Grassme H, Helfrich I, Gulbins E (2015) Regulation of hematogenous tumor metastasis by acid sphingomyelinase. EMBO Mol Med 7:714–734. https://doi.org/10.15252/emmm.201404571

Chaube R, Kallakunta VM, Espey MG, McLarty R, Faccenda A, Ananvoranich S, Mutus B (2012) Endoplasmic reticulum stress-mediated inhibition of NSMase2 elevates plasma membrane cholesterol and attenuates NO production in endothelial cells. Biochim Biophys Acta 1821:313–323. https://doi.org/10.1016/j.bbalip.2011.10.015

Chen Y, Zhang P, Xu SC, Yang L, Voss U, Ekblad E, Wu Y, Min Y, Hertervig E, Nilsson A, Duan RD (2015) Enhanced colonic tumorigenesis in alkaline sphingomyelinase (NPP7) knockout mice. Mol Cancer Ther 14:259–267. https://doi.org/10.1158/1535-7163.MCT-14-0468-T

Chen JY, Newcomb B, Zhou C, Pondick JV, Ghoshal S, York SR, Motola DL, Coant N, Yi JK, Mao C, Tanabe KK, Bronova I, Berdyshev EV, Fuchs BC, Hannun Y, Chung RT, Mullen AC (2017) Tricyclic antidepressants promote ceramide accumulation to regulate collagen production in human hepatic stellate cells. Sci Rep 7:44867. https://doi.org/10.1038/srep44867

Cheng Y, Tauschel HD, Nilsson A, Duan RD (1999) Ursodeoxycholic acid increases the activities of alkaline sphingomyelinase and caspase-3 in the rat colon. Scand J Gastroenterol 34:915–920

Cheng Y, Ohlsson L, Duan RD (2004) Psyllium and fat in diets differentially affect the activities and expressions of colonic sphingomyelinases and caspase in mice. Br J Nutr 91:715–723. https://doi.org/10.1079/BJN20041107

Cheng Y, Wu J, Hertervig E, Lindgren S, Duan D, Nilsson A, Duan RD (2007) Identification of aberrant forms of alkaline sphingomyelinase (NPP7) associated with human liver tumorigenesis. Br J Cancer 97:1441–1448. https://doi.org/10.1038/sj.bjc.6604013

Chung HY, Witt CJ, Jbeily N, Hurtado-Oliveros J, Giszas B, Lupp A, Graler MH, Bruns T, Stallmach A, Gonnert FA, Claus RA (2017) Acid sphingomyelinase inhibition prevents development of sepsis sequelae in the murine liver. Sci Rep 7:12348. https://doi.org/10.1038/s41598-017-11837-2

Clarke CJ, Cloessner EA, Roddy PL, Hannun YA (2011a) Neutral sphingomyelinase 2 (nSMase2) is the primary neutral sphingomyelinase isoform activated by tumour necrosis factor-alpha in MCF-7 cells. Biochem J 435:381–390. https://doi.org/10.1042/BJ20101752

Clarke CJ, Wu BX, Hannun YA (2011b) The neutral sphingomyelinase family: identifying biochemical connections. Adv Enzyme Regul 51:51–58. https://doi.org/10.1016/j.advenzreg.2010.09.016

Cogolludo A, Moreno L, Frazziano G, Moral-Sanz J, Menendez C, Castaneda J, Gonzalez C, Villamor E, Perez-Vizcaino F (2009) Activation of neutral sphingomyelinase is involved in acute hypoxic pulmonary vasoconstriction. Cardiovasc Res 82:296–302. https://doi.org/10.1093/cvr/cvn349

Corcoran CA, He Q, Ponnusamy S, Ogretmen B, Huang Y, Sheikh MS (2008) Neutral sphingomyelinase-3 is a DNA damage and nongenotoxic stress-regulated gene that is deregulated in human malignancies. Mol Cancer Res 6:795–807. https://doi.org/10.1158/1541-7786.MCR-07-2097

Dhami R, He X, Schuchman EH (2010) Acid sphingomyelinase deficiency attenuates bleomycin-induced lung inflammation and fibrosis in mice. Cell Physiol Biochem 26:749–760. https://doi.org/10.1159/000322342

Di Marzio L, Alesse E, Roncaioli P, Muzi P, Moretti S, Marcellini S, Amicosante G, De Simone C, Cifone MG (1997) Influence of L-carnitine on CD95 cross-lining-induced apoptosis and ceramide generation in human cell lines: correlation with its effects on purified acidic and neutral sphingomyelinases in vitro. Proc Assoc Am Physicians 109:154–163

Di Scala C, Mazzarino M, Yahi N, Varini K, Garmy N, Fantini J, Chahinian H (2017) Ceramide binding to anandamide increases its half-life and potentiates its cytotoxicity in human neuroblastoma cells. Chem Phys Lipids 205:11–17. https://doi.org/10.1016/j.chemphyslip.2017.04.001

Duan RD, Nilsson A (2009) Metabolism of sphingolipids in the gut and its relation to inflammation and cancer development. Prog Lipid Res 48:62–72. https://doi.org/10.1016/j.plipres.2008.04.003

Duan RD, Bergman T, Xu N, Wu J, Cheng Y, Duan J, Nelander S, Palmberg C, Nilsson A (2003) Identification of human intestinal alkaline sphingomyelinase as a novel ecto-enzyme related to the nucleotide phosphodiesterase family. J Biol Chem 278:38528–38536. https://doi.org/10.1074/jbc.M305437200

Duan RD, Hindorf U, Cheng Y, Bergenzaun P, Hall M, Hertervig E, Nilsson A (2014) Changes of activity and isoforms of alkaline sphingomyelinase (nucleotide pyrophosphatase phosphodiesterase 7) in bile from patients undergoing endoscopic retrograde cholangiopancreatography. BMC Gastroenterol 14:138. https://doi.org/10.1186/1471-230X-14-138

Ellegaard AM, Groth-Pedersen L, Oorschot V, Klumperman J, Kirkegaard T, Nylandsted J, Jaattela M (2013) Sunitinib and SU11652 inhibit acid sphingomyelinase, destabilize lysosomes, and inhibit multidrug resistance. Mol Cancer Ther 12:2018–2030. https://doi.org/10.1158/1535-7163.MCT-13-0084

Elojeimy S, Holman DH, Liu X, El-Zawahry A, Villani M, Cheng JC, Mahdy A, Zeidan Y, Bielwaska A, Hannun YA, Norris JS (2006) New insights on the use of desipramine as an inhibitor for acid ceramidase. FEBS Lett 580:4751–4756. https://doi.org/10.1016/j.febslet.2006.07.071

Essandoh K, Yang L, Wang X, Huang W, Qin D, Hao J, Wang Y, Zingarelli B, Peng T, Fan GC (2015) Blockade of exosome generation with GW4869 dampens the sepsis-induced inflammation and cardiac dysfunction. Biochim Biophys Acta 1852:2362–2371. https://doi.org/10.1016/j.bbadis.2015.08.010

Falcone S, Perrotta C, De Palma C, Pisconti A, Sciorati C, Capobianco A, Rovere-Querini P, Manfredi AA, Clementi E (2004) Activation of acid sphingomyelinase and its inhibition by the nitric oxide/cyclic guanosine 3′,5′-monophosphate pathway: key events in Escherichia coli-elicited apoptosis of dendritic cells. J Immunol 173:4452–4463

Figuera-Losada M, Stathis M, Dorskind JM, Thomas AG, Bandaru VV, Yoo SW, Westwood NJ, Rogers GW, McArthur JC, Haughey NJ, Slusher BS, Rojas C (2015) Cambinol, a novel inhibitor of neutral sphingomyelinase 2 shows neuroprotective properties. PLoS One 10: e0124481. https://doi.org/10.1371/journal.pone.0124481

Filosto S, Ashfaq M, Chung S, Fry W, Goldkorn T (2012) Neutral sphingomyelinase 2 activity and protein stability are modulated by phosphorylation of five conserved serines. J Biol Chem 287:514–522. https://doi.org/10.1074/jbc.M111.315481

Goggel R, Winoto-Morbach S, Vielhaber G, Imai Y, Lindner K, Brade L, Brade H, Ehlers S, Slutsky AS, Schutze S, Gulbins E, Uhlig S (2004) PAF-mediated pulmonary edema: a new role for acid sphingomyelinase and ceramide. Nat Med 10:155–160. https://doi.org/10.1038/nm977

Gorelik A, Heinz LX, Illes K, Superti-Furga G, Nagar B (2016a) Crystal structure of the acid sphingomyelinase-like phosphodiesterase SMPDL3B provides insights into determinants of substrate specificity. J Biol Chem 291:24054–24064. https://doi.org/10.1074/jbc.M116.755801

Gorelik A, Illes K, Heinz LX, Superti-Furga G, Nagar B (2016b) Crystal structure of mammalian acid sphingomyelinase. Nat Commun 7:12196. https://doi.org/10.1038/ncomms12196

Gorelik A, Illes K, Superti-Furga G, Nagar B (2016c) Structural basis for nucleotide hydrolysis by the acid sphingomyelinase-like phosphodiesterase SMPDL3A. J Biol Chem 291:6376–6385. https://doi.org/10.1074/jbc.M115.711085

Gorelik A, Liu F, Illes K, Nagar B (2017) Crystal structure of the human alkaline sphingomyelinase provides insights into substrate recognition. J Biol Chem 292:7087–7094. https://doi.org/10.1074/jbc.M116.769273

Groth-Pedersen L, Jaattela M (2013) Combating apoptosis and multidrug resistant cancers by targeting lysosomes. Cancer Lett 332:265–274. https://doi.org/10.1016/j.canlet.2010.05.021

Gu L, Huang B, Shen W, Gao L, Ding Z, Wu H, Guo J (2013) Early activation of nSMase2/ceramide pathway in astrocytes is involved in ischemia-associated neuronal damage via inflammation in rat hippocampi. J Neuroinflammation 10:109. https://doi.org/10.1186/1742-2094-10-109

Gulbins E, Palmada M, Reichel M, Luth A, Bohmer C, Amato D, Muller CP, Tischbirek CH, Groemer TW, Tabatabai G, Becker KA, Tripal P, Staedtler S, Ackermann TF, van Brederode J, Alzheimer C, Weller M, Lang UE, Kleuser B, Grassme H, Kornhuber J (2013) Acid sphingomyelinase-ceramide system mediates effects of antidepressant drugs. Nat Med 19:934–938. https://doi.org/10.1038/nm.3214

Gulbins A, Grassme H, Hoehn R, Wilker B, Soddemann M, Kohnen M, Edwards MJ, Kornhuber J, Gulbins E (2016) Regulation of neuronal stem cell proliferation in the hippocampus by endothelial ceramide. Cell Physiol Biochem 39:790–801. https://doi.org/10.1159/000447789

Guo BB, Bellingham SA, Hill AF (2016) Stimulating the release of exosomes increases the intercellular transfer of prions. J Biol Chem 291:5128–5137. https://doi.org/10.1074/jbc.M115.684258

Hamada M, Iikubo K, Ishikawa Y, Ikeda A, Umezawa K, Nishiyama S (2003) Biological activities of alpha-mangostin derivatives against acidic sphingomyelinase. Bioorg Med Chem Lett 13:3151–3153

Hannun YA, Obeid LM (1995) Ceramide: an intracellular signal for apoptosis. Trends Biochem Sci 20:73–77

Hannun YA, Obeid LM (2008) Principles of bioactive lipid signalling: lessons from sphingolipids. Nat Rev Mol Cell Biol 9:139–150. https://doi.org/10.1038/nrm2329

Hannun YA, Obeid LM (2011) Many ceramides. J Biol Chem 286:27855–27862. https://doi.org/10.1074/jbc.R111.254359

Heinz LX, Baumann CL, Koberlin MS, Snijder B, Gawish R, Shui G, Sharif O, Aspalter IM, Muller AC, Kandasamy RK, Breitwieser FP, Pichlmair A, Bruckner M, Rebsamen M, Bluml S, Karonitsch T, Fauster A, Colinge J, Bennett KL, Knapp S, Wenk MR, Superti-Furga G (2015) The lipid-modifying enzyme SMPDL3B negatively regulates innate immunity. Cell Rep 11:1919–1928. https://doi.org/10.1016/j.celrep.2015.05.006

Henry J, Guillotte A, Luberto C, Del Poeta M (2011) Characterization of inositol phospho-sphingolipid-phospholipase C 1 (Isc1) in Cryptococcus neoformans reveals unique biochemical features. FEBS Lett 585:635–640. https://doi.org/10.1016/j.febslet.2011.01.015

Hertervig E, Nilsson A, Nyberg L, Duan RD (1997) Alkaline sphingomyelinase activity is decreased in human colorectal carcinoma. Cancer 79:448–453

Hoehn R, Monse M, Pohl E, Wranik S, Wilker B, Keitsch S, Soddemann M, Kornhuber J, Kohnen M, Edwards MJ, Grassme H, Gulbins E (2016) Melatonin acts as an antidepressant by inhibition of the acid sphingomyelinase/ceramide system. Neurosignals 24:48–58. https://doi.org/10.1159/000442611

Hoehn RS, Jernigan PL, Japtok L, Chang AL, Midura EF, Caldwell CC, Kleuser B, Lentsch AB, Edwards MJ, Gulbins E, Pritts TA (2017) Acid sphingomyelinase inhibition in stored erythrocytes reduces transfusion-associated lung inflammation. Ann Surg 265:218–226. https://doi.org/10.1097/SLA.0000000000001648

Horres CR, Hannun YA (2012) The roles of neutral sphingomyelinases in neurological pathologies. Neurochem Res 37:1137–1149. https://doi.org/10.1007/s11064-011-0692-y

Hurwitz R, Ferlinz K, Sandhoff K (1994) The tricyclic antidepressant desipramine causes proteolytic degradation of lysosomal sphingomyelinase in human fibroblasts. Biol Chem Hoppe Seyler 375:447–450

Hwang SY, Kim TH, Lee HH (2015) Neutral sphingomyelinase and breast cancer research. J Menopausal Med 21:24–27. https://doi.org/10.6118/jmm.2015.21.1.24

Ito H, Tanaka K, Hagiwara K, Kobayashi M, Hoshikawa A, Mizutani N, Takagi A, Kojima T, Sobue S, Ichihara M, Suzuki M, Tamiya-Koizumi K, Nakamura M, Banno Y, Nozawa Y, Murate T (2012) Transcriptional regulation of neutral sphingomyelinase 2 in all-trans retinoic acid-treated human breast cancer cell line, MCF-7. J Biochem 151:599–610. https://doi.org/10.1093/jb/mvs037

Jana A, Pahan K (2010) Fibrillar amyloid-beta-activated human astroglia kill primary human neurons via neutral sphingomyelinase: implications for Alzheimer's disease. J Neurosci 30:12676–12689. https://doi.org/10.1523/JNEUROSCI.1243-10.2010

Jenkins RW, Canals D, Idkowiak-Baldys J, Simbari F, Roddy P, Perry DM, Kitatani K, Luberto C, Hannun YA (2010) Regulated secretion of acid sphingomyelinase: implications for selectivity of ceramide formation. J Biol Chem 285:35706–35718. https://doi.org/10.1074/jbc.M110.125609

Kanfer JN, Young OM, Shapiro D, Brady RO (1966) The metabolism of sphingomyelin. I. Purification and properties of a sphingomyelin-cleaving enzyme from rat liver tissue. J Biol Chem 241:1081–1084

Kim WJ, Okimoto RA, Purton LE, Goodwin M, Haserlat SM, Dayyani F, Sweetser DA, McClatchey AI, Bernard OA, Look AT, Bell DW, Scadden DT, Haber DA (2008) Mutations in the neutral sphingomyelinase gene SMPD3 implicate the ceramide pathway in human leukemias. Blood 111:4716–4722. https://doi.org/10.1182/blood-2007-10-113068

Kobayashi K, Ishizaki Y, Kojo S, Kikuzaki H (2016) Strong Inhibition of secretory sphingomyelinase by catechins, particularly by (−)-epicatechin 3-O-gallate and (−)-3′-O-methylepigallocatechin 3-O-gallate. J Nutr Sci Vitaminol (Tokyo) 62:123–129. doi: https://doi.org/10.3177/jnsv.62.123

Kolmakova A, Kwiterovich P, Virgil D, Alaupovic P, Knight-Gibson C, Martin SF, Chatterjee S (2004) Apolipoprotein C-I induces apoptosis in human aortic smooth muscle cells via recruiting neutral sphingomyelinase. Arterioscler Thromb Vasc Biol 24:264–269. https://doi.org/10.1161/01.ATV.0000112036.72200.ac

Kolzer M, Werth N, Sandhoff K (2004) Interactions of acid sphingomyelinase and lipid bilayers in the presence of the tricyclic antidepressant desipramine. FEBS Lett 559:96–98. https://doi.org/10.1016/S0014-5793(04)00033-X

Kong JN, He Q, Wang G, Dasgupta S, Dinkins MB, Zhu G, Kim A, Spassieva S, Bieberich E (2015) Guggulsterone and bexarotene induce secretion of exosome-associated breast cancer resistance protein and reduce doxorubicin resistance in MDA-MB-231 cells. Int J Cancer 137:1610–1620. https://doi.org/10.1002/ijc.29542

Kornhuber J, Tripal P, Reichel M, Muhle C, Rhein C, Muehlbacher M, Groemer TW, Gulbins E (2010) Functional inhibitors of acid sphingomyelinase (FIASMAs): a novel pharmacological group of drugs with broad clinical applications. Cell Physiol Biochem 26:9–20. https://doi.org/10.1159/000315101

Kornhuber J, Rhein C, Muller CP, Muhle C (2015) Secretory sphingomyelinase in health and disease. Biol Chem 396:707–736. https://doi.org/10.1515/hsz-2015-0109

Kosaka N, Iguchi H, Hagiwara K, Yoshioka Y, Takeshita F, Ochiya T (2013) Neutral sphingomyelinase 2 (nSMase2)-dependent exosomal transfer of angiogenic microRNAs regulate cancer cell metastasis. J Biol Chem 288:10849–10859. https://doi.org/10.1074/jbc.M112.446831

Kramer M, Quickert S, Sponholz C, Menzel U, Huse K, Platzer M, Bauer M, Claus RA (2015) Alternative splicing of SMPD1 in human sepsis. PLoS One 10:e0124503. https://doi.org/10.1371/journal.pone.0124503

Kruse AC, Huseby MJ, Shi K, Digre J, Ohlendorf DH, Earhart CA (2011) Structure of a mutant beta toxin from Staphylococcus aureus reveals domain swapping and conformational flexibility. Acta Crystallogr Sect F Struct Biol Cryst Commun 67:438–441. https://doi.org/10.1107/S1744309111005239

Krut O, Wiegmann K, Kashkar H, Yazdanpanah B, Kronke M (2006) Novel tumor necrosis factor-responsive mammalian neutral sphingomyelinase-3 is a C-tail-anchored protein. J Biol Chem 281:13784–13793. https://doi.org/10.1074/jbc.M511306200

Kuemmel TA, Schroeder R, Stoffel W (1997a) Light and electron microscopic analysis of the central and peripheral nervous systems of acid sphingomyelinase-deficient mice resulting from gene targeting. J Neuropathol Exp Neurol 56:171–179

Kuemmel TA, Thiele J, Schroeder R, Stoffel W (1997b) Pathology of visceral organs and bone marrow in an acid sphingomyelinase deficient knock-out mouse line, mimicking human Niemann-Pick disease type A. A light and electron microscopic study. Pathol Res Pract 193:663–671. https://doi.org/10.1016/S0344-0338(97)80025-8

Kuzu OF, Toprak M, Noory MA, Robertson GP (2017) Effect of lysosomotropic molecules on cellular homeostasis. Pharmacol Res 117:177–184. https://doi.org/10.1016/j.phrs.2016.12.021

Lee JK, Jin HK, Park MH, Kim BR, Lee PH, Nakauchi H, Carter JE, He X, Schuchman EH, Bae JS (2014) Acid sphingomyelinase modulates the autophagic process by controlling lysosomal biogenesis in Alzheimer's disease. J Exp Med 211:1551–1570. https://doi.org/10.1084/jem.20132451

Lim SM, Yeung K, Tresaugues L, Ling TH, Nordlund P (2015) The structure and catalytic mechanism of human sphingomyelin phosphodiesterase like 3a – an acid sphingomyelinase homologue with a novel nucleotide hydrolase activity. FEBS J 283:1107–1123. https://doi.org/10.1111/febs.13655

Liu B, Andrieu-Abadie N, Levade T, Zhang P, Obeid LM, Hannun YA (1998) Glutathione regulation of neutral sphingomyelinase in tumor necrosis factor-alpha-induced cell death. J Biol Chem 273:11313–11320

Liu F, Cheng Y, Wu J, Tauschel HD, Duan RD (2006) Ursodeoxycholic acid differentially affects three types of sphingomyelinase in human colon cancer Caco 2 cells. Cancer Lett 235:141–146. https://doi.org/10.1016/j.canlet.2005.04.016

Luberto C, Hassler DF, Signorelli P, Okamoto Y, Sawai H, Boros E, Hazen-Martin DJ, Obeid LM, Hannun YA, Smith GK (2002) Inhibition of tumor necrosis factor-induced cell death in MCF7 by a novel inhibitor of neutral sphingomyelinase. J Biol Chem 277:41128–41139. https://doi.org/10.1074/jbc.M206747200

McGovern MM, Wasserstein MP, Kirmse B, Duvall WL, Schiano T, Thurberg BL, Richards S, Cox GF (2016) Novel first-dose adverse drug reactions during a phase I trial of olipudase alfa (recombinant human acid sphingomyelinase) in adults with Niemann-Pick disease type B (acid sphingomyelinase deficiency). Genet Med 18:34–40. https://doi.org/10.1038/gim.2015.24

Milhas D, Clarke CJ, Idkowiak-Baldys J, Canals D, Hannun YA (2010) Anterograde and retrograde transport of neutral sphingomyelinase-2 between the Golgi and the plasma membrane. Biochim Biophys Acta 1801:1361–1374. https://doi.org/10.1016/j.bbalip.2010.08.001

Miller ME, Adhikary S, Kolokoltsov AA, Davey RA (2012) Ebolavirus requires acid sphingomyelinase activity and plasma membrane sphingomyelin for infection. J Virol 86:7473–7483. https://doi.org/10.1128/JVI.00136-12

Moylan JS, Smith JD, Wolf Horrell EM, McLean JB, Deevska GM, Bonnell MR, Nikolova-Karakashian MN, Reid MB (2014) Neutral sphingomyelinase-3 mediates TNF-stimulated oxidant activity in skeletal muscle. Redox Biol 2:910–920. https://doi.org/10.1016/j.redox.2014.07.006

Olmeda B, Garcia-Alvarez B, Perez-Gil J (2013) Structure-function correlations of pulmonary surfactant protein SP-B and the saposin-like family of proteins. Eur Biophys J 42:209–222. https://doi.org/10.1007/s00249-012-0858-9

Peng H, Li C, Kadow S, Henry BD, Steinmann J, Becker KA, Riehle A, Beckmann N, Wilker B, Li PL, Pritts T, Edwards MJ, Zhang Y, Gulbins E, Grassme H (2015) Acid sphingomyelinase inhibition protects mice from lung edema and lethal Staphylococcus aureus sepsis. J Mol Med (Berl) 93:675–689. https://doi.org/10.1007/s00109-014-1246-y

Perrotta C, Cervia D, De Palma C, Assi E, Pellegrino P, Bassi MT, Clementi E (2015) The emerging role of acid sphingomyelinase in autophagy. Apoptosis 20:635–644. https://doi.org/10.1007/s10495-015-1101-9

Perry DM, Newcomb B, Adada M, Wu BX, Roddy P, Kitatani K, Siskind L, Obeid LM, Hannun YA (2014) Defining a role for acid sphingomyelinase in the p38/interleukin-6 pathway. J Biol Chem 289:22401–22412. https://doi.org/10.1074/jbc.M114.589648

Petersen NH, Olsen OD, Groth-Pedersen L, Ellegaard AM, Bilgin M, Redmer S, Ostenfeld MS, Ulanet D, Dovmark TH, Lonborg A, Vindelov SD, Hanahan D, Arenz C, Ejsing CS, Kirkegaard T, Rohde M, Nylandsted J, Jaattela M (2013) Transformation-associated changes in sphingolipid metabolism sensitize cells to lysosomal cell death induced by inhibitors of acid sphingomyelinase. Cancer Cell 24:379–393. https://doi.org/10.1016/j.ccr.2013.08.003

Pitsinos EN, Wascholowski V, Karaliota S, Rigou C, Couladouros EA, Giannis A (2003) Synthesis and evaluation of three novel scyphostatin analogues as neutral sphingomyelinase inhibitors. ChemBioChem 4:1223–1225. https://doi.org/10.1002/cbic.200300667

Rajagopalan V, Canals D, Luberto C, Snider J, Voelkel-Johnson C, Obeid LM, Hannun YA (2015) Critical determinants of mitochondria-associated neutral sphingomyelinase (MA-nSMase) for mitochondrial localization. Biochim Biophys Acta 1850:628–639. https://doi.org/10.1016/j.bbagen.2014.11.019

Rao SS, Thompson C, Cheng J, Haimovitz-Friedman A, Powell SN, Fuks Z, Kolesnick RN (2014) Axitinib sensitization of high single dose radiotherapy. Radiother Oncol 111:88–93. https://doi.org/10.1016/j.radonc.2014.02.010

Revill K, Wang T, Lachenmayer A, Kojima K, Harrington A, Li J, Hoshida Y, Llovet JM, Powers S (2013) Genome-wide methylation analysis and epigenetic unmasking identify tumor suppressor genes in hepatocellular carcinoma. Gastroenterology 145:1424–1435, e1-e25. https://doi.org/10.1053/j.gastro.2013.08.055

Rhein C, Reichel M, Kramer M, Rotter A, Lenz B, Muhle C, Gulbins E, Kornhuber J (2017) Alternative splicing of SMPD1 coding for acid sphingomyelinase in major depression. J Affect Disord 209:10–15. https://doi.org/10.1016/j.jad.2016.09.019

Rodrigues-Lima F, Fensome AC, Josephs M, Evans J, Veldman RJ, Katan M (2000) Structural requirements for catalysis and membrane targeting of mammalian enzymes with neutral sphingomyelinase and lysophospholipid phospholipase C activities. Analysis by chemical modification and site-directed mutagenesis. J Biol Chem 275:28316–28325. https://doi.org/10.1074/jbc.M003080200

Romero-Ramirez L, Garcia-Alvarez I, Casas J, Barreda-Manso MA, Yanguas-Casas N, Nieto-Sampedro M, Fernandez-Mayoralas A (2015) New oleyl glycoside as anti-cancer agent that targets on neutral sphingomyelinase. Biochem Pharmacol 97:158–172. https://doi.org/10.1016/j.bcp.2015.07.009

Roth AG, Drescher D, Yang Y, Redmer S, Uhlig S, Arenz C (2009) Potent and selective inhibition of acid sphingomyelinase by bisphosphonates. Angew Chem Int Ed Engl 48:7560–7563. https://doi.org/10.1002/anie.200903288

Rutkute K, Karakashian AA, Giltiay NV, Dobierzewska A, Nikolova-Karakashian MN (2007) Aging in rat causes hepatic hyperresposiveness to interleukin-1beta which is mediated by neutral sphingomyelinase-2. Hepatology 46:1166–1176. https://doi.org/10.1002/hep.21777

Saftig P, Sandhoff K (2013) Cancer: Killing from the inside. Nature 502:312–313. https://doi.org/10.1038/nature12692

Sagy-Bross C, Hadad N, Levy R (2013) Cytosolic phospholipase A2alpha upregulation mediates apoptotic neuronal death induced by aggregated amyloid-beta peptide1-42. Neurochem Int 63:541–550. https://doi.org/10.1016/j.neuint.2013.09.007

Savic R, Schuchman EH (2013) Use of acid sphingomyelinase for cancer therapy. Adv Cancer Res 117:91–115. https://doi.org/10.1016/B978-0-12-394274-6.00004-2

Sawai H, Okamoto Y, Luberto C, Mao C, Bielawska A, Domae N, Hannun YA (2000) Identification of ISC1 (YER019w) as inositol phosphosphingolipid phospholipase C in Saccharomyces cerevisiae. J Biol Chem 275:39793–39798. https://doi.org/10.1074/jbc.M007721200

Schram AW, Dreissen M, Bastiaannet J, Donker-Koopman WE, Brouwer-Kelder EM, Weitz G, Barranger JA, Sandhoff K, Tager JM (1984) Immunological studies on lysosomal sphingomyelinase: identification of a 28 000-Da component deficient in urine from patients with Niemann-Pick disease types A and B. Biosci Rep 4:1051–1057

Schuchman EH (2007) The pathogenesis and treatment of acid sphingomyelinase-deficient Niemann-Pick disease. J Inherit Metab Dis 30:654–663. https://doi.org/10.1007/s10545-007-0632-9

Schuchman EH, Desnick RJ (2010) Chaperone-based therapy for Niemann-Pick disease. Google Patents. https://patentimages.storage.googleapis.com/41/7f/10/72633ad790eeae/US7750050.pdf

Schuchman EH, Desnick RJ (2017) Types A and B Niemann-Pick disease. Mol Genet Metab 120:27–33. https://doi.org/10.1016/j.ymgme.2016.12.008

Shamseddine AA, Airola MV, Hannun YA (2015a) Roles and regulation of neutral sphingomyelinase-2 in cellular and pathological processes. Adv Biol Regul 57:24–41. https://doi.org/10.1016/j.jbior.2014.10.002

Shamseddine AA, Clarke CJ, Carroll B, Airola MV, Mohammed S, Rella A, Obeid LM, Hannun YA (2015b) P53-dependent upregulation of neutral sphingomyelinase-2: role in doxorubicin-induced growth arrest. Cell Death Dis 6:e1947. https://doi.org/10.1038/cddis.2015.268

Singh R, Pochampally R, Watabe K, Lu Z, Mo YY (2014) Exosome-mediated transfer of miR-10b promotes cell invasion in breast cancer. Mol Cancer 13:256. https://doi.org/10.1186/1476-4598-13-256

Sjoqvist U, Hertervig E, Nilsson A, Duan RD, Ost A, Tribukait B, Lofberg R (2002) Chronic colitis is associated with a reduction of mucosal alkaline sphingomyelinase activity. Inflamm Bowel Dis 8:258–263

Smith EL, Schuchman EH (2008) The unexpected role of acid sphingomyelinase in cell death and the pathophysiology of common diseases. FASEB J 22:3419–3431. https://doi.org/10.1096/fj.08-108043

Sonoda K, Sakamoto T, Yoshikawa H, Ashizuka S, Ohshima Y, Kishihara K, Nomoto K, Ishibashi T, Inomata H (1998) Inhibition of corneal inflammation by the topical use of Ras farnesyltransferase inhibitors: selective inhibition of macrophage localization. Invest Ophthalmol Vis Sci 39:2245–2251

Soo I, Madsen KL, Tejpar Q, Sydora BC, Sherbaniuk R, Cinque B, Di Marzio L, Cifone MG, Desimone C, Fedorak RN (2008) VSL#3 probiotic upregulates intestinal mucosal alkaline sphingomyelinase and reduces inflammation. Can J Gastroenterol 22:237–242

Tani M, Hannun YA (2007a) Analysis of membrane topology of neutral sphingomyelinase 2. FEBS Lett 581:1323–1328. https://doi.org/10.1016/j.febslet.2007.02.046

Tani M, Hannun YA (2007b) Neutral sphingomyelinase 2 is palmitoylated on multiple cysteine residues. Role of palmitoylation in subcellular localization. J Biol Chem 282:10047–10056. https://doi.org/10.1074/jbc.M611249200

Tseng TH, Shen CH, Huang WS, Chen CN, Liang WH, Lin TH, Kuo HC (2014) Activation of neutral-sphingomyelinase, MAPKs, and p75 NTR-mediating caffeic acid phenethyl ester-induced apoptosis in C6 glioma cells. J Biomed Sci 21:61. https://doi.org/10.1186/1423-0127-21-61

van Hell AJ, Haimovitz-Friedman A, Fuks Z, Tap WD, Kolesnick R (2017) Gemcitabine kills proliferating endothelial cells exclusively via acid sphingomyelinase activation. Cell Signal 34:86–91. https://doi.org/10.1016/j.cellsig.2017.02.021

Volk BW, Adachi M, Schneck L (1972) The pathology of sphingolipidoses. Semin Hematol 9:317–348

Wheeler D, Knapp E, Bandaru VV, Wang Y, Knorr D, Poirier C, Mattson MP, Geiger JD, Haughey NJ (2009) Tumor necrosis factor-alpha-induced neutral sphingomyelinase-2 modulates synaptic plasticity by controlling the membrane insertion of NMDA receptors. J Neurochem 109:1237–1249. https://doi.org/10.1111/j.1471-4159.2009.06038.x

Wu J, Liu F, Nilsson A, Duan RD (2004) Pancreatic trypsin cleaves intestinal alkaline sphingomyelinase from mucosa and enhances the sphingomyelinase activity. Am J Physiol Gastrointest Liver Physiol 287:G967–G973. https://doi.org/10.1152/ajpgi.00190.2004

Wu J, Hansen GH, Nilsson A, Duan RD (2005) Functional studies of human intestinal alkaline sphingomyelinase by deglycosylation and mutagenesis. Biochem J 386:153–160. https://doi.org/10.1042/BJ20041455

Wu BX, Rajagopalan V, Roddy PL, Clarke CJ, Hannun YA (2010) Identification and characterization of murine mitochondria-associated neutral sphingomyelinase (MA-nSMase), the mammalian sphingomyelin phosphodiesterase 5. J Biol Chem 285:17993–18002. https://doi.org/10.1074/jbc.M110.102988

Wu BX, Clarke CJ, Matmati N, Montefusco D, Bartke N, Hannun YA (2011) Identification of novel anionic phospholipid binding domains in neutral sphingomyelinase 2 with selective binding preference. J Biol Chem 286:22362–22371. https://doi.org/10.1074/jbc.M110.156471

Xiong ZJ, Huang J, Poda G, Pomes R, Prive GG (2016) Structure of human acid sphingomyelinase reveals the role of the saposin domain in activating substrate hydrolysis. J Mol Biol 428:3026–3042. https://doi.org/10.1016/j.jmb.2016.06.012

Yokomatsu T, Takechi H, Akiyama T, Shibuya S, Kominato T, Soeda S, Shimeno H (2001) Synthesis and evaluation of a difluoromethylene analogue of sphingomyelin as an inhibitor of sphingomyelinase. Bioorg Med Chem Lett 11:1277–1280

Yu H, Zeidan YH, Wu BX, Jenkins RW, Flotte TR, Hannun YA, Virella-Lowell I (2009) Defective acid sphingomyelinase pathway with Pseudomonas aeruginosa infection in cystic fibrosis. Am J Respir Cell Mol Biol 41:367–375. https://doi.org/10.1165/rcmb.2008-0295OC

Yun SH, Park ES, Shin SW, Na YW, Han JY, Jeong JS, Shastina VV, Stonik VA, Park JI, Kwak JY (2012) Stichoposide C induces apoptosis through the generation of ceramide in leukemia and colorectal cancer cells and shows in vivo antitumor activity. Clin Cancer Res 18:5934–5948. https://doi.org/10.1158/1078-0432.CCR-12-0655

Zeidan YH, Jenkins RW, Hannun YA (2008) Remodeling of cellular cytoskeleton by the acid sphingomyelinase/ceramide pathway. J Cell Biol 181:335–350. https://doi.org/10.1083/jcb.200705060

Zhang L, Guo J (2013) Advance in research on regulatory mechanism and functions of neutral sphingomyelinse 2. Zhongguo Yi Xue Ke Xue Yuan Xue Bao 35:581–585. https://doi.org/10.3881/j.issn.1000-503X.2013.05.018

Zhou Y, Salker MS, Walker B, Munzer P, Borst O, Gawaz M, Gulbins E, Singh Y, Lang F (2016a) Acid sphingomyelinase (ASM) is a negative regulator of regulatory T cell (Treg) development. Cell Physiol Biochem 39:985–995. https://doi.org/10.1159/000447806

Zhou YF, Metcalf MC, Garman SC, Edmunds T, Qiu H, Wei RR (2016b) Human acid sphingomyelinase structures provide insight to molecular basis of Niemann-Pick disease. Nat Commun 7:13082. https://doi.org/10.1038/ncomms13082

Sphingosine Kinases as Druggable Targets

Susan Pyne, David R. Adams, and Nigel J. Pyne

Contents

Abstract

There is substantial evidence that the enzymes, sphingosine kinase 1 and 2, which catalyse the formation of the bioactive lipid sphingosine 1-phosphate, are

S. Pyne · N. J. Pyne (✉)
Strathclyde Institute of Pharmacy and Biomedical Sciences, University of Strathclyde, Glasgow, Scotland, UK
e-mail: n.j.pyne@strath.ac.uk

D. R. Adams
Institute of Chemical Sciences, Heriot-Watt University, Edinburgh, Scotland, UK

J. Gomez-Cambronero, M. A. Frohman (eds.), *Lipid Signaling in Human Diseases*, Handbook of Experimental Pharmacology 259, https://doi.org/10.1007/164_2018_96

involved in pathophysiological processes. In this chapter, we appraise the evidence that both enzymes are druggable and describe how isoform-specific inhibitors can be developed based on the plasticity of the sphingosine-binding site. This is contextualised with the effect of sphingosine kinase inhibitors in cancer, pulmonary hypertension, neurodegeneration, inflammation and sickling.

Keywords
Cancer · Inflammation · Neurodegeneration · Pulmonary hypertension · Sickling · Sphingosine 1-phosphate · Sphingosine kinase

1 Sphingosine Kinases

There are two isoforms of sphingosine kinase, termed SphK1 and SphK2, which catalyse the phosphorylation of sphingosine (Sph) to form the bioactive lipid, sphingosine 1-phosphate (S1P). SphK1 and SphK2 are encoded by different genes, are localised in distinct sub-cellular compartments and have different biochemical properties and inhibitor sensitivities (Pyne et al. 2016a). There are splice variants of both SphK1 (SphK1a–c) and SphK2 (SphK2a, b) that, for each isozyme, are distinguished by their N-terminal sequences. Although the relative expression, tissue distribution and function of the various splice variants are not well established, the differing N-terminal sequences are known to influence biochemical properties. Thus, the 36 amino acid N-terminally extended SphK2b isoform has higher activity compared with the SphK2a isoform, indicating that the N-terminus might regulate catalysis (Billich et al. 2003). Moreover, SphK1b, which contains an additional N-terminal 86 amino acids, is more resistant to SphK inhibitor-induced ubiquitin-proteasomal degradation compared with SphK1a (Loveridge et al. 2010). SphK1 and SphK2 exhibit some redundancy in function, as evident from studies in *sphk1*$^{-/-}$ or *sphk2*$^{-/-}$ mice, which are phenotypically healthy, while deletion of both genes is embryonic lethal (Mizugishi et al. 2005). In this regard, SphK1 and SphK2 appear to regulate discrete sub-cellular pools of S1P that govern both overlapping and/or non-overlapping biology (Pyne et al. 2016a). Levels of S1P are controlled both by SphK1/2, acting on pools of Sph that are coupled to ceramide biosynthesis (vide infra), and by the activity of S1P lyase and S1P phosphatases (Pyne et al. 2016a). S1P lyase catalyses the irreversible cleavage of S1P to form (*E*)-2-hexadecenal and phosphoethanolamine (Aguilar and Saba 2012) and represents the only exit point from the sphingolipid metabolic pathway, providing precursors for phospholipid biosynthesis (Nakahara et al. 2012). In contrast, S1P phosphatases, of which there are two isoforms, catalyse dephosphorylation of S1P to form Sph (Mandala 2001). Once formed, S1P can be released from cells by transporters [including Spns2 (Hisano et al. 2012), MFsd2b (Vu et al. 2017) and some ABC proteins (Kobayashi et al. 2009)] to subsequently bind to a family of S1P-specific G protein-coupled receptors (GPCRs), $S1P_{1-5}$, and thereby induce cellular responses (Blaho and Hla 2014). However, S1P also acts inside cells by binding to intracellular targets, such as histone deacetylase (HDAC1/2) (Hait et al. 2009) and telomerase reverse transcriptase (hTERT) (Panneer Selvam et al. 2015), to regulate epigenetic programmes and senescence. Therefore, S1P is a rather versatile bioactive lipid, being able to act both extracellularly and intracellularly to regulate biological processes.

2 Role of S1P and Ceramide

S1P is involved in regulating cardiovascular function, neuronal development and immune cell trafficking as well as other physiological processes (Pyne et al. 2016a). Not surprisingly, then, S1P is implicated in various pathophysiological conditions, including cardiovascular disease, autoimmune/inflammatory disease, neurodegeneration and cancer (Pyne et al. 2016a, 2017). Therefore, targeting the S1P signalling pathway is a potential therapeutic option for a number of diseases. There are two objectives here. The first is to suppress S1P signalling via its receptors and intracellular targets, either by antagonism of the receptors or by inhibition of SphK1/2 activity. The second, which is particularly relevant to cancer, is to promote an increase in cellular ceramide and Sph levels by blocking conversion of the latter to S1P, again by inhibition of SphK1/2 activity. Indeed, the physiological actions of ceramide and Sph generally oppose the actions of S1P and have been shown to promote senescence and induce apoptotic cell death in mammalian cells (Hannun and Obeid 2008, 2011). In contrast, S1P is involved in promoting cell growth (Spiegel and Milstien 2011). Therefore, the aim in elevating ceramide levels is to induce cytotoxicity in cancer cells.

3 Sphingolipid Biosynthesis

De novo synthesis of ceramide begins with the condensation of serine and palmitoyl CoA, catalysed by serine palmitoyltransferase, to form 3-ketosphinganine as the rate limiting step in ceramide biosynthesis (Hannun and Obeid 2008). 3-Ketosphinganine reductase then converts 3-ketosphinganine into dihydrosphingosine (sphinganine), which is acylated to produce dihydroceramide by ceramide synthases (CerS). Finally dihydroceramide desaturase (Degs1) catalyses the formation of ceramide by introduction of a 4,5-*trans* double bond. Ceramide can also be formed by the hydrolysis of sphingomyelin, catalysed by sphingomyelinase, which is part of the 'salvage pathway'. Ceramide is deacylated to Sph by ceramidase, and finally Sph can be either phosphorylated by SphK1 or SphK2, to form S1P, or it can be converted back into ceramide, catalysed by CerS (Fig. 1).

4 The Sphingolipid Rheostat

The dynamic interconversion of ceramide, Sph and S1P has been termed the 'sphingolipid rheostat' (Pyne et al. 1996; Cuvillier et al. 1996). In order for this pathway to be considered a rheostat the forward reactions (ceramide → Sph → S1P) and backward reactions (S1P → Sph → ceramide) should be regulated in a

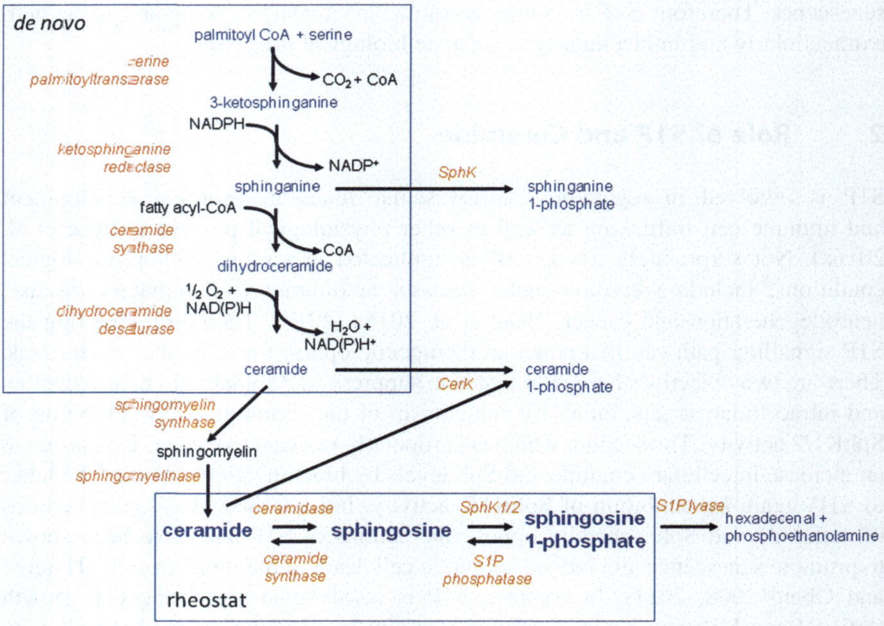

Fig. 1 Schematic of the sphingolipid metabolic pathway

reciprocal manner. In order to achieve this it is probable that the enzymes involved in the interconversion of ceramide, Sph and S1P are allosterically regulated. Indeed, it has been reported that S1P inhibits CerS2 by binding to two residues that are part of an S1P receptor-like motif found only in CerS2 (Laviad et al. 2008). This might therefore provide the essential molecular regulation that enables a rheostat to function. Inhibition of CerS2 by S1P would bias the rheostat toward the synthesis of S1P. In addition, the inhibition of CerS2 by S1P is expected to reduce de novo synthesis of long chain ceramides by redirecting dihydrosphingosine toward dihydrosphingosine 1-phosphate formation where SphK1 negatively regulates de novo ceramide synthesis (Siow et al. 2015). Regulation of SphK1 by ERK-1/2 catalysed phosphorylation (Pitson et al. 2003) stimulated by extracellular mediators is a mechanism by which the forward flux can be enhanced. In addition, regulation of the rheostat might be achieved by an unidentified sensor that can modulate forward and backward fluxes to determine the position of the rheostat, thereby programming cell death versus survival. Indeed, homeostatic sensors have been identified for regulating de novo ceramide synthesis (Siow et al. 2015). Thus, SphK inhibitors are expected to increase ceramide synthesis through modulation of both de novo and salvage pathways.

However, the sphingolipid rheostat model has additional complexity. For example, different molecular species of ceramide do not always promote cell death and, in some cases, can promote cell survival (Saddoughi and Ogretmen 2013). In addition, ceramide can be converted by ceramide kinase into ceramide 1-phosphate (C1P)

(Hoeferlin et al. 2013), which is a pro-survival signal. Moreover, the presence or absence of the key enzymes in various cellular compartments will determine whether the rheostat can operate in the manner expected, and distinct enzyme forms appear to regulate discrete lipid pools. Thus, at the plasma membrane, neutral sphingomyelinase catalyses the formation of ceramide (Hannun and Obeid 2008), which can then be converted into Sph which is used by SphK1 to produce S1P. However, the Sph substrate for SphK2 at the endoplasmic reticulum (ER) derives, at least in part, from the action of acid sphingomyelinase in the lysosome to generate ceramide, which is then deacylated by acid ceramidase (Hannun and Obeid 2008). Ceramide is also formed by the de novo pathway in the ER (Hannun and Obeid 2008). A ceramide transporter protein (CERT) transfers ceramide from the ER to the Golgi apparatus, where it is converted into complex sphingolipids, e.g. sphingomyelin and glycosphingolipids, which are then transported to various cellular compartments, including the plasma membrane (Yamaji and Hanada 2015). Therefore, there is both spatial and temporal regulation in the interconversion of ceramide, Sph and S1P in mammalian cells, which can influence cellular fate and offer opportunities for therapeutic intervention.

S1P-dependent signalling might enable cells to undergo positive selection by conferring enhanced survival. Therefore, the sphingolipid rheostat might have evolved in order to endow organisms with the capacity to use sphingolipids in interconverted and branched pathways to induce pleiotropy, thereby providing a wider repertoire of biological functions that enhance cell renewal and survival. In this regard, the ability of cancer cells to up-regulate SphK1 expression as part of a 'non-oncogenic addiction' (Vadas et al. 2008) and to drive the forward reaction of the sphingolipid rheostat might enable positive selection of a clonally expanded cancer cell population with replicative immortality. Therefore, pharmacological inhibition of SphK activity in cancer, for example, is geared to subverting the gain in cell survival achieved by enhancing ceramide formation to shift the balance toward cell death. This requires the development of effective isoform selective inhibitors of SphK1 and SphK2 that exhibit minimal or no 'off-target' effects.

5 Concept of Modulation of the Sphingolipid Rheostat

It is not immediately obvious why inhibition of SphK should necessarily increase ceramide levels with a pro-apoptotic outcome. One mechanistic explanation might involve dis-inhibition of the allosteric effects of S1P on CerS2. This enzyme has no activity using C16:0-CoA and very low activity using C18:0 CoA, but instead utilises longer acyl-chain CoAs (C20–C26) for ceramide synthesis (Laviad et al. 2008). In contrast to C16:0 ceramide, which has been shown to promote growth, longer chain species of ceramide are apoptotic (Saddoughi and Ogretmen 2013). Therefore, enhanced activity of CerS2 in the sphingolipid rheostat, due to a blockade of S1P formation by SphK inhibitors, could potentially bias synthesis toward apoptotic ceramides. A second possibility is that the conversion of ceramide to Sph, catalysed by ceramidase, might be inhibited by Sph that has accumulated as a consequence of inhibiting SphK activity, and there is evidence for product inhibition of epidermal ceramidase (Yada et al. 1995). Furthermore, rectifying sensors or relief of allosteric inhibition of enzymes involved in S1P and dihydrosphingosine 1-phosphate metabolism might induce a 'rippling effect' throughout the de novo ceramide, 'salvage' and complex sphingolipid biosynthetic pathways, adding complexity to therapeutic approaches that target sphingolipids. In addition, other conceptual considerations require evaluation, such as whether the sphingolipid rheostat involves graded or switch responses, involving 'threshold' levels of specific sphingolipids.

6 Sub-Cellular Localisation of SphK1 and SphK2

SphK1 is predominantly localised in the cytoplasm and is recruited to the plasma membrane in response to receptor stimulation by extracellular ligands, e.g. growth factors, TNFα and S1P (Pyne et al. 2016a). Once localised at the plasma membrane, SphK1 is thought to access its lipid substrate via a gating mechanism that involves opening of a flap-like lid to the substrate binding site (Adams et al. 2016). The surface of this lid, denoted lipid binding loop-1 (LBL-1), contains a hydrophobic patch that has been implicated in recruitment of SphK1 to membranes and may potentially insert into the plasma membrane (Adams et al. 2016). Recruitment of SphK1 to the plasma membrane is promoted by the action of extracellular signal-regulated kinases, ERK-1/2, which catalyse phosphorylation of a serine (Ser225) within an extended surface-exposed regulatory loop (the 'R-loop') (Pitson et al. 2003, 2005). Translocation of SphK1 to the plasma membrane also requires the calcium and integrin-binding protein 1, CIB1, which functions as a molecular chaperone (Jarman et al. 2010). SphK1 is additionally recruited to the plasma membrane in an ERK-1/2-independent manner involving G_q-coupled GPCRs (ter Braak et al. 2009). Thus, a Ser225Ala SphK1 mutant retains the capacity to translocate to the plasma membrane in response to muscarinic receptor stimulation. Both wild type (WT) and constitutively activated forms of G_q (e.g. $G\alpha_q^{R183C}$, $G\alpha_q^{Q209L}$-EE) promote this alternative mode of translocation (ter Braak et al. 2009), which might potentially involve association of G_q with the SphK1 C-terminal tail sequence (Adams et al. 2016). Indeed, this region of SphK1 is known to facilitate binding to other proteins, namely TNF receptor-associated factor 2 (TRAF2, in response to TNFα stimulation) and protein phosphatase 2 (PP2A, for dephosphorylation of Ser225) (Xia et al. 2002; Barr et al. 2008). Moreover, SphK1 adopts a dimeric quaternary structure that might allow coordinated coupling of plasma membrane association with phosphorylation of Ser225 in the R-loop, catalytic activity and protein–protein interaction (Lim et al. 2011b; Adams et al. 2016). Thus, the regulation of catalytic activity is likely to be more complex than a simple targeting of the protein to its substrate pool, potentially involving direct structural modulation of the enzyme's phosphoryl transfer capacity. In particular, the catalytic centre of the enzyme features a key loop, the 'T-loop', that presents the ATP co-substrate to the lipid. The T-loop is located at the N-terminal end of a short helix, α5, and exhibits structural plasticity that is likely to be important for kinase activity. The C-terminal end of helix-α5 lies proximal to and may be capped by the SphK1 C-terminal protein-binding sequence, deletion of which results in constitutive activation (Hengst et al. 2010a). It is therefore possible that protein binding to the C-terminal sequence modulates capping and thence T-loop structure to regulate activity (Adams et al. 2016).

In contrast, SphK2 is localised at the endoplasmic reticulum or is associated with mitochondria (Maceyka et al. 2005). In this regard, SphK2 contains both a nuclear localisation sequence (NLS) and a nuclear export signal sequence (NES) that enable the enzyme to shuttle in and out of the nucleus and to be exported from the nucleus after phosphorylation of the NLS by protein kinase D (Ding et al. 2007). S1P generated in the nucleus can regulate epigenetic programmes via the inhibition of HDAC1/2 activity (Hait et al. 2009). In addition, S1P binds to other intracellular targets that affect gene expression, such as the transcription factor, peroxisome proliferator-activated receptor gamma (PPARγ) (Parham et al. 2015).

7 S1P Receptors

S1P-specific GPCRs, $S1P_1$–$S1P_5$ (Chun et al. 2002; Kihara et al. 2014) are involved in numerous physiological processes in the cardiovascular, immune and nervous systems and can participate in regulating vascular barrier integrity, trafficking of lymphocytes and astrocyte function (Blaho and Hla 2014). However, S1P receptors also participate in the pathophysiology of autoimmune/inflammatory diseases and cancer. Therefore, members of the S1P receptor family are of significant interest as therapeutic targets, with drug discovery most advanced for ligands acting via $S1P_1$, such as fingolimod (FTY720) and ozanimod (Gonzalez-Cabrera et al. 2014). The latter and phosphorylated FTY720 serve as agonists for $S1P_1$ but trigger internalisation of the receptor, resulting in a functional antagonism that inhibits T-cell trafficking (Hla and Brinkmann 2011). FTY720 is currently licensed for treatment of multiple sclerosis (MS), while ozanimod is in Phase III and Phase II clinical trials for MS and ulcerative colitis, respectively. FTY720 phosphate, acting via S1P receptors, also regulates astrogliosis and nerve remyelination (Bigaud et al. 2014). Therefore, in terms of the development and utility of SphK inhibitors, a key question is whether these compounds can reduce the bioavailability of S1P at S1P receptors as a pharmacologically useful alternative to ligands targeting the receptors themselves. There is a substantial literature that relates to the release of S1P formed by SphK1 from cells and action on S1P receptors, both in terms of autocrine (termed 'inside-out' signalling) and paracrine mechanisms (Takabe et al. 2008). However, there is far less evidence that SphK2 can perform a similar function. Nevertheless, SphK2 catalyses the phosphorylation of FTY720, and phosphorylated FTY720 is released from cells to functionally antagonise $S1P_1$ on T-cells. This underlies, in part, the pharmacological action of fingolimod and, additionally, suggests that SphK2 can indirectly regulate S1P receptor function.

8 Intracellular Actions of S1P

In addition to its action on S1P receptors, there is evidence that S1P binds to and regulates intracellular target proteins to induce cell responses (Fig. 2). These represent additional targets for therapeutic intervention. However, at present there is a paucity of information concerning binding affinities for S1P and the stoichiometry at putative targets. Current understanding is further compromised by the lack of information concerning the concentration of S1P in various sub-cellular compartments. Nevertheless, intracellular targets of S1P have been directly related to fundamental biological processes that can potentially contribute to disease pathology. For instance, S1P formed by SphK1 has been reported to confer E3 ligase activity on TRAF2, where S1P is modelled to bind to its RING finger (Alvarez et al. 2010). TRAF2 has been shown to associate with SphK1 (Xia et al. 2002), thereby enabling the S1P formed to be in close proximity with its target. TRAF2 mediates the K63 polyubiquitination of RIP1, which participates in regulating pro-inflammatory TNFα/NFκB signalling. However, other reports have suggested that while TNFα-stimulated NF-κB activation is indeed reduced in *traf2*$^{-/-}$ keratinocytes,

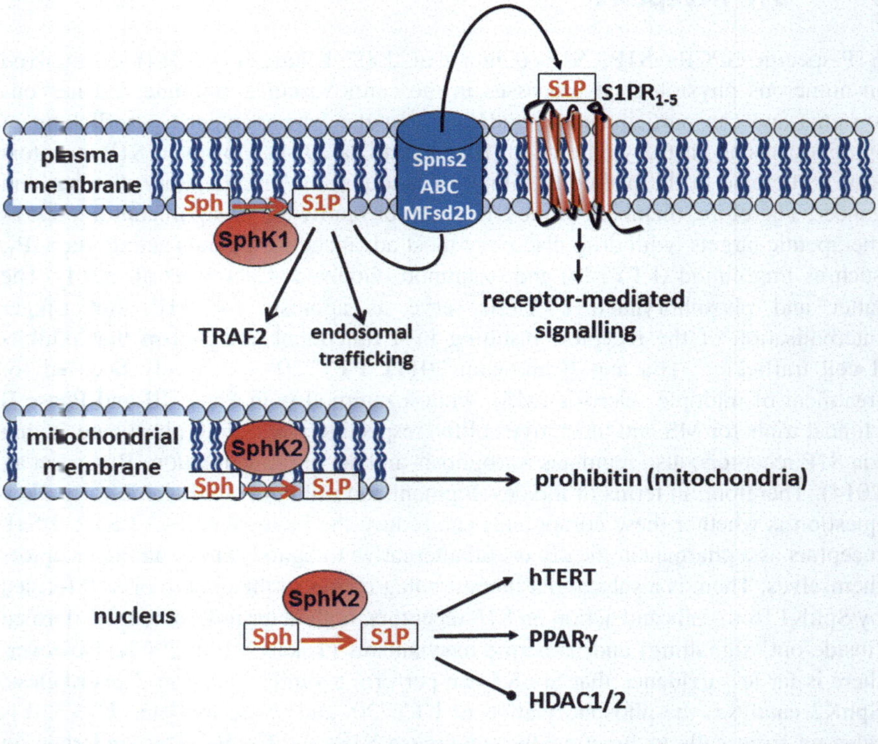

Fig. 2 Schematic illustrating various known targets of S1P as possible points of therapeutic intervention by blockade of S1P signalling through receptors or intracellular targets such as HDAC-1/2, PPARγ, TERT and prohibitin

it is not affected by the loss of SphK1 (Etemadi et al. 2015). An additional intracellular role for SphK1 is in endosomal processing/endocytic signalling and neurotransmission (Shen et al. 2014). Indeed, knockdown of SphK1 modulates endocytic recycling and results in dysfunctional neurotransmission, an outcome that is rescued by WT SphK1 but not by SphK1 that is mutated in the hydrophobic LBL-1 patch implicated in membrane targeting (V268Q-SphK1) (Shen et al. 2014).

S1P formed by SphK2 also has intracellular roles. For example, nuclear localised SphK2 forms a complex with histone H3 and HDAC1/2 in the promoters of *c-fos* and *p21* genes (Hait et al. 2009). The S1P formed by SphK2 inhibits HDAC1/2 to preserve histone acetylation at specific lysine residues, thereby enhancing gene transcription and implicating SphK2 in epigenetic regulation. S1P has also been shown to bind to the transcription factor PPARγ to enhance expression of genes in endothelial cells linked with neovascularisation (Parham et al. 2015). In addition, S1P formed by SphK2 binds to prohibitin 2 (PHB2), which regulates mitochondrial assembly and function (Strub et al. 2011). SphK2-derived S1P also stabilises hTERT; this catalytic subunit of telomerase maintains telomeres and its activity is increased in cancer cells (Panneer Selvam et al. 2015). Finally, S1P activates the β-site amyloid precursor protein (APP) cleaving enzyme-1 (BACE1), suggesting a role for S1P formed by SphK2 in β amyloid accumulation and synaptic spread in neurodegenerative disease (Takasugi et al. 2011).

9 Role of SphK1 and SphK2 in Disease and Utility of Inhibitors

The case for pharmacological development of SphK1 and SphK2 inhibitors is dependent largely on whether unequivocal target validation can be demonstrated. Therefore, the following sections describe a number of instances where SphK1 or SphK2 play key roles in diseases. Figure 3 summarises isoform-selective and dual inhibitors of SphK1 and SphK2, which have recently been reviewed (Pitman et al. 2016).

9.1 S1P Levels in Blood

Kharel et al. (2012) reported that the treatment of mice with the SphK2 inhibitor, SRL080811, increased blood S1P levels. This contrasts with the effect of SphK2 inhibitor, ABC294640, which lowers S1P levels (Beljanski et al. 2011). However, the latter might be attributed to indirect effects on SphK1 expression, as ABC294640 has been shown to induce the proteasomal degradation of SphK1 in cancer cells (McNaughton et al. 2016). Significantly, SRL080811 recapitulated the elevation of blood S1P levels observed in *sphk2*$^{-/-}$ mice, suggesting that SphK2 might exhibit additional activities in regulating S1P uptake into cells (Kharel et al. 2012).

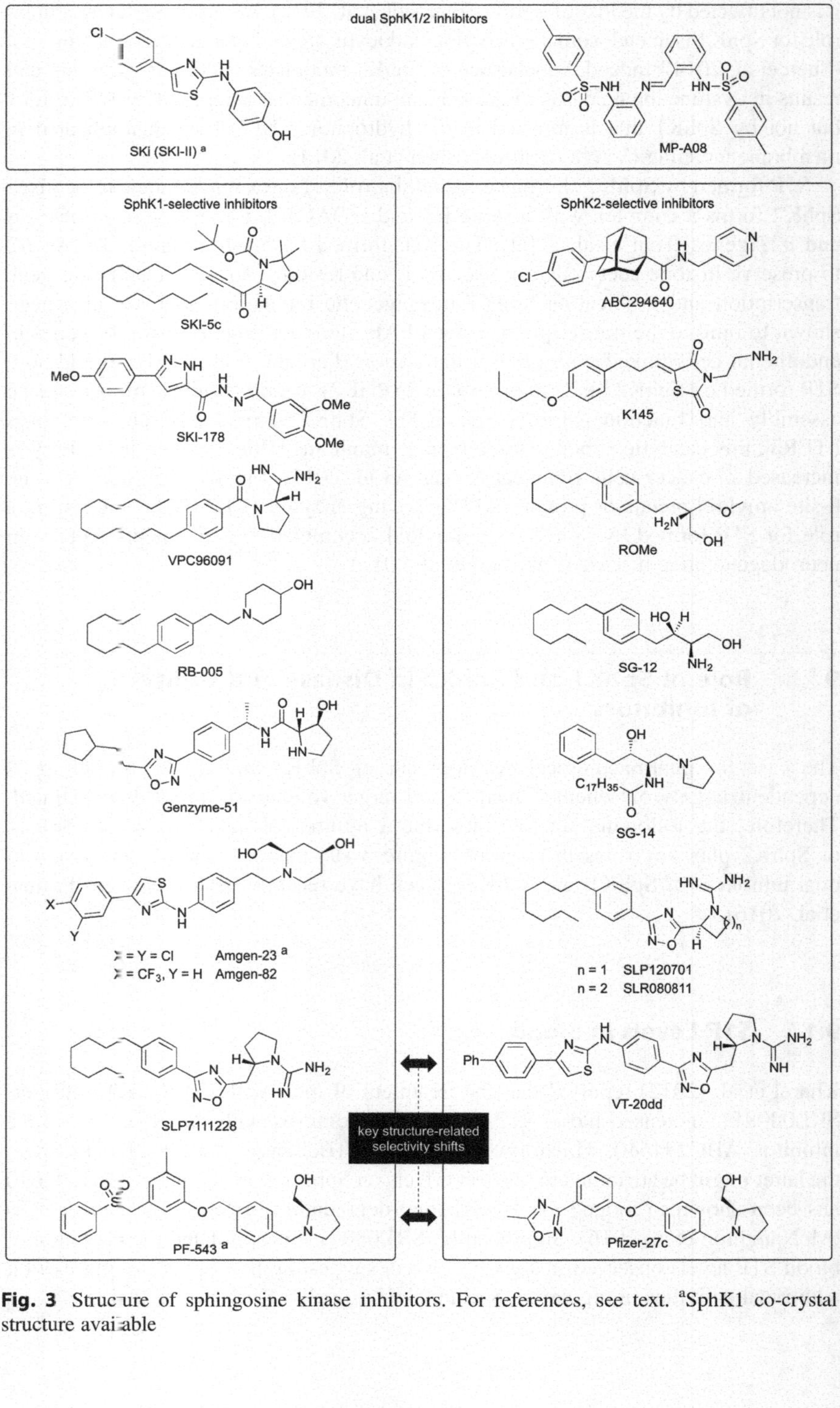

Fig. 3 Structure of sphingosine kinase inhibitors. For references, see text. [a]SphK1 co-crystal structure available

9.2 Role of SphK1 and SphK2 in Cancer

In patients, SphK1 expression levels are higher in tumours compared with normal tissue and this is associated with poor prognosis in breast (Watson et al. 2010; Ohotski et al. 2013), colon (Tan et al. 2014), head and neck carcinoma (Facchinetti et al. 2010), prostate (Malavaud et al. 2010) and other cancers (Pyne and Pyne 2010). Indeed, there are numerous examples of a role for SphK1 in cancer. For instance, the over-expression of the K-RasG12V oncogene stimulates translocation and activation of SphK1 and this promotes cellular transformation (Gault et al. 2012). SphK1 also participates in stimulating neovascularisation of tumours involving paracrine signalling by S1P leading to angiogenesis and lymphangiogenesis (Anelli et al. 2010). In addition, cross-regulation between SphK1, $S1P_3$ and Notch promotes cancer stem cell proliferation to increase tumorigenesis (Hirata et al. 2014). Significantly, *sphk1*$^{-/-}$ mice have reduced S1P levels and decreased tumour multiplicity and volume in 4-NQO-induced head and neck squamous cell carcinoma carcinogenesis (Shirai et al. 2011).

Furthermore, the stability of Bcr-Abl1 (a fusion gene involved in promoting haematological cancers) is reduced upon siRNA knockdown of SphK1 in imatinib-resistant K562/IMA-3 chronic myeloid leukaemia (CML) cells or in *sphk1*$^{-/-}$ mouse embryonic fibroblasts (Salas et al. 2011). In addition, treatment of a murine model of breast cancer metastasis with the selective SphK1 inhibitor, SPHK1-I ((2*R*,3*S*,4*E*)-*N*-methyl-5-(4-pentylphenyl)-2-aminopent-4-ene-1,3-diol (BML-258)), suppresses S1P levels, reduces metastasis to lymph nodes and lungs and decreases overall tumour burden (Nagahashi et al. 2012). Loss of systemic, but not tumour SphK1 prevents S1P elevation and inhibits TRAMP-induced prostate cancer growth in *TRAMP*$^{+/+}$ *sphk1*$^{-/-}$ mice or lung metastasis of multiple cancer cell types in *sphk1*$^{-/-}$ mice (Ponnusamy et al. 2012). SphK1 is also over-expressed and constitutively activate in primary acute myeloid leukaemia (AML) patient blasts but not in normal mononuclear cells (Powell et al. 2017). Inhibition of SphK1 with the dual SphK1/SphK2 inhibitor, MP-A08, or shRNA knockdown reduced AML cancer cell survival (Powell et al. 2017). In addition, MP-A08 induces caspase-dependent cell death via down-regulation of Mcl-1 in AML cell lines, primary AML patient blasts and isolated AML patient leukemic progenitor/stem cells. MP-A08 also reduced tumour burden and increased overall survival in orthotopic AML patient-derived xenografts (Powell et al. 2017).

There is also evidence for a role for SphK2 in cancer. Indeed, low-level SphK2 expression has been shown to enhance cell survival and proliferation and promote neoplastic transformation in vivo and this is associated with plasma membrane localised SphK2, while high expression promoted cell death (Neubauer et al. 2016). The reason why both localisation and function of SphK2 are altered is unknown, but these are clearly concentration-dependent. This might reflect competition for binding partners, such that high concentrations of SphK2 via its BH3 domain can sequester and inactivate the anti-apoptotic protein, Bcl2 (Liu et al. 2003). Therefore, SphK2 inhibitors have utility in cancer. For example, treatment of early stage and advanced prostate cancer cells with the SphK2-selective inhibitor, ABC294640, reduces growth, proliferation and cell cycle progression.

Furthermore, oral treatment of mice with ABC294640 reduced xenograft tumour growth (Schrecengost et al. 2015). In addition, the SphK2 selective inhibitor, (*R*)-FTY720 methyl ether (ROMe), induces the autophagic death of T cell acute lymphoblastic leukaemia (T-ALL) cell lines and patient lymphoblasts (Evangelisti et al. 2014). SphK2 also confers an ability on tumour cells to evade the immune system. Thus, *SPHK2*$^{-/-}$ MCF-7 breast cancer cells display retarded growth in vivo and tumour associated macrophages exhibit an anti-tumour phenotype (Weigert et al. 2009).

Analysis of a large gene expression data set from CD138^{+} bone marrow plasma cells from newly diagnosed myeloma patients revealed increased *SPHK2* expression compared to healthy controls (Wallington-Beddoe et al. 2017). In addition, the SphK2 inhibitors, K145 and ABC294640, induce a caspase-3-dependent apoptosis of multiple myeloma (MM) cells via an ER stress/sustained unfolded protein response (UPR), and non-lethal concentrations of K145 and bortezomib synergise to promote sustained UPR and CCAAT-enhancer-binding protein homologous protein (CHOP)-induced apoptosis of MM cells (Wallington-Beddoe et al. 2017; Pyne and Pyne 2017).

9.3 Role of SphK1 in Pulmonary Hypertension

A variety of evidence clearly supports a significant role for SphK1 in pulmonary hypertension. For instance, SphK1 expression is increased in the lungs and pulmonary artery smooth muscle cells from patients with pulmonary arterial hypertension (Chen et al. 2014). Increased SphK1 expression is also evident in remodelled pulmonary arteries of patients with idiopathic pulmonary arterial hypertension and in the Suger5416/hypoxia/normoxia (Su/Hx/Nx PAH) rat model of occlusive pulmonary hypertension (Gairhe et al. 2016). The potential of SphK1 as a therapeutic target in pulmonary hypertension is further supported by studies with *sphk1*$^{-/-}$ mice, which exhibit lower right ventricular systolic pressure, decreased right ventricular hypertrophy (RVH) and less severe pulmonary vascular remodelling in response to chronic hypoxia (Chen et al. 2014). Additionally, the SphK1/2 inhibitor, SKi (SKI-II), prevented the development of hypoxia-dependent pulmonary hypertension (Chen et al. 2014). The utility of SphK1 inhibitors is also evident in other disease models. Thus, the SphK1 inhibitor, SLP7111228, reduced plasma S1P levels and the percentage of occluded pulmonary arteries, while increasing the percentage of non-occluded pulmonary arteries in the Su/Hx/Nx PAH rat model (Gairhe et al. 2016). Finally, administration of the highly selective SphK1 inhibitor, PF-543, in a mouse hypoxic model of pulmonary hypertension reduced RVH (MacRitchie et al. 2016), thereby suggesting that the SphK1 inhibitor might be protective in heart failure. In this regard, PF-543 also reduced chronic cardiac inflammation and ameliorated cardiac remodelling and dysfunction in vivo following myocardial infarction in mice (Zhang et al. 2016).

9.4 Role of SphK1 and SphK2 in the Central Nervous System

SphK2-derived S1P promotes the survival of dopaminergic neurons that are involved in the development of Parkinson's disease. In this regard, SphK2 expression is decreased in the *substantia nigra* region in a 1-methyl-4-phenyl-1,2,3,6-tetrahydropyridine (MPTP)-induced Parkinson's disease mouse model (Sivasubramanian et al. 2015). The localisation of SphK2 to the mitochondria might be important here, as mitochondrial dysfunction is a feature of Parkinson's disease. Indeed, the inhibition of SphK2 activity reduces the expression of peroxisome proliferator-activated receptor gamma coactivator 1-alpha (PGC-1α, the co-activator of PPARγ), nuclear respiratory factor 1 (NRF-1) and mitochondrial transcription factor A (TFAM) (Sivasubramanian et al. 2015). There is also evidence for a role for SphK in Alzheimer's disease (AD). In this regard, β-amyloid peptide fragment 25–35 (Aβ25–35) toxicity is associated with a marked down-regulation of SphK1 expression (Yang et al. 2014). Moreover, siRNA knockdown of SphK1 expression increased Aβ load and worsened learning and memory ability in *APP/PS1* transgenic mice, a model for AD (Zhang et al. 2013). SphK2 activity is also up-regulated in brains from patients with AD and S1P formed by SphK2 activates BACE1 (Takasugi et al. 2011).

9.5 Role of SphK1 and SphK2 in Inflammation

SphK1 has a pro-inflammatory role in cancer (Liang et al. 2013; Pyne and Pyne 2013) and rheumatoid arthritis (Baker et al. 2010) but is protective in neuro-inflammation (Grinkina et al. 2012). For instance, colitis-associated cancer is linked to an amplification loop involving SphK1, $S1P_1$, NFκB, STAT3 and IL-6 (Liang et al. 2013), and *sphk1*$^{-/-}$ mice are protected from dextran sulphate sodium-induced ulcerative colitis (Snider et al. 2009). Similarly, *sphk1*$^{-/-}$ mice are protected against development of TNFα-induced arthritis (Baker et al. 2010). Furthermore, enforced over-expression of SphK1 increases IL-12 formation from dendritic cells and siRNA knockdown of SphK1 in these cells prevents IFN-γ formation from Th1 cells (Jung et al. 2007). However, administration of the SphK1 inhibitor, PF-543, to mice increased disease progression in the experimental auto-immune encephalomyelitis (EAE) model of MS with enhanced infiltration of $CD4^+$ T-cells, $CD11b^+$ monocytes and $F4/80^+$ macrophages in the spinal cord (Pyne et al. 2016b).

In contrast with deletion of *sphk1*, *sphk2* deficiency does not affect the severity of inflammatory arthritis, even though the SphK2-inhibitory compound, ABC294640, worsens hTNFα-induced arthritis (Baker et al. 2013). The explanation for this apparent paradox may lie in the fact that ABC294640 does not have a pharmacologically clean profile, but also induces proteasomal degradation of SphK1 and inhibits Degs1 in cancer cells (McNaughton et al. 2016). However, a pro-inflammatory role for SphK2 is evident from studies demonstrating that the number of infiltrating $CD3^+$ T cells, $CD11b^+$ neutrophils and macrophages are reduced in the fibrotic kidney from *sphk2*$^{-/-}$ mice compared with WT mice (Bajwa et al. 2016). In addition, increased mRNA expression levels of CXCL1 and CXCL2 were evident in WT and *sphk1*$^{-/-}$ mice but not in *sphk2*$^{-/-}$ mice (Bajwa et al. 2016). Furthermore, *sphk2*$^{-/-}$ mice are protected against EAE (Imeri et al. 2016), and the SphK2 inhibitor, (*R*)-FTY720 methyl ether (ROMe), prevents inflammatory cell infiltration into the spinal cord and reduces disease progression in this model (Barbour et al. 2017). Further evidence that SphK2 has a pro-inflammatory function was obtained in studies demonstrating that the SphK2 inhibitor, ABC294640, can produce anti-inflammatory outcomes in rodent models of inflammatory bowel disease (IBD) (French et al. 2010; Maines et al. 2008, 2010) and collagen-induced arthritis (Fitzpatrick et al. 2011).

Therefore, there is sufficient evidence to suggest that both SphK1 and SphK2 inhibitors could have utility for treatment of inflammatory disease. However, isoform-specific inhibitors may be important for any future clinical deployment in order to maintain homeostatic control of S1P through compensatory effects exerted by the SphK isoform that is not targeted. Dual SphK1/SphK2 inhibitors, whilst potentially exhibiting pharmacological activity, may carry a risk of undesirable effects arising from blanket, unmitigated reduction in cellular S1P.

9.6 S1P and Sickling

S1P levels are substantially increased in the blood of humans with sickle cell disease (SCD) and in SCD transgenic mice. SphK1, the expression of which is increased in this condition, is responsible for the elevation of S1P in the blood in a murine model of SCD, but was found to promote sickling in an S1P receptor-independent manner in isolated erythrocytes (Zhang et al. 2014). A direct role for elevated S1P levels as a driving factor in SCD was shown by the fact that the SphK1 inhibitor, PF-543, reduced sickling, haemolysis and inflammation in SCD mice (Zhang et al. 2014). Circulating IL-2, IL-6 and IL-17A were also significantly reduced in SCD mice. Moreover, shRNA knockdown of SphK1 in hematopoietic stem cells decreased erythrocyte sickling and reticulocytes in SCD chimeras (Zhang et al. 2014). Therefore, in terms of targeting SphK1 it is necessary to consider the specific disease context. For instance, PF-543 lowers IL-6/IL-17A in SCD mice but worsens disease progression in an EAE mouse model (Zhang et al. 2014).

10 Significance and Questions Concerning the Sphingolipid Rheostat

As discussed above, pharmacologically active SphK inhibitors can increase the ceramide/S1P ratio in cells. Conversely, elevated levels and/or activity of SphK is expected to decrease the ceramide/S1P ratio. Consistent with this, enforced expression of SphK1 reduces the C18-ceramide/S1P ratio in K-562 human erythroleukemia cells and prevents imatinib-induced apoptosis (Baran et al. 2007). In addition, the ceramide/S1P ratio is increased in response to imatinib in imatinib-sensitive LAMA84 cells, while the ratio is unaltered in imatinib-resistant cells.

Similarly, daunorubicin-sensitive but not -insensitive leukaemia cells (CML, AML and ALL) exhibit an elevated ceramide/S1P ratio, and sensitivity to daunorubicin is restored by inhibiting SphK1 activity (Sobue et al. 2008). There are other examples (e.g. MP-A08 in multiple myeloma) where SphK inhibitors increase ceramide and reduce S1P levels, with subsequent induction of apoptosis (Wallington-Beddoe et al. 2017). However, controversy has arisen over whether the sphingolipid rheostat is modulated by SphK1 inhibitors and whether these compounds have utility in the treatment of cancer. These questions arise because the nanomolar-potent selective SphK1 inhibitor, PF-543 (K_i 3.6 nM), fails to induce cytotoxicity in head and neck cancer cells (Schnüte et al. 2012). However, in this study PF-543 failed to increase ceramide levels (but did reduce S1P levels), unless cells were incubated with Sph (Schnüte et al. 2012). An assessment of whether PF-543 induces apoptosis of cancer cells in the presence of Sph was not undertaken. In principle, the lack of effect of PF-543 on ceramide levels might also be due to its potential modulation of other targets involved in sphingolipid metabolism so as to rebalance the changes in ceramide levels caused by inhibition of SphK1. These issues require further investigation. In addition, certain SphK inhibitors (e.g. SKi, ABC294640) also indirectly inhibit Degs1 and we have proposed that combined inhibition of Degs1 and SphK1 activity might be necessary to arrest growth and/or kill certain types of cancer cells (McNaughton et al. 2016). Thus, SphK1 inhibition alone might not be sufficient, and in order to kill cancer cells it might be necessary to modulate both de novo ceramide and sphingolipid rheostat pathways. In addition, the N-terminal SphK1b splice variant (with an additional 86 amino acids, Mr. = 51 kDa) can exhibit resistance to SphK1 inhibitors in terms of proteasomal degradation (Loveridge et al. 2010). Proteasomal degradation of SphK1 might be required in order to disrupt the sphingolipid rheostat to increase ceramide levels and to promote growth arrest and/or kill cancer cells.

11 SphK Inhibitor-Induced Proteasomal Degradation of SphK1

In addition to reversible inhibition of catalytic activity, SphK inhibitors induce the ubiquitin-proteasomal degradation of SphK1, which occurs through two distinct mechanisms. First, inhibitors, such as PF-543, appear to bind to SphK1 to induce a conformational change that promotes proteasomal degradation of the enzyme (Byun et al. 2013). In this regard, there is a strong correlation between the concentrations of inhibitor required to induce proteasomal degradation in cells and the K_i for inhibition of purified SphK1 (Byun et al. 2013). Second, relatively weak inhibitors of SphK1, such as SKi (K_i 17 μM, Lim et al. 2011b), activate the proteasome to remove SphK1 (along with c-Myc and cyclin D1) in human prostate cancer cells (Loveridge et al. 2010; Watson et al. 2013). In this regard, SKi induces the proteasomal degradation of both SphK1a (42 kDa) and SphK1b (51 kDa) in androgen-sensitive LNCaP prostate cancer cells, and this is associated with increased C22:0 and C24:0 ceramide and Sph levels, reduced S1P levels and the activation of apoptosis (Loveridge et al. 2010). In contrast, androgen-independent LNCaP-AI cells fail to undergo apoptosis in response to SKi, and this is associated with the proteasomal degradation of SphK1a, but not SphK1b, with no change in ceramide levels (Loveridge et al. 2010). The resistance of SphK1b might be a consequence of a compensatory enhanced expression of SphK1b and/or post-translational-dependent stabilisation of SphK1b in androgen-independent prostate cancer cells. Thus, treatment of LNCaP-AI cells with siRNA (to reduce SphK1 expression) in combination with SKi (to promote proteasomal degradation) is able remove SphK1b and thereby induce apoptosis of these cells (Loveridge et al. 2010). Activation of the proteasome involves additional inhibition of Degs1 by SKi (McNaughton et al. 2016). Therefore, we have proposed that Degs1 might function to limit protein degradation flux through the proteasome in cancer cells. Indeed, SKi increases the levels of multiple molecular species of dihydroceramide in prostate cancer cells (Loveridge et al. 2010). Interestingly, the SphK2 selective inhibitor ABC294640 also inhibits Degs1 (Venant et al. 2015; McNaughton et al. 2016) and induces proteasomal degradation of SphK1a in LNCaP-AI cells (McNaughton et al. 2016). Both ABC294640 and SKi induce an increase in p53 and p21 expression levels in these cells, indicative of an enhanced senescent programme. The mechanism of action of these inhibitors is validated by siRNA knockdown of Degs1, which increases p53 expression, while siRNA knockdown of SphK1 and Degs1 increases p21 expression in these cancer cells (McNaughton et al. 2016).

12 Progress Towards Isoform-Selective SphK1 and SphK2 Inhibitors

Although ATP-competitive inhibitors have recently been discovered (MP-A08, Fig. 3) (Powell et al. 2017), work to develop SphK inhibitors to date has been heavily focused on compounds that are competitive for the lipid substrate binding site. A number of SphK1-selective inhibitor chemotypes have been developed, some with inhibitory potency in the nanomolar range. Notable representatives of these that have proved useful as tool compounds include SKI-5c (Li et al. 2016), SKI-178 (Hengst et al. 2010b), VPC96091 (Lynch et al. 2016), RB-005 (Baek et al. 2013), Genzyme-51 (Xiang et al. 2010), Amgen-23/82 (Gustin et al. 2013), SLP7111228 (Patwardhan et al. 2015) and PF-543 (Schnüte et al. 2012) (Fig. 3) (reviewed in Pitman et al. 2016). Since 2013, the development of SphK1-selective inhibitors has been assisted by the emergence of co-crystal structures for this isozyme, firstly with the non-selective inhibitor, SKi (also referred to as SKI-II) (Wang et al. 2013), and a representative (Amgen-23) of a derivative series (Gustin et al. 2013), and more recently with PF-543 (Wang et al. 2014). This latter compound has risen to prominence in biochemical and pharmacological studies by virtue of its low nanomolar potency for SphK1 inhibition (K_i 3.6 nM) coupled with greater than 100-fold selectivity over SphK2 (Schnüte et al. 2012). The development of correspondingly potent and selective inhibitors for SphK2 has lagged behind that of SphK1 inhibitors, and, until very recently, the most selective compounds – ABC294640

(French et al. 2010), K145 (Liu et al. 2013), ROMe (Lim et al. 2011a), SG-12/14 (Kim et al. 2005), SLP120701 (Patwardhan et al. 2015) and SLR080811 (Congdon et al. 2015) (Fig. 3) – have been limited to activity in the micromolar range and with only modest levels of selectivity in several cases. Examples of nanomolar potent SphK2-selective inhibitors are now just beginning to emerge as seen with VT-20dd (Childress et al. 2017) and Pfizer-27c (Schnüte et al. 2017) suggesting that efforts to develop SphK2 inhibitors are gaining traction at last. The most advanced SphK2 inhibitor to date, in terms of clinical development, remains ABC294640 (Yeliva®), although (as noted above) its pharmacological profile is undoubtedly complicated by actions on other proteins, limiting its utility as a tool to fully explore the potential of SphK2 as a target. Thus, the development of clean, potent SphK2-selective inhibitors remains a key objective in the field, with ongoing efforts in our own laboratory and elsewhere to unlock the structural determinants for rational design of such compounds. As yet there are no SphK2 crystal structures available to assist this effort, although there is strong sequence homology between the two isozymes, thereby permitting the development of reasonable structural models based on the available SphK1 crystal structures.

We have recently reviewed the structure of SphK1 and discussed current structure–function hypotheses in detail elsewhere (Adams et al. 2016; Pyne et al. 2017). In brief, the enzyme comprises two domains, a C-terminal domain (CTD) that hosts the lipid substrate binding site and an ATP-binding N-terminal domain (Fig. 4a). The CTD folds as a two-layer β-sandwich, with three 'lipid binding loops' (LBL-1 to LBL-3) occupying one face; a fourth loop, the regulatory R-loop, contains the ERK phosphorylation site for SphK1 and packs on the opposite face of the CTD β-sandwich (occluded from view in Fig. 4a). The cognate loop in SphK2 is greatly extended and contains the phosphorylation-dependent NES sequence. The different R-loops provide one of the main features of distinction between SphK1 and SphK2. In contrast, the three lipid binding loops are identical in length and exhibit 43–62% sequence identity across the isozymes (see Supplementary Fig. S1 in Adams et al. (2016) for sequence alignment). These loops pack so as to encapsulate a curved cavity, termed the 'J-channel', as binding site both for Sph substrate and the majority of inhibitors.

Ligand access to the J-channel is postulated (Adams et al. 2016) to involve hinged opening and closure of LBL-1, which comprises two reverse-paired helices (α7/α8). Residues in this loop together with LBL-2 provide the contact surface for the polar head group of the lipid and its central region. The majority of SphK inhibitors are substrate-mimetic and also comprise a polar, frequently basic, head group that is thought to engage the same region of the protein. Like LBL-1, LBL-3 is flap-like in structure; it contains an additional helix (α9) that packs antiparallel against α8, and this folding of LBL-3 provides much of the enclosure for the lipid tail (yellow surface in Fig. 4b). Some 20 residues contribute to the direct ligand contact surface of the J-channel, and, of these, SphK2 differs from SphK1 in only three – Val304, Leu517 and Cys533, corresponding respectively to Ile174, Met272 and Phe288 in SphK1 (Fig. 4b/4c). In the SphK1 co-crystal structure with PF-543, Ile174 and Met272 flank the inhibitor's *p*-xylylene subunit; in principle, their replacement by

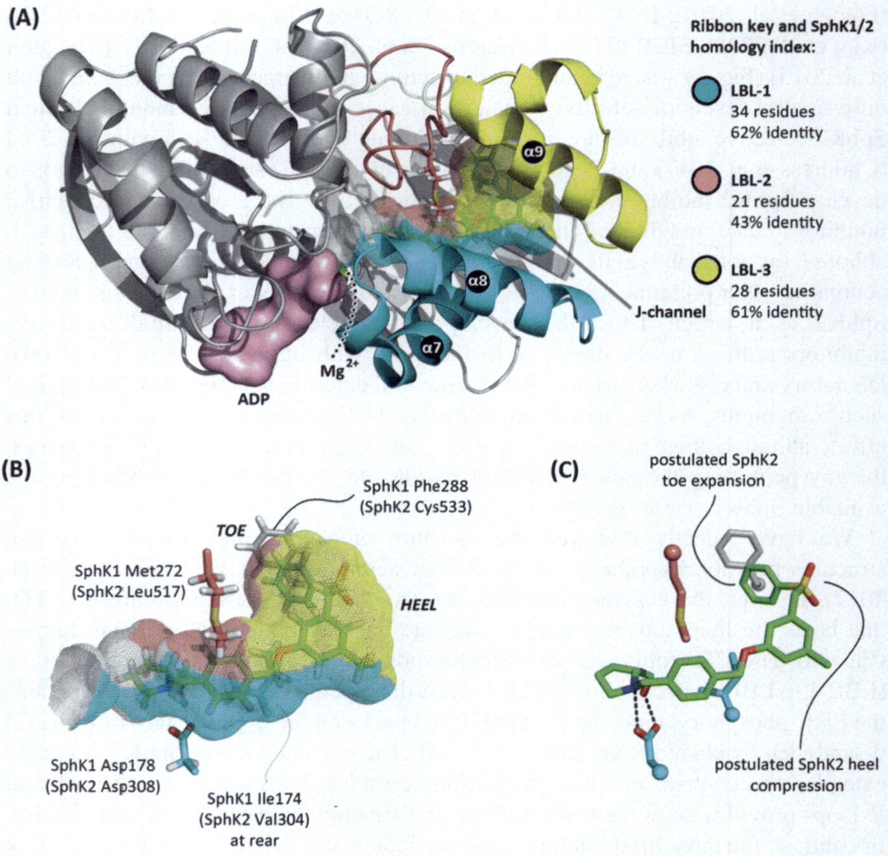

Fig. 4 Structure of SphK1 and the lipid binding J-channel. (**a**) The co-crystal structure of SphK1 with bound PF-543 (PDB: 4V24) is shown, with the nucleotide-binding site marked by superimposition of ADP (pink surface) from the SphK1 co-crystal structure (3VZD) with Mg-ADP. Three lipid binding loops (LBL-1 to LBL-3, colour coded as indicated in the key) fold across a β-sandwich core to generate the Sph-binding J-channel (coloured mesh). (**b**) Detail of the J-channel surface (mesh) extracted from (**a**) and highlighting three isozyme differences in surface-contributory residues (SphK1: Ile174, Met272, Phe288); a fourth residue (Asp178) is conserved in SphK2 and plays a key role in anchoring the polar head groups of many SphK inhibitors. (**c**) As (**b**), but with surface removal to highlight the organisation of residues relative to PF-543 (green stick); key regions of likely J-channel surface expansion and compression in SphK2 are marked

Val and Leu in SphK2 might lead to isozyme distinguishing differences in the J-channel surface in this region. The third direct contact residue difference lies in the toe of the J-channel, which is stoppered by Phe288 in SphK1. Clearly, the replacement of this residue by a smaller one, Cys533 in SphK2, might generate a longer J-channel, a notion that has influenced the direction of a number of recent chemistry programmes that have usefully examined probing inhibitor tail subunits directed to the J-channel toe (Schnüte et al. 2017; Childress et al. 2017; Xi et al. 2016; Congdon et al. 2015, 2016).

The structural basis for discrimination of the SphK isozymes by ligands remains under-addressed to date however and, we suggest, is likely to be more complex and subtle than simply a rigidly extended J-channel as a consequence of a single residue interchange in the toe. In particular, we hypothesise that differences in neighbouring non-contact residues are likely to exert a significant impact in modulating the J-channel surface in both the toe and heel regions. For that reason, work is currently underway in our laboratory with ligand probes designed to explore the structural differences between the isozymes in these regions, and as part of this programme we have explored ligand docking to SphK2 homology models based on the structure of SphK1. These models do indeed suggest that toe expansion in SphK2 is likely to be a significant determinant of distinguishing ligand-binding preferences and that increased steric demand by ligands in the toe may discriminate against SphK1. This is the case with ABC294640 (Fig. 5a), where the chlorine atom on the terminal phenyl group is predicted to be packed against Cys533 in SphK2. However, our models also suggest that the toe in SphK2 may not necessarily be rigidly expanded, rather that it may exhibit greater surface plasticity than in the case of SphK1. Thus, the toe surface in SphK2 is generated both by Cys533 and an adjacent side chain, Leu506. This latter residue is conserved in SphK1 (as Leu261) but is packed against two other non-conserved residues – Val304 (SphK1 Ile174) and Ile508 (SphK1 Leu263). Our models suggest that loosened packing of Leu506 may conspire with Phe/Cys exchange in the isozymes so as to allow SphK2 to accommodate more demanding ligand substituents in this region than SphK1, whilst still providing flexibility for good surface contact with tail subunits of similar size to those that fit SphK1 well.

In contrast to the toe region, however, our models suggest that the J-channel heel surface may be more contracted in SphK2 than in SphK1. Thus, the prediction here is that increased steric demand by ligands will discriminate against SphK2, whilst a combination of enhanced demand in the toe and reduced demand in the heel will favour binding to SphK2. This may be a factor in the remarkable selectivity switching seen between the two structurally related ligands, PF-543 and Pfizer-27c (Fig. 3), where a reported ninefold loss in potency against SphK1 coupled with a 148-fold gain in potency against SphK2 (IC_{50} for SK2 is 2.4 nM and for SK1, it is 25 nM) results in a swing to net tenfold SphK2-selective inhibition for Pfizer-27c (Schnüte et al. 2017). The co-crystal structure of PF-543 reveals that the inhibitor's sulphonyl group is tightly fitted to the heel region in SphK1 (Fig. 4b), a binding locus that we propose will experience significant steric compression in SphK2. Our models (Fig. 5b) suggest that replacement of the phenylsulphonylmethyl tail of PF-543 by the terminal 5-methyl-1,2,4-oxadiazoly-3-yl group will alleviate compression in the SphK2 heel, whilst the methyl substituent, which is likely to be a little tight against toe residue Phe288 in SphK1, will be more comfortably accommodated by the cysteine (Cys533) in SphK2.

Another notable example of isozyme selectivity switching has been reported recently by Childress et al., where tail replacement in the potent SphK1-selective inhibitor, SLP7111228 (K_i 48 nM, >200-fold selectivity over SphK2) (Patwardhan et al. 2015), strongly enhanced activity against SphK2 but weakened activity against

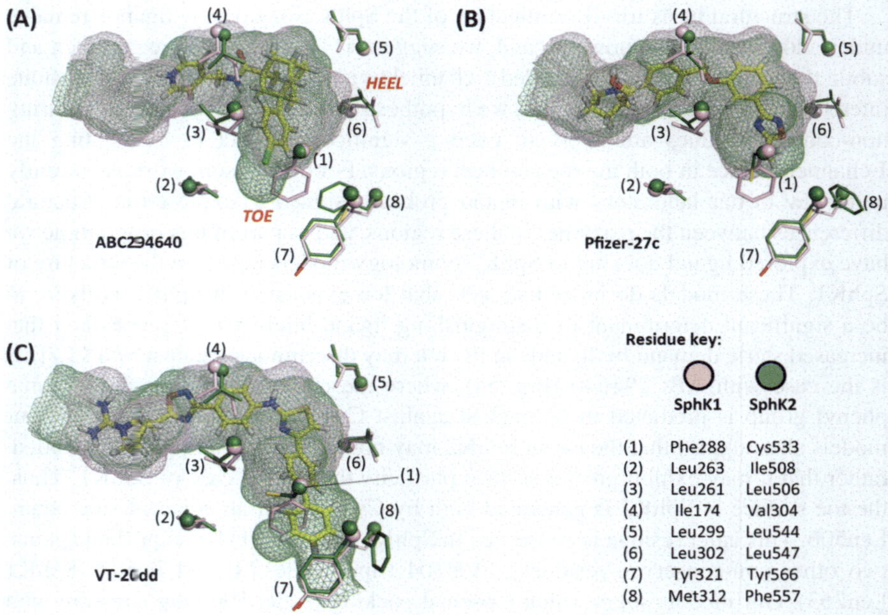

Fig. 5 SphK2 binding models suggest probable determinants of isozyme selectivity for inhibitors. (**a**) A model of ABC294640 (yellow stick) is shown docked into the J-channel of a SphK2 homology model (green mesh/green stick) with the SphK1 J-channel (pink mesh/pink stick) superimposed from its co-crystal structure (3VZD) with inhibitor, SKi. Residues (1)–(8) are identified in the key (bottom right). Plasticity in the J-channel toe for SphK2 is postulated to be a key feature of distinction from SphK1, where residue differences in (2) and (4) may allow greater mobility in conserved Leu (3). This, coupled with the Phe-to-Cys exchange at (1), is proposed to allow accommodation of the Cl atom of SphK2-selective inhibitor ABC294640; in SphK1 the Cl atom would be compressed against residues (1) and (3). (**b**) As (**a**), but showing a model of Pfizer-27c (yellow stick) docked to the SphK2 homology model (green mesh/stick). SphK2 is postulated to have a contracted heel surface proximal to Leu (6) as a second key feature of distinction from SphK1. The sulphonyl oxygens of structurally related SphK1-selective inhibitor, PF-543, known to occupy the expanded heel of SphK1, may compromise binding to SphK2, thereby conferring SphK1 selectivity. The modified tail of Pfizer-27c may circumvent the heel compression, consistent with a substantial gain in binding affinity and inhibitory potency against SphK2. Compression of the terminal methyl group of Pfizer-27c against Phe (1) in SphK1 is additionally predicted to contribute to the isozyme selectivity switch between PF-543 and Pfizer-27c. (**c**) As (**a**), but showing a model of VT-20dd (yellow stick) docked to the SphK2 homology model (green mesh/stick). Conformational mobility in SphK2 Cys (1) coupled with rotation of Phe (8) may allow 'tunnelling' and accommodation of the long biphenyl tail of VT-20dd as an additional aspect of SphK2 toe plasticity. Limited conformational freedom for Phe (1) in SphK1 is likely to preclude such tunnelling, requiring more substantial structural perturbation for binding to SphK1

SphK1 to give pronounced overall SphK2-selective inhibition in VT-20dd (IC_{50} 90 nM, 100-fold selectivity over SphK1) (Fig. 3) (Childress et al. 2017). The remarkable feature with VT-20dd is the compound's very long biphenyl tail subunit, which our models suggest cannot fit along the J-channel toe expansion trajectory postulated for accommodation of ABC294640, notwithstanding the proposed toe plasticity in that region. The very strong implication of this is that there is a second direction of expansion in the J-channel of SphK2 that is not readily accessible in SphK1. Our models suggest that this may involve rotation of phenylalanine Phe557 on LBL-3 to allow tunnelling of the inhibitor's biphenyl group between LBL-2 and LBL-3 (Fig. 5c). Toe plasticity in SphK2 is predicted to assist such tunnelling, with the Cys588 side chain being displaced into the expansion region postulated to host the ABC294640 chlorine atom. SphK1 differs from SphK2 in a number of LBL-3 residues proximal to the proposed tunnelling interface, and these differences, combined with the presence of the large conformationally restricted Phe288 toe residue, may require a higher degree of structural perturbation in SphK1 for adoption of a similar binding mode. The associated energy penalty for such structural perturbation may account for the strong SphK2 selectivity with VT-20dd.

13 Conclusion

In this review, we have not attempted to comprehensively detail the field of SphK inhibitor development; others have recently reviewed the area (Lynch et al. 2016; Pitman et al. 2016). Rather, the intention has been to focus on a possible structural rationale for achieving isozyme-selective inhibition by exploitation of hypothesised structural differences between SphK1 and SphK2 in the toe and heel regions of the lipid substrate binding J-channel. Potent and selective SphK1 inhibitors are now relatively well established, at least at the level of tool compounds. However, the corresponding availability of SphK2-selective inhibitors has been problematic, with examples of nanomolar potent inhibitors with good selectivity over SphK1 only just beginning to be reported. Whilst the development of SphK1 inhibitors has been structurally enabled by protein crystallography in recent years, no SphK2 crystal structures have emerged to date. Nevertheless, homology models of SphK2 suggest plausible approaches for achieving SphK2-over-SphK1 selectivity with compounds that exhibit increased steric demand in the J-channel toe and reduced demand in the heel. The outlook for developing nanomolar potent SphK2 inhibitors with at least two orders of magnitude selectivity over SphK1 is encouraging, therefore, and may provide the tools for a more thorough exploration of the pharmacological potential of SphK2 as a target to complement ongoing investigations with SphK1 and the biochemical interplay between these two isozymes. This will also enable realisation of the therapeutic potential of inhibiting either one or both isoforms for a variety of pathophysiological conditions.

References

Adams DR, Pyne S, Pyne NJ (2016) Sphingosine kinases: emerging structure-function insights. Trends Biochem Sci 41(5):395–409

Aguilar A, Saba JD (2012) Truth and consequences of sphingosine-1-phosphate lyase. Adv Biol Regul 52:17–30

Alvarez SE, Harikumar KB, Hait NC, Allegood J, Strub GM, Kim EY, Maceyka M, Jiang H, Luo C, Kordula T, Milstien S, Spiegel S (2010) Sphingosine-1-phosphate is a missing cofactor for the E3 ubiquitin ligase TRAF2. Nature 465:1084–1088

Anelli V, Gault CR, Snider AJ, Obeid LM (2010) Role of sphingosine kinase-1 in paracrine/transcellular angiogenesis and lymphangiogenesis in vitro. FASEB J 24:2727–2738

Baek DJ, MacRitchie N, Pyne NJ, Pyne S, Bittman R (2013) Synthesis of selective inhibitors of sphingosine kinase 1. Chem Commun (Camb) 49(21):2136–2138

Bajwa A, Huang L, Kurmaeva E, Ye H, Dondeti KR, Chroscicki P, Foley LS, Balogun ZA, Alexander KJ, Park H, Lynch KR, Rosin DL, Okusa MD (2016) Sphingosine kinase 2 deficiency attenuates kidney fibrosis via IFN-γ. J Am Soc Nephrol 28(4):1145–1161

Baker DA, Barth J, Chang R, Obeid LM, Gilkeson GS (2010) Genetic sphingosine kinase 1 deficiency significantly decreases synovial inflammation and joint erosions in murine TNF-alpha-induced arthritis. J Immunol 185:2570–2579

Baker DA, Eudaly J, Smith CD, Obeid LM, Gilkeson GS (2013) Impact of sphingosine kinase 2 deficiency on the development of TNF-alpha-induced inflammatory arthritis. Rheumatol Int 33(10):2677–2681

Baran Y, Salas A, Senkal CE, Gunduz U, Bielawski J, Obeid LM, Ogretmen B (2007) Alterations of ceramide/sphingosine 1-phosphate rheostat involved in the regulation of resistance to imatinib-induced apoptosis in K562 human chronic myeloid leukemia cells. J Biol Chem 282(15):10922–10934

Barbour M, McNaughton M, Boomkamp SD, MacRitchie N, Jiang HR, Pyne NJ, Pyne S (2017) Effect of sphingosine kinase modulators on interleukin-1β release, sphingosine 1-phosphate receptor 1 expression and experimental autoimmune encephalomyelitis. Br J Pharmacol 174(2):210–222

Barr RK, Lynn HE, Moretti PA, Khew-Goodall Y, Pitson SM (2008) Deactivation of sphingosine kinase 1 by protein phosphatase 2A. J Biol Chem 283:4994–35002

Beljanski V, Lewis CS, Smith CD (2011) Antitumor activity of sphingosine kinase 2 inhibitor ABC294640 and sorafenib in hepatocellular carcinoma xenografts. Cancer Biol Ther 11:524–534

Bigaud M, Guerini D, Billich A, Bassilana F, Brinkmann V (2014) Second generation S1P pathway modulators: research strategies and clinical developments. Biochim Biophys Acta 1841:745–758

Billich A, Bornancin F, Devay P, Mechtcheriakova D, Urtz N, Baumruker T (2003) Phosphorylation of the immunomodulatory drug FTY720 by sphingosine kinases. J Biol Chem 278:47408–47415

Blaho VA, Hla T (2014) An update on the biology of sphingosine 1-phosphate receptors. J Lipid Res 55:1596–1608

Byun HS, Pyne S, Macritchie N, Pyne NJ, Bittman R (2013) Novel sphingosine-containing analogues selectively inhibit sphingosine kinase (SK) isozymes, induce SK1 proteasomal degradation and reduce DNA synthesis in human pulmonary arterial smooth muscle cells. Med Chem Commun 4(10):1394

Chen J, Tang H, Sysol JR, Moreno-Vinasco L, Shioura KM, Chen T, Gorshkova I, Wang L, Huang LS, Usatyuk PV, Sammani S, Zhou G, Raj JU, Garcia JG, Berdyshev E, Yuan JX, Natarajan V, Machado RF (2014) The sphingosine kinase 1/sphingosine-1-phosphate pathway in pulmonary arterial hypertension. Am J Respir Crit Care Med 190:1032–1043

Childress ES, Kharel Y, Brown AM, Bevan DR, Lynch KR, Santos WL (2017) Transforming Sphingosine kinase 1 inhibitors into dual and Sphingosine kinase 2 selective inhibitors: design, synthesis, and in vivo activity. J Med Chem 60(9):3933–3957

Chun J, Goetzl EJ, Hla T, Igarashi Y, Lynch KR, Moolenaar W, Pyne S, Tigyi G (2002) International union of pharmacology. XXXIV. Lysophospholipid receptor nomenclature. Pharmacol Rev 54:265–269

Congdon MD, Childress ES, Patwardhan NN, Gumkowski J, Morris EA, Kharel Y, Lynch KR, Santos WL (2015) Structure-activity relationship studies of the lipophilic tail region of sphingosine kinase 2 inhibitors. Bioorg Med Chem Lett 25(21):4956–4960

Congdon MD, Kharel Y, Brown AM, Lewis SN, Bevan DR, Lynch KR, Santos WL (2016) Structure-activity relationship studies and molecular modeling of naphthalene-based Sphingosine kinase 2 inhibitors. ACS Med Chem Lett 7(3):229–234

Cuvillier O, Pirianov G, Kleuser B, Vanek PG, Coso OA, Gutkind S, Spiegel S (1996) Suppression of ceramide-mediated programmed cell death by sphingosine-1-phosphate. Nature 381:800–803

Ding G, Sonoda H, Yu H, Kajimoto T, Goparaju SK, Jahangeer S, Okada T, Nakamura S (2007) Protein kinase D-mediated phosphorylation and nuclear export of sphingosine kinase 2. J Biol Chem 282:27493–27502

Etemadi N, Chopin M, Anderton H, Tanzer MC, Rickard JA, Abeysekera W, Hall C, Spall SK, Wang B, Xiong Y, Hla T, Pitson SM, Bonder CS, Wong WW, Ernst M, Smyth GK, Vaux DL, Nutt SL, Nachbur U, Silke J (2015) TRAF2 regulates TNF and NF-κB signalling to suppress apoptosis and skin inflammation independently of Sphingosine kinase 1. Elife 4. pii: e10592

Evangelisti C, Evangelisti C, Teti G, Chiarini F, Falconi M, Melchionda F, Pession A, Bertaina A, Locatelli F, McCubrey JA, Beak DJ, Bittman R, Pyne S, Pyne NJ, Martelli AM (2014) Assessment of the effect of sphingosine kinase inhibitors on apoptosis,unfolded protein response and autophagy of T-cell acute lymphoblastic leukemia cells; indications for novel therapeutics. Oncotarget 5:7886–7901

Facchinetti MM, Gandini NA, Fermento ME, Sterin-Speziale NB, Ji Y, Patel V, Gutkind JS, Rivadulla MG, Curino AC (2010) The expression of sphingosine kinase-1 in head and neck carcinoma. Cells Tissues Organs 192(5):314–324

Fitzpatrick LR, Green C, Frauenhoffer EE, French KJ, Zhuang Y, Maines LW, Upson JJ, Paul E, Donahue H, Mosher TJ, Smith CD (2011) Attenuation of arthritis in rodents by a novel orally-available inhibitor of sphingosine kinase. Inflammopharmacology 19(2):75–87

French KJ, Zhuang Y, Maines LW, Gao P, Wang W, Beljanski V, Upson JJ, Green CL, Keller SN, Smith CD (2010) Pharmacology and antitumor activity of ABC294640, a selective inhibitor of sphingosine kinase-2. J Pharmacol Exp Ther 333(1):129–139

Gairhe S, Joshi SR, Bastola MM, McLendon JM, Oka M, Fagan KA, McMurtry IF (2016) Sphingosine-1-phosphate is involved in the occlusive arteriopathy of pulmonary arterial hypertension. Pulm Circ 6:369–380

Gault CR, Eblen ST, Neumann CA, Hannun YA, Obeid LM (2012) Oncogenic K-Ras regulates bioactive sphingolipids in a sphingosine kinase 1-dependent manner. J Biol Chem 287:31794–31803

Gonzalez-Cabrera P, Brown S, Studer SM, Rosen H (2014) S1P signaling: new therapies and opportunities. F1000Prime Rep 6:109

Grinkina NM, Karnabi EE, Damania D, Wadgaonkar S, Muslimov IA, Wadgaonkar R (2012) Sphingosine kinase 1 deficiency exacerbates LPS-induced neuroinflammation. PLoS One 7:e36475

Gustin DJ, Li Y, Brown ML, Min X, Schmitt MJ, Wanska M, Wang X, Connors R, Johnstone S, Cardozo M, Cheng AC, Jeffries S, Franks B, Li S, Shen S, Wong M, Wesche H, Xu G, Carlson TJ, Plant M, Morgenstern K, Rex K, Schmitt J, Coxon A, Walker N, Kayser F, Wang Z (2013) Structure guided design of a series of sphingosine kinase (SphK) inhibitors. Bioorg Med Chem Lett 23(16):4608–4616

Hait NC, Allegood J, Maceyka M, Strub GM, Harikumar KB, Singh SK, Luo C, Marmorstein R, Kordula T, Milstien S, Spiegel S (2009) Regulation of histone acetylation in the nucleus by sphingosine-1-phosphate. Science 325:1254–1257

Hannun YA, Obeid LM (2008) Principles of bioactive lipid signalling: lessons from sphingolipids. Nat Rev Mol Cell Biol 9:139–150

Hannun YA, Obeid LM (2011) Many ceramides. J Biol Chem 286:27855–27862

Hengst JA, Guilford JM, Conroy EJ, Wang X, Yun JK (2010a) Enhancement of sphingosine kinase 1 catalytic activity by deletion of 21 amino acids from the COOH-terminus. Arch Biochem Biophys 494:23–31

Hengst JA, Wang X, Sk UH, Sharma AK, Amin S, Yun JK (2010b) Development of a sphingosine kinase 1 specific small-molecule inhibitor. Bioorg Med Chem Lett 20(24):7498–7502

Hirata N, Yamada S, Shoda T, Kurihara M, Sekino Y, Kanda Y (2014) Sphingosine-1-phosphate promotes expansion of cancer stem cells via S1PR3 by a ligand-independent notch activation. Nat Commun 5:4806

Hisano Y, Kobayashi N, Yamaguchi A, Nishi T (2012) Mouse SPNS2 functions as a sphingosine-1-phosphate transporter in vascular endothelial cells. PLoS One 7:e38941

Hla T, Brinkmann V (2011) Sphingosine 1-phosphate (S1P): physiology and the effects of S1P receptor modulation. Neurology 76(8 Suppl 3):S3–S8

Hoeferlin LA, Wijesinghe DS, Chalfant CE (2013) The role of ceramide-1-phosphate in biological functions. Handb Exp Pharmacol 215:153–166

Imeri F, Schwalm S, Lyck R, Zivkovic A, Stark H, Engelhardt B, Pfeilschifter J, Huwiler A (2016) Sphingosine kinase 2 deficient mice exhibit reduced experimental autoimmune encephalomyelitis: resistance to FTY720 but not ST-968 treatments. Neuropharmacology 105:341–350

Jarman KE, Moretti PA, Zebol JR, Pitson SM (2010) Translocation of sphingosine kinase 1 to the plasma membrane is mediated by calcium- and integrin-binding protein 1. J Biol Chem 285:483–492

Jung ID, Lee JS, Kim YJ, Jeong YI, Lee CM, Baumruker T, Billlich A, Banno Y, Lee MG, Ahn SC, Park WS, Han J, Park YM (2007) Sphingosine kinase inhibitor suppresses a Th1 polarization via the inhibition of immunostimulatory activity in murine bone marrow-derived dendritic cells. Int Immunol 19:411–426

Kharel Y, Raje M, Gao M, Gellett AM, Tomsig JL, Lynch KR, Santos WL (2012) Sphingosine kinase type 2 inhibition elevates circulating sphingosine 1-phosphate. Biochem J 447(1):149–157

Kihara Y, Maceyka M, Spiegel S, Chun J (2014) Lysophospholipid receptor nomenclature review: IUPHAR review 8. Br J Pharmacol 171:3575–3594

Kim JW, Kim YW, Inagaki Y, Hwang YA, Mitsutake S, Ryu YW, Lee WK, Ha HJ, Park CS, Igarashi Y (2005) Synthesis and evaluation of sphingoid analogs as inhibitors of sphingosine kinases. Bioorg Med Chem 13(10):3475–3485

Kobayashi N, Kobayashi N, Yamaguchi A, Nishi T (2009) Characterization of the ATP dependent sphingosine 1-phosphate transporter in rat erythrocytes. J Biol Chem 284:21192–21200

Laviad EL, Albee L, Pankova-Kholmyansky I, Epstein S, Park H, Merrill AH Jr, Futerman AH (2008) Characterization of ceramide synthase 2: tissue distribution, substrate specificity, and inhibition by sphingosine 1-phosphate. J Biol Chem 283(9):5677–5684

Li ZH, Tao YF, Xu LX, Zhao H, Li XL, Fang F, Wu Y, Lu J, Li YH, Du WW, Ren JL, Li YP, Xu YY, Feng X, Wang J, He WQ, Pan J (2016) A novel sphingosine kinase 1 inhibitor (SKI-5C) induces cell death of Wilms' tumor cells in vitro and in vivo. Am J Transl Res 8(11):4548–4563

Liang J, Nagahashi M, Kim EY, Harikumar KB, Yamada A, Huang WC, Hait NC, Allegood JC, Price MM, Avni D, Takabe K, Kordula T, Milstien S, Spiegel S (2013) Sphingosine-1-phosphate links persistent STAT3 activation, chronic intestinal inflammation, and development of colitis-associated cancer. Cancer Cell 23:107–120

Lim KG, Sun C, Bittman R, Pyne NJ, Pyne S (2011a) (*R*)-FTY720 methyl ether is a specific sphingosine kinase 2 inhibitor: effect on sphingosine kinase 2 expression in HEK 293 cells and actin rearrangement and survival of MCF-7 breast cancer cells. Cell Signal 23(10):1590–1595

Lim KG, Tonelli F, Li Z, Lu X, Bittman R, Pyne S, Pyne NJ (2011b) FTY720 analogues as sphingosine kinase 1 inhibitors: enzyme inhibition kinetics, allosterism, proteasomal degradation, and actin rearrangement in MCF-7 breast cancer cells. J Biol Chem 286(21):18633–18640

Liu H, Toman RE, Goparaju SK, Maceyka M, Nava VE, Sankala H, Payne SG, Bektas M, Ishii I, Chun J, Milstien S, Spiegel S (2003) Sphingosine kinase type 2 is a putative BH3-only protein that induces apoptosis. J Biol Chem 278(41):40330–40336

Liu K, Guo TL, Hait NC, Allegood J, Parikh HI, Xu W, Kellogg GE, Grant S, Spiegel S, Zhang S (2013) Biological characterization of 3-(2-amino-ethyl)-5-[3-(4-butoxyl-phenyl)-propylidene]-thiazolidine-2,4-dione (K145) as a selective sphingosine kinase-2 inhibitor and anticancer agent. PLoS One 8(2):e56471

Loveridge C, Tonelli F, Leclercq T, Lim KG, Long JS, Berdyshev E, Tate RJ, Natarajan V, Pitson SM, Pyne NJ, Pyne S (2010) The sphingosine kinase 1 inhibitor 2-(p-hydroxyanilino)-4-(p-chlorophenyl)thiazole induces proteasomal degradation of sphingosine kinase 1 in mammalian cells. J Biol Chem 285(50):38841–38852

Lynch KR, Thorpe SB, Santos WL (2016) Sphingosine kinase inhibitors: a review of patent literature (2006-2015). Expert Opin Ther Pat 26(12):1409–1416

Maceyka M, Sankala H, Hait NC, Le Stunff H, Liu H, Toman R, Collier C, Zhang M, Satin LS, Merrill AH Jr, Milstien S, Spiegel S (2005) SphK1 and SphK2, sphingosine kinase isoenzymes with opposing functions in sphingolipid metabolism. J Biol Chem 280:37118–37129

MacRitchie N, Volpert G, Al Washih M, Watson DG, Futerman AH, Kennedy S, Pyne S, Pyne NJ (2016) Effect of the sphingosine kinase 1 selective inhibitor, PF-543 on arterial and cardiac remodeling in a hypoxic model of pulmonary arterial hypertension. Cell Signal 28:946–955

Maines LW, Fitzpatrick LR, French KJ, Zhuang Y, Xia Z, Keller SN, Upson JJ, Smith CD (2008) Suppression of ulcerative colitis in mice by orally available inhibitors of sphingosine kinase. Dig Dis Sci 53(4):997–1012

Maines LW, Fitzpatrick LR, Green CL, Zhuang Y, Smith CD (2010) Efficacy of a novel sphingosine kinase inhibitor in experimental Crohn's disease. Inflammopharmacology 18(2):73–85

Malavaud B, Pchejetski D, Mazerolles C, de Paiva GR, Calvet C, Doumerc N, Pitson S, Rischmann P, Cuvillier O (2010) Sphingosine kinase-1 activity and expression in human prostate cancer resection specimens. Eur J Cancer 46(18):3417–3424

Mandala SM (2001) Sphingosine-1-phosphate phosphatases. Prostaglandins Other Lipid Mediat 64(1–4):143–156

McNaughton M, Pitman M, Pitson SM, Pyne NJ, Pyne S (2016) Proteasomal degradation of sphingosine kinase 1 and inhibition of dihydroceramide desaturase by the sphingosine kinase inhibitors, SKi or ABC294640, induces growth arrest in androgen-independent LNCaP-AI prostate cancer cells. Oncotarget 7(13):16663–16675

Mizugishi K, Yamashita T, Olivera A, Miller GF, Spiegel S, Proia RL (2005) Essential role for sphingosine kinases in neural and vascular development. Mol Cell Biol 25:11113–11121

Nagahashi M, Ramachandran S, Kim EY, Allegood JC, Rashid OM, Yamada A, Zhao R, Milstien S, Zhou H, Spiegel S, Takabe K (2012) Sphingosine-1-phosphate produced by sphingosine kinase 1 promotes breast cancer progression by stimulating angiogenesis and lymphangiogenesis. Cancer Res 72:726–735

Nakahara K, Ohkuni A, Kitamura T, Abe K, Naganuma T, Ohno Y, Zoeller RA, Kihara A (2012) The Sjögren-Larsson syndrome gene encodes a hexadecenal dehydrogenase of the sphingosine 1-phosphate degradation pathway. Mol Cell 46(4):461–471

Neubauer HA, Pham DH, Zebol JR, Moretti PA, Peterson AL, Leclercq TM, Chan H, Powell JA, Pitman MR, Samuel MS, Bonder CS, Creek DJ, Gliddon BL, Pitson SM (2016) An oncogenic role for sphingosine kinase 2. Oncotarget 7(40):64886–64899

Ohotski J, Edwards J, Elsberger B, Watson C, Orange C, Mallon E, Pyne S, Pyne NJ (2013) Identification of novel functional and spatial associations between sphingosine kinase 1, sphingosine 1-phosphate receptors and other signalling proteins that affect prognostic outcome in estrogen receptor-positive breast cancer. Int J Cancer 132(3):605–616

Panneer Selvam S, De Palma RM, Oaks JJ, Oleinik N, Peterson YK, Stahelin RV, Skordalakes E, Ponnusamy S, Garrett-Mayer E, Smith CD, Ogretmen B (2015) Binding of the sphingolipid S1P to hTERT stabilizes telomerase at the nuclear periphery by allosterically mimicking protein phosphorylation. Sci Signal 8:ra58

Parham KA, Zebol JR, Tooley KL, Sun WY, Moldenhauer LM, Cockshell MP, Gliddon BL, Moretti PA, Tigyi G, Pitson SM, Bonder CS (2015) Sphingosine 1-phosphate is a ligand for peroxisome proliferator-activated receptor-γ that regulates neoangiogenesis. FASEB J 29:3638–3653

Patwardhan NN, Morris EA, Kharel Y, Raje MR, Gao M, Tomsig JL, Lynch KR, Santos WL (2015) Structure-activity relationship studies and in vivo activity of guanidine-based sphingosine kinase inhibitors: discovery of SphK1- and SphK2-selective inhibitors. J Med Chem 58(4):1879–1899

Pitman MR, Costabile M, Pitson SM (2016) Recent advances in the development of sphingosine kinase inhibitors. Cell Signal 28(9):1349–1363

Pitson SM, Moretti PA, Zebol JR, Lynn HE, Xia P, Vadas MA, Wattenberg BW (2003) Activation of sphingosine kinase 1 by ERK1/2-mediated phosphorylation. EMBO J 22:5491–5500

Pitson SM, Xia P, Leclercq TM, Moretti PA, Zebol JR, Lynn HE, Wattenberg BW, Vadas MA (2005) Phosphorylation-dependent translocation of sphingosine kinase to the plasma membrane drives its oncogenic signalling. J Exp Med 201:49–54

Ponnusamy S, Selvam SP, Mehrotra S, Kawamori T, Snider AJ, Obeid LM, Shao Y, Sabbadini R, Ogretmen B (2012) Communication between host organism and cancer cells is transduced by systemic sphingosine kinase 1/sphingosine 1-phosphate signalling to regulate tumour metastasis. EMBO Mol Med 4:761–775

Powell JA, Lewis AC, Zhu W, Toubia J, Pitman MR, Wallington-Beddoe CT, Moretti PA, Iarossi D, Samaraweera SE, Cummings N, Ramshaw HS, Thomas D, Wei AH, Lopez AF, D'Andrea RJ, Lewis ID, Pitson SM (2017) Targeting sphingosine kinase 1 induces MCL1-dependent cell death in acute myeloid leukemia. Blood 129(6):771–782

Pyne NJ, Pyne S (2010) Sphingosine 1-phosphate and cancer. Nat Rev Cancer 10(7):489–503

Pyne NJ, Pyne S (2013) Sphingosine 1-phosphate is a missing link between chronic inflammation and colon cancer. Cancer Cell 23:5–7

Pyne NJ, Pyne S (2017) Sphingosine kinase 2 and multiple myeloma. Oncotarget 8(27):43596–43597

Pyne S, Chapman J, Steele L, Pyne NJ (1996) Sphingomyelin-derived lipids differentially regulate the extracellular signal-regulated kinase 2 (ERK-2) and c-Jun N-terminal kinase (JNK) signal cascades in airway smooth muscle. Eur J Biochem 237:819–826

Pyne S, Adams DR, Pyne NJ (2016a) Sphingosine 1-phosphate and sphingosine kinases in health and disease: recent advances. Prog Lipid Res 62:93–106

Pyne NJ, McNaughton M, Boomkamp S, MacRitchie N, Evangelisti C, Martelli AM, Jiang HR, Ubhi S, Pyne S (2016b) Role of sphingosine 1-phosphate receptors, sphingosine kinases and sphingosine in cancer and inflammation. Adv Biol Regul 60:151–159

Pyne NJ, Adams DR, Pyne S (2017) Sphingosine kinase 2 in autoimmune/inflammatory disease and the development of Sphingosine kinase 2 inhibitors. Trends Pharmacol Sci 38(7):581–591

Saddoughi SA, Ogretmen B (2013) Diverse functions of ceramide in cancer cell death and proliferation. Adv Cancer Res 117:37–58

Salas A, Ponnusamy S, Senkal CE, Meyers-Needham M, Selvam SP, Saddoughi SA, Apohan E, Sentelle RD, Smith C, Gault CR, Obeid LM, El-Shewy HM, Oaks J, Santhanam R, Marcucci G, Baran Y, Mahajan S, Fernandes D, Stuart R, Perrotti D, Ogretmen B (2011) Sphingosine kinase-1 and sphingosine 1-phosphate receptor 2 mediate Bcr-Abl1 stability and drug resistance by modulation of protein phosphatase 2A. Blood 117:5941–5952

Schnüte ME, McReynolds MD, Kasten T, Yates M, Jerome G, Rains JW, Hall T, Chrencik J, Kraus M, Cronin CN, Saabye M, Highkin MK, Broadus R, Ogawa S, Cukyne K, Zawadzke LE, Peterkin V, Iyanar K, Scholten JA, Wendling J, Fujiwara H, Nemirovskiy O, Wittwer AJ, Nagiec MM (2012) Modulation of cellular S1P levels with a novel, potent and specific inhibitor of sphingosine kinase-1. Biochem J 444(1):79–88

Schnüte ME, McReynolds MD, Carroll J, Chrencik J, Highkin MK, Iyanar K, Jerome G, Rains JW, Saabye M, Scholten JA, Yates M, Nagiec MM (2017) Discovery of a potent and selective sphingosine kinase 1 inhibitor through the molecular combination of chemotype-distinct screening hits. J Med Chem 60(6):2562–2572

Schrecengost RS, Keller SN, Schiewer MJ, Knudsen KE, Smith CD (2015) Downregulation of critical oncogenes by the selective SK2 inhibitor ABC294640 hinders prostate cancer progression. Mol Cancer Res 13:1591–1601

Shen H, Giordano F, Wu Y, Chan J, Zhu C, Milosevic I, Wu X, Yao K, Chen B, Baumgart T, Sieburth D, De Camilli P (2014) Coupling between endocytosis and sphingosine kinase 1 recruitment. Nat Cell Biol 16:652–662

Shirai K, Kaneshiro T, Wada M, Furuya H, Bielawski J, Hannun YA, Obeid LM, Ogretmen B, Kawamori T (2011) A role of sphingosine kinase 1 in head and neck carcinogenesis. Cancer Prev Res (Phila) 4:454–462

Siow D, Sunkara M, Morris A, Wattenberg B (2015) Regulation of *de novo* sphingolipid biosynthesis by the ORMDL proteins and sphingosine kinase-1. Adv Biol Regul 57:42–54

Sivasubramanian M, Kanagaraj N, Dheen ST, Tay SS (2015) Sphingosine kinase 2 and sphingosine-1-phosphate promotes mitochondrial function in dopaminergic neurons of mouse model of Parkinson's disease and in MPP+ -treated MN9D cells in vitro. Neuroscience 290:636–648

Snider AJ, Kawamori T, Bradshaw SG, Orr KA, Gilkeson GS, Hannun YA, Obeid LM (2009) A role for sphingosine kinase 1 in dextran sulfate sodium-induced colitis. FASEB J 23:143–152

Sobue S, Nemoto S, Murakami M, Ito H, Kimura A, Gao S, Furuhata A, Takagi A, Kojima T, Nakamura M, Ito Y, Suzuki M, Banno Y, Nozawa Y, Murate T (2008) Implications of sphingosine kinase 1 expression level for the cellular sphingolipid rheostat: relevance as a marker for daunorubicin sensitivity of leukemia cells. Int J Hematol 87(3):266–275

Spiegel S, Milstien S (2011) The outs and the ins of sphingosine-1-phosphate in immunity. Nat Rev Immunol 11:403–415

Strub GM, Paillard M, Liang J, Gomez L, Allegood JC, Hait NC, Maceyka M, Price MM, Chen Q, Simpson DC, Kordula T, Milstien S, Lesnefsky EJ, Spiegel S (2011) Sphingosine-1-phosphate produced by sphingosine kinase 2 in mitochondria interacts with prohibitin 2 to regulate complex IV assembly and respiration. FASEB J 25:600–612

Takabe K, Paugh SW, Milstien S, Spiegel S (2008) "Inside-out" signaling of sphingosine-1-phosphate: therapeutic targets. Pharmacol Rev 60:181–195

Takasugi N, Sasaki T, Suzuki K, Osawa S, Isshiki H, Hori Y, Shimada N, Higo T, Yokoshima S, Fukuyama T, Lee VM, Trojanowski JQ, Tomita T, Iwatsubo T (2011) BACE1 activity is modulated by cell-associated sphingosine-1-phosphate. J Neurosci 31:6850–6857

Tan SS, Khin LW, Wong L, Yan B, Ong CW, Datta A, Salto-Tellez M, Lam Y, Yap CT (2014) Sphingosine kinase 1 promotes malignant progression in colon cancer and independently predicts survival of patients with colon cancer by competing risk approach in South Asian population. Clin Transl Gastroenterol 5:e51

ter Braak M, Danneberg K, Lichte K, Liphardt K, Ktistakis NT, Pitson SM, Hla T, Jakobs KH, Meyer zu Heringdorf D (2009) Galpha(q)-mediated plasma membrane translocation of sphingosine kinase-1 and cross-activation of S1P receptors. Biochim Biophys Acta 1791:357–370

Vadas M, Xia P, McCaughan G, Gamble J (2008) The role of sphingosine kinase 1 in cancer: oncogene or non-oncogene addiction? Biochim Biophys Acta 1781(9):442–447

Venant H, Rahmaniyan M, Jones EE, Lu P, Lilly MB, Garrett-Mayer E, Drake RR, Kraveka JM, Smith CD, Voelkel-Johnson C (2015) The Sphingosine kinase 2 inhibitor ABC294640 reduces the growth of prostate cancer cells and results in accumulation of dihydroceramides in vitro and in vivo. Mol Cancer Ther 14(12):2744–2752

Vu TM, Ishizu AN, Foo JC, Toh XR, Zhang F, Whee DM, Torta F, Cazenave-Gassiot A, Matsumura T, Kim S, Toh SES, Suda T, Silver DL, Wenk MR, Nguyen LN (2017) Mfsd2b is essential for the sphingosine-1-phosphate export in erythrocytes and platelets. Nature 550 (7677):524–528

Wallington-Beddoe CT, Bennett MK, Vandyke K, Davies L, Zebol JR, Moretti PAB, Pitman MR, Hewett DR, Zannettino ACW, Pitson SM (2017) Sphingosine kinase 2 inhibition synergises with bortezomib to target myeloma by enhancing endoplasmic reticulum stress. Oncotarget 8(27):43602–43616

Wang Z, Min X, Xiao SH, Johnstone S, Romanow W, Meininger D, Xu H, Liu J, Dai J, An S, Thibault S, Walker N (2013) Molecular basis of sphingosine kinase 1 substrate recognition and catalysis. Structure 21(5):798–809

Wang J, Knapp S, Pyne NJ, Pyne S, Elkins JM (2014) Crystal structure of Sphingosine kinase 1 with PF-543. ACS Med Chem Lett 5(12):1329–1333

Watson C, Long JS, Orange C, Tannahill CL, Mallon E, McGlynn LM, Pyne S, Pyne NJ, Edwards J (2010) High expression of sphingosine 1-phosphate receptors, S1P1 and S1P3, sphingosine kinase 1, and extracellular signal-regulated kinase-1/2 is associated with development of tamoxifen resistance in estrogen receptor-positive breast cancer patients. Am J Pathol 177(5):2205–2215

Watson DG, Tonelli F, Alossaimi M, Williamson L, Chan E, Gorshkova I, Berdyshev E, Bittman R, Pyne NJ, Pyne S (2013) The roles of sphingosine kinases 1 and 2 in regulating the Warburg effect in prostate cancer cells. Cell Signal 25(4):1011–1017

Weigert A, Schiffmann S, Sekar D, Ley S, Menrad H, Werno C, Grosch S, Geisslinger G, Brüne B (2009) Sphingosine kinase 2 deficient tumor xenografts show impaired growth and fail to polarize macrophages towards an anti-inflammatory phenotype. Int J Cancer 125:2114–2121

Xi M, Ge J, Wang X, Sun C, Liu T, Fang L, Xiao Q, Yin D (2016) Development of hydroxy-based sphingosine kinase inhibitors and anti-inflammation in dextran sodium sulfate induced colitis in mice. Bioorg Med Chem 24(14):3218–3230

Xia P, Wang L, Moretti PA, Albanese N, Chai F, Pitson SM, D'Andrea RJ, Gamble JR, Vadas MA (2002) Sphingosine kinase interacts with TRAF2 and dissects tumor necrosis factor-alpha signalling. J Biol Chem 277:7996–8003

Xiang Y, Hirth B, Kane JL Jr, Liao J, Noson KD, Yee C, Asmussen G, Fitzgerald M, Klaus C, Booker M (2010) Discovery of novel sphingosine kinase-1 inhibitors. Part 2. Bioorg Med Chem Lett 20(15):4550–4554

Yada Y, Higuchi K, Imokawa G (1995) Purification and biochemical characterisation of membrane-bound epidermal ceramidase from guinea pig skin. J Biol Chem 270(20):12677–12684

Yamaji T, Hanada K (2015) Sphingolipid metabolism and interorganellar transport: localization of sphingolipid enzymes and lipid transfer proteins. Traffic 16(2):101–212

Yang Y, Wang M, Lv B, Ma R, Hu J, Dun Y, Sun S, Li G (2014) Sphingosine kinase-1 protects differentiated N2a cells against beta-amyloid25-35-induced neurotoxicity via the mitochondrial pathway. Neurochem Res 39:932–940

Zhang Y, Yu Q, Lai TB, Yang Y, Li G, Sun SG (2013) Effects of small interfering RNA targeting sphingosine kinase-1 gene on the animal model of Alzheimer's disease. J Huazhong Univ Sci Technolog Med Sci 33:427–432

Zhang Y, Berka V, Song A, Sun K, Wang W, Zhang W, Ning C, Li C, Zhang Q, Bogdanov M, Alexander DC, Milburn MV, Ahmed MH, Lin H, Idowu M, Zhang J, Kato GJ, Abdulmalik OY, Zhang W, Dowhan W, Kellems RE, Zhang P, Jin J, Safo M, Tsai AL, Juneja HS, Xia Y (2014) Elevated sphingosine-1-phosphate promotes sickling and sickle cell disease progression. J Clin Invest 124(6):2750–2761

Zhang F, Xia Y, Yan W, Zhang H, Zhou F, Zhao S, Wang W, Zhu D, Xin C, Lee Y, Zhang L, He Y, Gao E, Tao L (2016) Sphingosine 1-phosphate signaling contributes to cardiac inflammation, dysfunction, and remodeling following myocardial infarction. Am J Physiol Heart Circ Physiol 310:H250–H261

Part II

Phospholipase D and Mitogen Phosphatidic Acid in Human Disease

Prospects for PLD Inhibition in Cancer and Thrombotic Disease

Christian Salazar and Michael A. Frohman

Contents

Abstract

Functions for phospholipase D1 and D2 (PLD1 and PLD2), the canonical isoforms of the PLD superfamily in mammals, have been explored using cell biological and animal disease models for two decades. PLD1 and PLD2, which are activated as a consequence of extracellular signaling events and generate the second messenger signaling lipid phosphatidic acid (PA), have been reported to play roles in settings ranging from platelet activation to the response to cardiac ischemia, viral infection, neurodegenerative disease, and cancer. Of these, the most tractable as therapeutic targets may be thrombotic disease and cancer, as will be discussed here in the context of ongoing efforts to develop small molecule PLD inhibitors.

Keywords

Cancer · Phosphatidic acid · Phospholipase D · Small molecule inhibitors · Thrombotic disease

C. Salazar · M. A. Frohman (✉)
Center for Developmental Genetics and the Department of Pharmacological Sciences, Stony Brook University School of Medicine, Stony Brook, NY, USA
e-mail: Michael.Frohman@Stonybrook.edu

J. Gomez-Cambronero, M. A. Frohman (eds.), *Lipid Signaling in Human Diseases*, Handbook of Experimental Pharmacology 259, https://doi.org/10.1007/164_2019_244

1 Introduction

The mammalian phospholipase D (PLD) superfamily consists of six isoforms, PLD1–PLD6 (Frohman 2015). Cloning and characterization of PLD1 (Hammond et al. 1995) and PLD2 (Colley et al. 1997) identified two highly conserved sequences, HxKxxxDGSxN, which became denoted as the "HKD" motifs (Morris et al. 1996). Each motif forms half of the mature catalytic site (Leiros et al. 2004; Sung et al. 1997, 1999), and the charged residues, in particular the histidines, mediate PLD1 and PLD2's enzymatic hydrolysis of phosphatidylcholine, the most abundant cellular phospholipid, to yield choline and the signaling lipid phosphatidic acid (PA). PLD3 and PLD4 were recently reported to be single-stranded 5′ DNA exonucleases (Gavin et al. 2018), PLD5 has not been reported to have activity, and PLD6 has been reported to both cleave the mitochondrial lipid cardiolipin to generate PA (Choi et al. 2006) and to be a single-stranded RNA endonuclease (Nishimasu et al. 2012).

PLD1 and PLD2 exhibit low-level basal activity in cells but are best known for increasing their activity as a consequence of extracellular stimulatory events such as engagement of G-protein-coupled receptors or receptor tyrosine kinases with their ligands (Bruntz et al. 2014; Jenkins and Frohman 2005). PLD1 and PLD2 are not thought to be activated directly by these receptors but rather to respond to the downstream activation of small GTPases, such as RhoA and ARF family members, and protein kinase C. Many other regulatory mechanisms including phosphorylation, the availability of the lipid cofactor phosphoinositide 4,5 bisphosphate, and other protein activators have been proposed, leading to the view that PLD1 and PLD2 are both complex signaling hubs (Jang et al. 2012) and coincidence detectors (Du et al. 2000).

PA, the product of PLD action, is pleiotropic in action, both altering membrane curvature and charge and serving as a lipid anchor for scores of proteins with well-characterized PA-binding domains. PA can also be converted, through action of other enzymes, to the important bioactive lipids diacylglycerol and lysophosphatidic acid. Together, these direct and indirect consequences of the generation of PA have been shown, in cell culture settings, to affect a large number of cell biological functions including virtually all types of vesicular trafficking and cytoskeletal organization. Many of these findings are reviewed in detail in other chapters in this volume (Egea-Jimenez and Zimmermann 2019; Shah and Gomez-Cambronero 2019; Tanguy et al. 2019).

It was accordingly surprising, then, that mice lacking PLD1 (Elvers et al. 2010), PLD2 (Oliveira et al. 2010), or both isoforms (Stegner et al. 2013) are viable and overtly normal in the controlled setting of an animal facility. Nonetheless, phenotypes have been identified in mice lacking one or both PLD isoforms that present potential therapeutic opportunities for thrombotic disease (Elvers et al. 2010; Stegner et al. 2013) and cancer (Chen et al. 2012; Wang et al. 2017a), as will be subsequently discussed. Moreover, some of the findings reported for mice lacking PLD1 and/or PLD2 have been mimicked using small molecule PLD inhibitors (Stegner et al. 2013; Chen et al. 2012), supporting the prospects for therapeutic

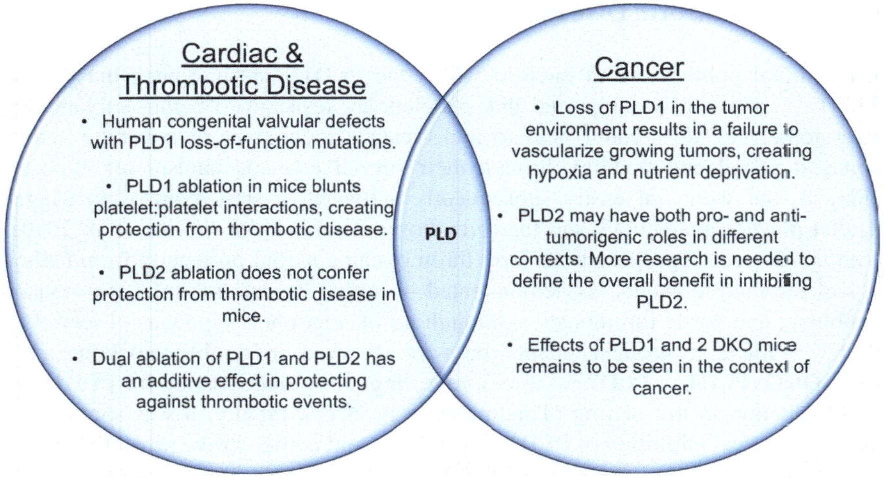

Fig. 1 Proposed therapeutic settings for PLD1 and PLD2 inhibition. As discussed in the text, PLD1 and PLD2 have partially unique and partially redundant roles in two short- and long-term disease settings that represent potential opportunities for small molecule therapeutic inhibition

intervention. There can, however, also be undesirable consequences that result from the loss of PLD1 and/or PLD2 function (Ali et al. 2013; Ngo Thai Bich et al. 2018; Nelson et al. 2017) – thus, therapeutic applications will best take place in acute settings for which long-term consequences of PLD loss-of-function are not manifested (e.g., ongoing thrombotic events) or are of less concern than the underlying disease process (e.g., cancer and possibly Alzheimer's disease) (Frohman 2015) (Fig. 1).

Finally, it was also unexpected when PLD1 loss-of-function mutations were linked to human pathophysiology in a context that had not been reported for PLD1-deficient mice, despite the mice having been studied for a decade by multiple groups. In an elegant study, Ta-Shma and colleagues employed whole-exome analysis to identify PLD1 mutations as being causative for congenital valvular defects (Ta-Shma et al. 2017). Subsequent reexamination of PLD1-deficient mice revealed that they exhibited tricuspid regurgitation, right atrial enlargement, and increased flow velocity, narrowing and thickened leaflets of the pulmonic valve. Interestingly, these changes were not obviously associated with viability or activity issues during development or adulthood in mice, whereas all six human patients with loss of PLD1 function were strongly affected, with two dying in infancy, three requiring corrective surgery, and the last medical treatment. It is not clear why the loss of PLD1 is more physiologically damaging in humans than in mice. However, since the underlying mechanism appears to involve formation of the cardiac valves during development, there isn't currently any basis for being concerned that use of a PLD1 small molecule inhibitor would elicit valvular disease in genetically normal adult humans.

2 Thrombotic Disease

In the initial publication on mice in which the PLD1 gene had been inactivated ($PLD1^{-/-}$ mice), it was reported that platelets are resistant to being activated by sheer force, i.e., they could bind to and create a monolayer of coverage across damaged vessel endothelium through their surveillance mechanism for exposed collagen, but were not easily subsequently activated, a step required to trigger platelet-platelet interactions and the formation of a blood clot (Elvers et al. 2010). With the decreased propensity to form thrombi came partial protection from pathological thrombotic events, as demonstrated in mouse models of stoke, pulmonary embolism, and aortic thrombosis. Although no platelet phenotype was observed in $PLD2^{-/-}$ mice, a stronger phenotype was observed in double-knockout mice (PLD-DKO; $PLD1^{-/-}PLD2^{-/-}$ mice), revealing partial redundancy for PLD1 and PLD2 function in this setting (Thielmann et al. 2012). Finally, it was shown that pharmacological inhibition of PLD1 and PLD2 could confer stroke protection equal in magnitude to that seen in the PLD-DKO mice, although as a limitation of the study, the mice needed to be dosed with the inhibitor prior to the thrombo-inflammatory brain infarction event, since protocols for use of the inhibitor (i.p. injection) did not inhibit PLD inhibition in platelets fast enough to prevent thrombus formation (Stegner et al. 2013). Nonetheless, PLD inhibition even in this setting was proposed to be a potential therapeutic opportunity for conditions such as evolving stroke or for patients otherwise at elevated risk of thrombotic events, since the pathological thrombus formation was blunted without adverse effects on hemostasis.

These findings have recently been extended to studies of human platelets (Lu et al. 2018), where similar but not identical findings have been reported. For human platelets, pharmacological inhibition solely of PLD1 seemed less effective than was observed for mice; but more broadly, optimal results were again seen when both isoforms were inhibited.

3 Small Molecule PLD Inhibitors

PLD activity "inhibition" was achieved for several decades by taking advantage of PLD's propensity to use primary alcohols as the enzymatic reaction nucleophile over water, leading to formation of a relatively biologically inert phosphatidyl alcohol at the expense of production of PA. However, the concentrations of alcohol required to fully block PA production had many unconnected effects on cellular functions, resulting in PLD activity being causally linked to many phenomena, such as fMLP-triggered mast cell degranulation or glucose-stimulated insulin release, which in retrospect were due solely to an unrelated action of the alcohol (Su et al. 2009; Sato et al. 2013). Identification of small molecule inhibitors, use of RNAi, and studies with PLD knockout mice and cells procured from them led to re-evaluation of many of these earlier reports.

Many ultimately unsuccessful attempts to screen for small molecule PLD inhibitors were initiated by large pharmaceutical companies after the cloning of PLD1 and PLD2 in the 1990s. A breakthrough finally came from an unconventional approach used for PLD2 at Novartis (Monovich et al. 2007), which identified the psychotropic drug and dopamine receptor antagonist halopemide as being a PLD2 inhibitor. Reportedly, halopemide was used for psychosis at a dose high enough to inhibit PLD2, raising the intriguing question of whether PLD2 inhibition might have contributed to the symptomatic relief. Monovich and colleagues also synthetized halopemide analogs with increased potency against PLD2 and no inhibitory activity on dopamine receptors, generating the first compound (5-Fluoro-2-indolyl des-chlorohalopemide, FIPI) that could be used for PLD2 inhibition in cells and even in animal models, given the 5.5 h half-life and acceptable bioavailability of the inhibitor. Subsequent studies demonstrated that the halopemide analogs were actually potent inhibitors of both PLD1 and PLD2 (Su et al. 2009; Scott et al. 2009), and much subsequent effort was employed to develop isoform-selective inhibitors and dual PLD1-PLD2 inhibitors with improved pharmacokinetics (Waterson et al. 2018), while in parallel, FIPI was employed in a number of cell biological and animal disease models as proof of principle for the utility of PLD inhibition (e.g., Stegner et al. 2013; Chen et al. 2012; Nishikimi et al. 2009; Tsukahara et al. 2010; Dall'Armi et al. 2010; Oguin et al. 2014). The current state of the field is that an ideal inhibitor suitable for clinical testing does not yet exist, although considerable progress has been made toward that goal (Waterson et al. 2018), and there do exist isoform-selective or dual inhibitors that can be used for cellular or animal studies to complement RNAi and knockout animal approaches.

One note of caution concerns how the inhibitors have been employed in many reports. Some of the initial isoform-preferring halopemide analogs generated by the Brown and Lindsley labs (Scott et al. 2009) had reduced potency (IC_{50}s = 350 nM) that necessitated using them at concentrations approaching 10 μM to achieve full inhibition. Many subsequent analogs generated by this group had vastly better potency (4–20 nM IC_{50}s), similar to that of FIPI (1–10 nM). However, many independent groups have continued to use a concentration of 10 μM (or higher) in studies in which the highly potent compounds are being employed, and it is not known whether they have off-target effects at concentrations 20–250 times that needed for full inhibition. A number of groups have also employed the compounds generated by the Brown and Lindsley labs in vivo in animal studies without taking their pharmacokinetic properties into consideration, which is problematic since all but the most recently published compounds (Waterson et al. 2018) are cleared on first pass through the liver and hence have very short half-lives. Given the large variety of commercially available PLD inhibitors with highly differing IC_{50}s and pharmacokinetics, investigators should carefully consider the choice of compound and concentration to assure isoform selectivity (if that is desired), minimize the chance of off-target effects, and ensure duration of action in vivo as appropriate in a particular experimental setting, and should keep these issues in mind when assessing the published literature. Reports in which phenomena are observed only with excessively high concentrations of inhibitor are particularly at risk for ascribing off-target effects to PLD function.

4 Phospholipase D and Cancer

Hundreds of reports have linked phospholipase D function to one or more aspects of cancer progression, as detailed in several recent reviews (Brown et al. 2017; Roth and Frohman 2018) and another article in this volume (Shah and Gomez-Cambronero 2019). In this section, we will touch on some recent findings and summarize results from preclinical studies.

PLD1 and/or PLD2 are frequently found to be upregulated in many types of cancer, including prostate (Utter et al. 2018; Noble et al. 2018), breast (Gozgit et al. 2007), ovarian (Harel-Dassa et al. 2017), lung (Pazhouhandeh et al. 2017), osteosarcoma (Wang et al. 2017b), and pancreatic adenocarcinoma (Hu et al. 2016), and in many cases, the degree of elevated expression correlates with invasiveness and metastatic potential.

There are many mechanisms through which PLD1 and PLD2 may have pro-tumorigenic effects (Brown et al. 2017; Roth and Frohman 2018). Recent mechanisms proposed that are based on cell culture studies include promoting the formation of exosomes that prepare the metastatic tumor site environment (Gomez-Cambronero 2018; Egea-Jimenez and Zimmermann 2018) or affect the local tumor microenvironment (Munoz-Galvan et al. 2019), enabling the metabolism of endomembrane lipids through autophagy to support tumor metabolism (Cai et al. 2016), preventing apoptosis (Liu et al. 2016), or positively regulating the Hippo pathway (Han et al. 2018) or mTORC1 activity (Yoon et al. 2011, 2015).

Studies combining cell culture approaches and preclinical mouse models have suggested several important functions in which PLD activity may be important, both in tumor cells and in the tumor microenvironment. PLD1 activity in the tumor microenvironment was shown to be important for melanoma and lung cancer primary tumor growth and metastasis (Chen et al. 2012). The role in primary tumor growth was evidenced by a lack of neoangiogenic vascular growth into the expanding tumor, resulting in hypoxia and nutrient deficiency once the tumors acquired a size too large for surface diffusion of oxygen and nutrients; PLD1$^{-/-}$ vascular endothelial cells were shown to have aberrant responses to VEGF, which is secreted as the tumors reach this stage. The role in metastasis was linked to the platelet phenotype described earlier; tumor cells, which require interaction with activated platelets for efficient metastatic seeding, were hindered by the blunted activation of PLD1$^{-/-}$ platelets. Given the otherwise absence of overt phenotypes seen for PLD1$^{-/-}$ mice, this raised the prospects for using a PLD1 inhibitor as a cancer therapeutic, which was supported through demonstrating that short-term use of FIPI could phenocopy the inhibition of tumor neoangiogenesis and decreased metastatic seeding seen in the PLD1$^{-/-}$ mice. PLD1 may play roles in the tumor cells as well, based on a report that it regulates proliferation, migration, and invasion of hepatocellular carcinoma cells, in addition to promoting EMT (Xiao et al. 2016).

The role of PLD2 is more complicated. Chen et al. (2012) found that PLD2 did not appear to be important in the tumor environment for tumor growth or vascularization, which was confirmed by two other groups (Wang et al. 2017a; Ngo Thai Bich et al. 2018); however, a separate group found that PLD2 activity in the tumor environment was important for primary tumor growth and neoangiogenesis, albeit to a lesser degree than PLD1 (Ghim et al. 2014). It is not clear why differing results were obtained. One possibility might be that Ghim and colleagues (2014) used mice in which PLD2 was deleted only in the vascular endothelial cells, whereas the other groups all used mice with whole-body ablation of PLD2, which perhaps resulted in compensatory pro-angiogenic pathways of unknown mechanism. One other difference in these studies is that whereas Chen et al. (2012) and Wang et al. (2017a) saw no effect of PLD2 ablation on the growth of the primary tumor, Ngo Thai Bich et al. (2018) observed *increased* primary tumor volumes, which they linked to immunosuppression due to decreased CD8+ T-cell proliferation and recruitment to the tumor site. It is not clear why increased tumor size was seen only in this study. The balance of PLD effects on the immune system in relationship to tumor progression is complicated. Ablation of either PLD1 or PLD2 affects macrophage function (Ali et al. 2013), and PLD small molecule inhibitors have been reported to decrease the numbers of tumor-associated macrophages and neutrophils in breast tumors and lung and liver metastases (Henkels et al. 2016); hence there are potentially both pro- and anti-tumorigenic effects on the immune system in the absence of PLD1 or PLD2 activity. Perhaps most dramatically, PLD2 ablation in breast tumor cells has a significant effect on their ability to metastasize and has been proposed to ensue from roles for PLD2 in promoting kinesin-1-driven cell surface localization of membrane type 1 matrix metalloproteinase, with the loss of PLD2 function resulting in emigration of fewer circulating tumor cells and decreased metastatic seeding (Wang et al. 2017a). Other groups using siRNA or PLD2 small molecule inhibitors have similarly reported that breast tumor cell PLD2 may promote cell invasion and metastasis (Henkels et al. 2013).

5 Therapeutic Considerations

Ultimately, the utility of PLD inhibitors for cancer will depend on weighing the prospective benefits against risk. Clearly, mice lacking either or even both isoforms are without overt phenotypes, although there are numerous physiological and pathophysiological differences that have been elicited upon more in-depth testing. These findings suggest that it should be possible to use PLD inhibitors as therapeutics. Nonetheless, there are also many suggestions that PLD functions, while similar in mice and humans, may nonetheless play out different in detail, including the fact that PLD1 deficiency has a nearly 100% penetrant lethal phenotype for cardiac valvular disease only in humans, and that while human platelets require PLD1 similarly to mouse platelets, the specifics of the phenotype in the absence of PLD1 activity are partially different in detail. It is likely that PLD inhibitors will have effects on the human immune system, which could be either pro- or anti-tumorigenic, and there are other PLD roles, such as the role of PLD2 in preventing hypertension in mice (Nelson et al. 2017), which could be less or more dramatic in humans. Development of clean inhibitors with acceptable PK/PD will need to proceed with these potential outcomes in mind to determine the clinical settings in which they can be employed (Fig. 1).

Acknowledgments Supported by a Carol Baldwin Breast Cancer award to MAF.

References

Ali WH et al (2013) Deficiencies of the lipid-signaling enzymes phospholipase D1 and D2 alter cytoskeletal organization, macrophage phagocytosis, and cytokine-stimulated neutrophil recruitment. PLoS One 8(1):e55325

Brown HA, Thomas PG, Lindsley CW (2017) Targeting phospholipase D in cancer, infection and neurodegenerative disorders. Nat Rev Drug Discov 16(5):351–367

Bruntz RC, Lindsley CW, Brown HA (2014) Phospholipase D signaling pathways and phosphatidic acid as therapeutic targets in cancer. Pharmacol Rev 66(4):1033–1079

Cai M et al (2016) Phospholipase D1-regulated autophagy supplies free fatty acids to counter nutrient stress in cancer cells. Cell Death Dis 7(11):e2448

Chen Q et al (2012) Key roles for the lipid signaling enzyme phospholipase D1 in the tumor microenvironment during tumor angiogenesis and metastasis. Sci Signal 5(249):ra79

Choi SY et al (2006) A common lipid links Mfn-mediated mitochondrial fusion and SNARE-regulated exocytosis. Nat Cell Biol 8(11):1255–1262

Colley WC et al (1997) Phospholipase D2, a distinct phospholipase D isoform with novel regulatory properties that provokes cytoskeletal reorganization. Curr Biol 7(3):191–201

Dall'Armi C et al (2010) The phospholipase D1 pathway modulates macroautophagy. Nat Commun 1:142

Du G et al (2000) Dual requirement for rho and protein kinase C in direct activation of phospholipase D1 through G protein-coupled receptor signaling. Mol Biol Cell 11(12):4359–4368

Egea-Jimenez AL, Zimmermann P (2018) Phospholipase D and phosphatidic acid in the biogenesis and cargo loading of extracellular vesicles. J Lipid Res 59(9):1554–1560

Egea-Jimenez AL, Zimmermann P (2019) Lipids in exosome biology. Handb Exp Pharmacol. https://doi.org/10.1007/164_2019_220

Elvers M et al (2010) Impaired alpha(IIb)beta(3) integrin activation and shear-dependent thrombus formation in mice lacking phospholipase D1. Sci Signal 3(103):ra1

Frohman MA (2015) The phospholipase D superfamily as therapeutic targets. Trends Pharmacol Sci 36(3):137–144

Gavin AL et al (2018) PLD3 and PLD4 are single-stranded acid exonucleases that regulate endosomal nucleic-acid sensing. Nat Immunol 19(9):942–953

Ghim J et al (2014) Endothelial deletion of phospholipase D2 reduces hypoxic response and pathological angiogenesis. Arterioscler Thromb Vasc Biol 34(8):1697–1703

Gomez-Cambronero J (2018) Lack of effective translational regulation of PLD expression and exosome biogenesis in triple-negative breast cancer cells. Cancer Metastasis Rev 37 (2–3):491–507

Gozgit JM et al (2007) PLD1 is overexpressed in an ER-negative MCF-7 cell line variant and a subset of phospho-Akt-negative breast carcinomas. Br J Cancer 97(6):809–817

Hammond SM et al (1995) Human ADP-ribosylation factor-activated phosphatidylcholine-specific phospholipase D defines a new and highly conserved gene family. J Biol Chem 270 (50):29640–29643

Han H et al (2018) Regulation of the hippo pathway by phosphatidic acid-mediated lipid-protein interaction. Mol Cell 72(2):328–340.e8
Harel-Dassa K et al (2017) Phospholipase D messenger RNA expression and clinical role in high-grade serous carcinoma. Hum Pathol 62:115–121
Henkels KM et al (2013) Phospholipase D (PLD) drives cell invasion, tumor growth and metastasis in a human breast cancer xenograph model. Oncogene 32(49):5551–5562
Henkels KM, Muppani NR, Gomez-Cambronero J (2016) PLD-specific small-molecule inhibitors decrease tumor-associated macrophages and neutrophils infiltration in breast tumors and lung and liver metastases. PLoS One 11(11):e0166553
Hu J et al (2016) Simultaneous high expression of PLD1 and Sp1 predicts a poor prognosis for pancreatic ductal adenocarcinoma patients. Oncotarget 7(48):78557–78565
Jang JH et al (2012) Understanding of the roles of phospholipase D and phosphatidic acid through their binding partners. Prog Lipid Res 51(2):71–81
Jenkins GM, Frohman MA (2005) Phospholipase D: a lipid centric review. Cell Mol Life Sci 62(19–20):2305–2316
Leiros I, McSweeney S, Hough E (2004) The reaction mechanism of phospholipase D from Streptomyces sp strain PMF. Snapshots along the reaction pathway reveal a pentacoordinate reaction intermediate and an unexpected final product. J Mol Biol 339(4):805–820
Liu M et al (2016) Inhibition of phospholipaseD2 increases hypoxia-induced human colon cancer cell apoptosis through inactivating of the PI3K/AKT signaling pathway. Tumour Biol 37(5):6155–6168
Lu WJ et al (2018) An antithrombotic strategy by targeting phospholipase D in human platelets. J Clin Med 7(11):E440
Monovich L et al (2007) Optimization of halopemide for phospholipase D2 inhibition. Bioorg Med Chem Lett 17(8):2310–2311
Morris AJ, Engebrecht J, Frohman MA (1996) Structure and regulation of phospholipase D. Trends Pharmacol Sci 17(5):182–185
Munoz-Galvan S et al (2019) Tumor cell-secreted PLD increases tumor stemness by senescence-mediated communication with microenvironment. Oncogene 38(8):1309–1323
Nelson RK et al (2017) Phospholipase D2 loss results in increased blood pressure via inhibition of the endothelial nitric oxide synthase pathway. Sci Rep 7(1):9112
Ngo Thai Bich V et al (2018) Physiological function of phospholipase D2 in anti-tumor immunity: regulation of CD8(+) T lymphocyte proliferation. Sci Rep 8(1):6283
Nishikimi A et al (2009) Sequential regulation of DOCK2 dynamics by two phospholipids during neutrophil chemotaxis. Science 324(5925):384–387
Nishimasu H et al (2012) Structure and function of Zucchini endoribonuclease in piRNA biogenesis. Nature 491(7423):284–287
Noble AR et al (2018) Phospholipase D inhibitors reduce human prostate cancer cell proliferation and colony formation. Br J Cancer 118(2):189–199
Oguin TH 3rd et al (2014) Phospholipase D facilitates efficient entry of influenza virus, allowing escape from innate immune inhibition. J Biol Chem 289(37):25405–25417
Oliveira TG et al (2010) Phospholipase D2 ablation ameliorates Alzheimer's disease-linked synaptic dysfunction and cognitive deficits. J Neurosci 30(49):16419–16428
Pazhouhandeh M et al (2017) Comparative network analysis of patients with non-small cell lung cancer and smokers for representing potential therapeutic targets. Sci Rep 7(1):13812
Roth E, Frohman MA (2018) Proliferative and metastatic roles for phospholipase D in mouse models of cancer. Adv Biol Regul 67:134–140
Sato T et al (2013) Molecular mechanisms of N-formyl-methionyl-leucyl-phenylalanine-induced superoxide generation and degranulation in mouse neutrophils: phospholipase D is dispensable. Mol Cell Biol 33(1):136–145
Scott SA et al (2009) Design of isoform-selective phospholipase D inhibitors that modulate cancer cell invasiveness. Nat Chem Biol 5(2):108–117

Shah KN, Gomez-Cambronero J (2019) Phospholipase D and the mitogen phosphatidic acid in human disease – inhibitors of PLD at the crossroads of phospholipid biology and cancer. Handb Exp Pharmacol. https://doi.org/10.1007/164_2019_216

Stegner D et al (2013) Pharmacological inhibition of phospholipase D protects mice from occlusive thrombus formation and ischemic stroke-brief report. Arterioscler Thromb Vasc Biol 33 (9):2212–2217

Su W et al (2009) 5-Fluoro-2-indolyl des-chlorohalopemide (FIPI), a phospholipase D pharmacological inhibitor that alters cell spreading and inhibits chemotaxis. Mol Pharmacol 75 (3):437–446

Sung TC et al (1997) Mutagenesis of phospholipase D defines a superfamily including a trans-Golgi viral protein required for poxvirus pathogenicity. EMBO J 16(15):4519–4530

Sung TC et al (1999) Structural analysis of human phospholipase D1. J Biol Chem 274 (6):3659–3666

Tanguy E, Wang Q, Vitale N (2019) Role of phospholipase D-derived phosphatidic acid in regulated exocytosis and neurological disease. Handb Exp Pharmacol. https://doi.org/10.1007/164_2018_180

Ta-Shma A et al (2017) Congenital valvular defects associated with deleterious mutations in the PLD1 gene. J Med Genet 54(4):278–286

Thielmann I et al (2012) Redundant functions of phospholipases D1 and D2 in platelet alpha-granule release. J Thromb Haemost 10(11):2361–2372

Tsukahara T et al (2010) Phospholipase D2-dependent inhibition of the nuclear hormone receptor PPARgamma by cyclic phosphatidic acid. Mol Cell 39(3):421–432

Utter M et al (2018) Elevated phospholipase D activity in androgen-insensitive prostate cancer cells promotes both survival and metastatic phenotypes. Cancer Lett 423:28–35

Wang Z et al (2017a) Binding of PLD2-generated phosphatidic acid to KIF5B promotes MT1-MMP surface trafficking and lung metastasis of mouse breast cancer cells. Dev Cell 43 (2):186–197.e7

Wang XX et al (2017b) Tissue microarray staining reveals PLD1 and Sp1 have a collaborative, pro-tumoral effect in patients with osteosarcomas. Oncotarget 8(43):74340–74347

Waterson AG et al (2018) Isoform selective PLD inhibition by novel, chiral 2,8-diazaspiro[4.5] decan-1-one derivatives. Bioorg Med Chem Lett 28(23–24):3670–3673

Xiao J et al (2016) Therapeutic inhibition of phospholipase D1 suppresses hepatocellular carcinoma. Clin Sci (Lond) 130(13):1125–1136

Yoon MS et al (2011) Class III PI-3-kinase activates phospholipase D in an amino acid-sensing mTORC1 pathway. J Cell Biol 195(3):435–447

Yoon MS et al (2015) Rapid mitogenic regulation of the mTORC1 inhibitor, DEPTOR, by phosphatidic acid. Mol Cell 58(3):549–556

Phospholipase D and the Mitogen Phosphatidic Acid in Human Disease: Inhibitors of PLD at the Crossroads of Phospholipid Biology and Cancer

Julian Gomez-Cambronero and Krushangi N. Shah

Contents

Gomez-Cambronero was deceased at the time of publication.

K. N. Shah (✉)
Department of Biochemistry and Molecular Biology, Boonshoft School of Medicine, Wright State University, Dayton, OH, USA
e-mail: shah.222@wright.edu

J. Gomez-Cambronero, M. A. Frohman (eds.), *Lipid Signaling in Human Diseases*, Handbook of Experimental Pharmacology 259, https://doi.org/10.1007/164_2019_216

Abstract

Lipids are key building blocks of biological membranes and are involved in complex signaling processes such as metabolism, proliferation, migration, and apoptosis. Extracellular signaling by growth factors, stress, and nutrients is transmitted through receptors that activate lipid-modifying enzymes such as the phospholipases, sphingosine kinase, or phosphoinositide 3-kinase, which then modify phospholipids, sphingolipids, and phosphoinositides. One such important enzyme is phospholipase D (PLD), which cleaves phosphatidylcholine to yield phosphatidic acid and choline. PLD isoforms have dual role in cells. The first involves maintaining cell membrane integrity and cell signaling, including cell proliferation, migration, cytoskeletal alterations, and invasion through the PLD product PA, and the second involves protein-protein interactions with a variety of binding partners. Increased evidence of elevated PLD expression and activity linked to many pathological conditions, including cancer, neurological and inflammatory diseases, and infection, has motivated the development of dual- and isoform-specific PLD inhibitors. Many of these inhibitors are reported to be efficacious and safe in cells and mouse disease models, suggesting the potential for PLD inhibitors as therapeutics for cancer and other diseases. Current knowledge and ongoing research of PLD signaling networks will help to evolve inhibitors with increased efficacy and safety for clinical studies.

Keywords

Cancer · Infections · Inflammation · Neurological disorders · Phosphatidic acid (PA) · Phospholipase D (PLD)

1 Phospholipase D Biochemistry and Cell Biology

Phospholipase D (PLD) hydrolyzes the phosphodiester bond in structural phospholipids, primarily phosphatidylcholine (PC) in mammals, to form phosphatidic acid (PA) and choline (Fig. 1). Choline diffuses in the cytosol and has little second messenger activity, while PA is a second messenger and a well-characterized mitogen in cancer. Biochemically, PLD is a transphosphatidylase that mediates the exchange of the polar head group present in membrane-bound lipids by using water as a nucleophile (primary alcohols can also be used) to catalyze the cleavage of the phosphodiester bond.

1.1 Isoforms of PLD and Their Domains

The phospholipase D (PLD) superfamily contains six mammalian isoforms, all of which have the characteristic HxKxxxxD (His-Lys-Asp) motif in their catalytic domain (gray bars in Fig. 1). PLD1 (Hammond et al. 1995) and PLD2 (Colley et al. 1997) are the classical isoforms that possess two HKD motifs and phosphoinositide binding (PX) and pleckstrin homology (PH) domains, whereas PLD3–6 lack PX and PH domains and have either one or two HKD motifs (Frohman 2015). The PX and PH domains play major roles in regulating PLD subcellular

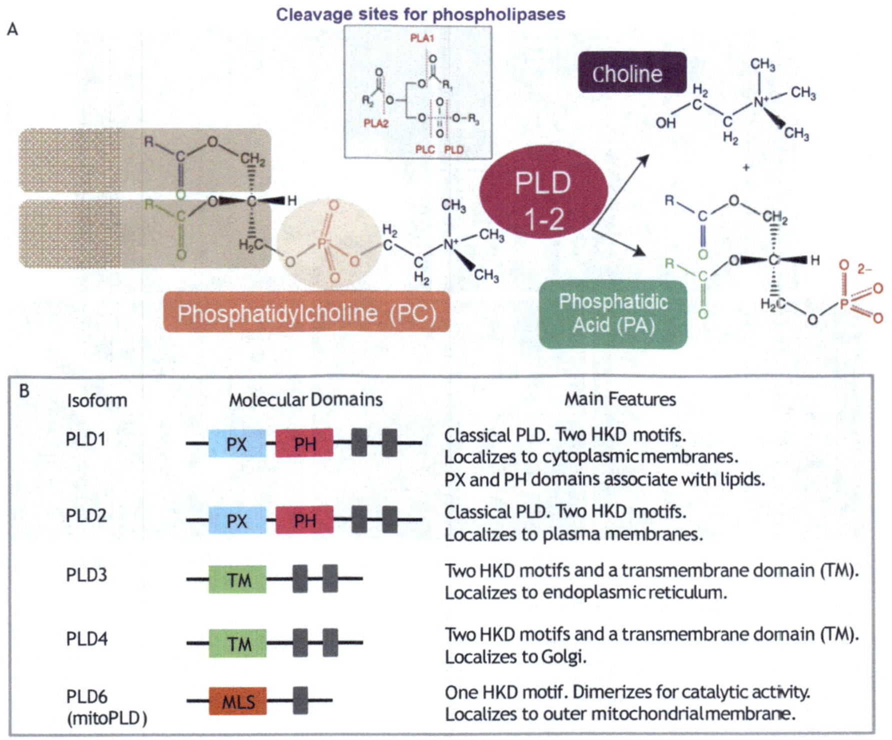

Fig. 1 Chemical reaction of PLD lipase activity and characteristics of mammalian phospholipase D. (**a**) The lipase activity of PLD1 and PLD2 mediates hydrolysis of the membrane lipid phosphatidylcholine into free choline and phosphatidic acid. The small box demonstrates lipid bonds cleaved by several phospholipases. (**b**) All PLD isoforms contain at least one HKD catalytic motif. The classical PLD isoforms are PLD1 and PLD2. Their PH and PX domains associate PLD to the membrane via interaction with lipids and other proteins. PLD3 and PLD4 are transmembrane proteins localizing to the ER and Golgi, respectively. PLD5 is not well-studied. PLD6, also termed MitoPLD, is the smallest isoform and localizes to the outer mitochondrial membrane. It dimerizes and functions as a lipase, hydrolyzing cardiolipin to phosphatidic acid, and also functions as a 3′ endonuclease in the maturation of piRNAs

localization and activity, whereas PLD's catalytic activity is mediated by HKD motif half-catalytic sites that juxtapose structurally. PLD-mediated cleavage of phospholipids occurs in two stages: (1) stabilization of an intermediate and release of choline and (2) formation of phosphatidic acid due to nucleophilic attack by a water molecule. Briefly, the histidine from the HKD I motif, with help from the aspartic acid, nucleophilically attacks the phosphate group of the phospholipid, leading to the formation of a tetrahedral phosphatidyl enzyme intermediate (Ponting and Kerr 1996; Sung et al. 1997). The HKD II histidine and the lysines from both HKD motifs help to stabilize the intermediate. Lysine, due to its positive charge, may stabilize the charge on the oxygen molecules of the phosphate group, while histidine does so by donating a proton, leading to dissociation of choline. The HKD

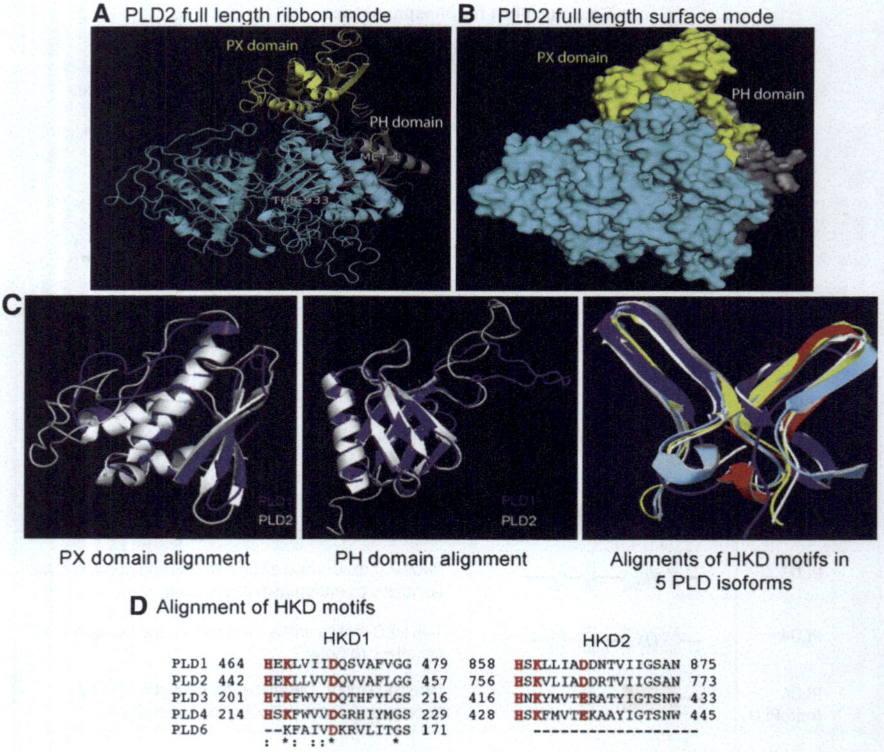

Fig. 2 Full-length hypothetical structure of PLD2 and sequence alignment of domains of mammalian PLD isoforms. (**a**, **b**) Hypothetical PLD2 3D structure in ribbon (**a**) and surface (**b**) modes. PX and PH domains of the protein are shown in yellow and gray, respectively, while the rest of the protein containing the HKD motif is shown in blue. (**c**) Three-dimensional structural alignment of PX (left image) and PH (center image) domains of PLD1 (white) and PLD2 (purple). Catalytic HKD motifs of PLD1–PLD6 show perfect alignment three-dimensionally (right image). (**d**) Sequence alignment of HKD motifs of the known mammalian PLD isoforms (PLD1–4 and 6)

II histidine also activates water with the help of a nearby tyrosine residue, and the activated water molecule acts as a nucleophile to form phosphatidic acid (Figs. 2 and 3) (Gottlin et al. 1998; Leiros et al. 2004; Lerchner et al. 2006). Mutation of the HKD motif histidine and/or lysine completely inactivates PLD lipase activity (Sung et al. 1997; Gottlin et al. 1998). *The PX domain* in classical PLD isoforms contains a conserved proline-rich region that can bind to several phosphoinositides like phosphatidylinositol 5-phosphate (PtdIns(5)P), phosphatidylinositol-3-phosphate (PtdIns(3)P), phosphatidylinositol 3,4-bisphosphate (PtdIns(3,4)P_2), and phosphatidylinositol 3,4,5-triphosphate (PtdIns(3,4,5)P_3) (Hodgkin et al. 2000a; Li et al. 2007; Du et al. 2003; Stahelin et al. 2004). The ability of the PX domain to bind to these phosphoinositides increases the affinity of PLD1 and PLD2 toward membranes, facilitating the translocation of PLD1/2 toward endocytosis sites in response to extracellular signals (Lee et al. 2005). RSK2, a kinase, has also been

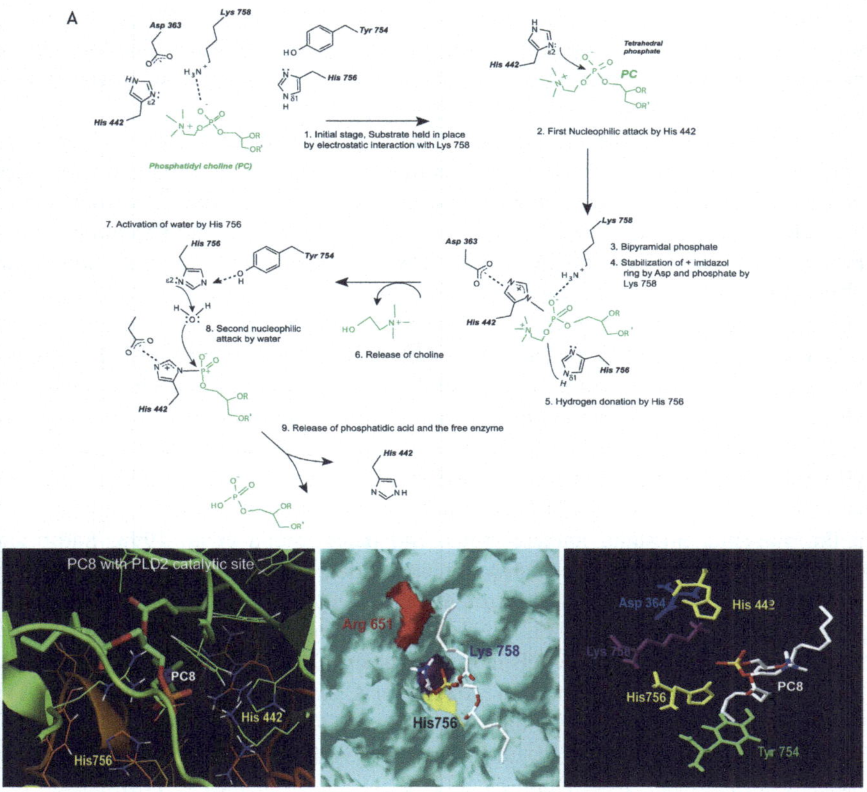

Fig. 3 Proposed mechanism of PLD lipase activity and PC8 alignment in the catalytic groove of PLD2. (**a**) Histidine 442 exerts a nucleophilic attack on phosphate moiety of PC with the help of aspartate 363. His 756 and lysines 444 and 758 might be involved in stabilizing the tetrahedral intermediate. In the final step, histidine 756 donates hydrogen to the tetrahedral intermediate and activates water, which then exerts a second nucleophilic attack, ultimately leading to the release of choline and phosphatidic acid (PA). (**b**) Catalytic site groove of PLD2 with the substrate PC8 (left image), orientation of key amino acids in the active site of PLD2 toward the substrate PC8 (center image), and PLD2 HKD catalytic site with the PC8 in surface mode that shows orientation of PC8 in such a way as to facilitate choline release from the HKD groove (right image)

shown to phosphorylate PLD1 on Thr147 within the PX domain and regulate neurosecretion (Zeniou-Meyer et al. 2008) and neuronal growth (Ammar et al. 2013). The PH domain in PLD1 and PLD2 possesses high selectivity for phosphatidylinositol 4,5-biphosphate (PtdIns(4,5)P_2) (Sciorra et al. 2002). This binding was reported to be required for PLD activity, with PIP_2 acting as a cofactor for PLD activity. However, point mutations in this region do not influence the activity in vitro but rather suppress the activity only in vivo (Sciorra et al. 1999, 2002; Du et al. 2004; Hodgkin et al. 2000b). In addition to regulation by PIP_2 binding, palmitoylation of cysteine residues in the PH domain also helps in translocation to membranes (Sugars et al. 1999; Xie et al. 2001). PLD1 also possesses a unique loop region which is absent in other isoforms. This loop region contains cleavage sites for many caspases and may be a reason for lower in vitro activity of PLD1 as compared to PLD2 (Sung et al. 1999).

The PLD1 gene is present on the q arm of chromosome 3 (3q26) (Park et al. 1998a) and has 31 exons (Redina and Frohman 1998a), 27 of which yield expression of four splice variants, PLD1a, PLD1a2, PLD1b, and PLD1b2 (Hammond et al. 1997; Katayama et al. 1998). PLD1 primarily localizes to endomembranes and is transported to the plasma membrane upon extracellular signaling (Hammond et al. 1995; Du et al. 2003). On the other hand, the PLD2 gene (Redina and Frohman 1998b) is located on the p arm of chromosome 17 (17p13) and has two splice variants, PLD2a and PLD2b (Park et al. 1998b; Steed et al. 1998). PLD2 encodes a 933 amino acid protein and is found mainly in the plasma membrane (Colley et al. 1997). PLD1 and PLD2 are expressed in almost all tissues and cell types to various levels (Colley et al. 1997). PLD1a is expressed in the lung, heart, and spleen, whereas PLD1b is found at the greatest levels in the kidney, small intestine, and liver (Katayama et al. 1998). PLD2 is ubiquitously expressed, with the highest levels in the placenta, prostate, lung, thymus, and heart (Steed et al. 1998; Saqib and Wakelam 1997). PLD3 and PLD4 are embedded in the endoplasmic reticulum (ER) membrane with a short, N-terminal transmembrane region and the rest of the protein in the ER lumen. PLD3, which has no reported lipid hydrolysis enzymatic activity, is expressed at high levels in many tissues (Osisami et al. 2012), and the loss of its function was implicated in Alzheimer's disease (Cruchaga et al. 2014), although this remains controversial (Cacace et al. 2015). PLD4 is largely found in the spleen, thymus, liver, and lungs, and its dysfunction leads to autoimmune diseases (Jung et al. 2014; Otani et al. 2011; Terao et al. 2013; Yoshikawa et al. 2010). Very recently, PLD3 and PLD4 have been identified as 5′ exonucleases that oppose TLR9 signaling, offering an explanation for the IL6-driven autoimmune disease that occurs in the absence of PLD4 and that is exasperated in the dual absence of PLD3 (Gavin et al. 2018). PLD5 remains poorly studied. While all other isoforms of PLD contain two HKD motifs, PLD6 only contains one, and therefore it homodimerizes to form an active site at the dimer interface (Choi et al. 2006; Nureki 2014). Moreover, the classical PLD isoforms contain PX and PH lipid-binding domains to associate with membranes, while PLD6 contains an N-terminal mitochondrial localization signal and transmembrane domain (Gao and Frohman 2012). It is anchored in the outer mitochondrial membrane facing the cytosol (hence also known as MitoPLD) and is the smallest member of the PLD family (28 kDa). As a lipase, it cleaves cardiolipin to generate PA. It also acts as an endonuclease and cleaves phosphodiester bonds present in the backbone of nucleic acids (Nureki 2014; Gao and Frohman 2012). Physiologically, the targets of PLD6 action are piRNAs, an ancestral third type of RNAi that has a critical role during spermatogenesis in mammals (Huang et al. 2011).

1.2 Regulation of PLD and Downstream Molecular Signaling

PLD is activated by nutrients (Yoon et al. 2011; Xu et al. 2011), growth signals (Chen et al. 2003), and stress (Fite et al. 2016; Gomez-Cambronero 2014a) via signaling through GPCRs and receptor tyrosine kinases. PLD activity is regulated by a variety of factors such as the level of phosphoinositides, fatty acids, protein kinase C (PKC), ADP ribosylation factor (ARF), Rho family GTPases (Rac1 and Cdc42), and protein phosphorylation (Brown et al. 1993, 1995). PLD, once activated, exerts its actions in two ways: (1) via protein-protein interactions (GAP and GEF activity) independent of its catalytic activity and (2) via PA, produced due to its lipase activity (Fig. 4).

1. PLD's PX domain is involved in the recruitment of the growth factor receptor-binding protein 2 (Grb2)/son of sevenless protein (SOS) complex, ultimately activating the Ras/MAPK signaling pathway (Di Fulvio et al. 2006; Sorkin et al. 2000). PLD can also interact with dynamin via its PH domain, and the activated dynamin is involved in EGF receptor recycling that contributes to MAPK signaling (Lee et al. 2006; Orth and McNiven 2006).
2. PA is produced via three pathways by three different enzymes, lysophosphatidic acid acyltransferase (LPAAT), diacylglycerol kinase (DGK), and PLD. PA produced by LPAAT (pathway 1) is converted to CDP-DAG (cytidine 5′-diphosphate diacylglycerol), which is mainly used for general phospholipid synthesis (Foster et al. 2014). DAG also acts as a second messenger, so only a smaller proportion of DAG gets converted to PA by PLC-DAG pathway (pathway 2). Therefore, most of the PA which acts as second messenger is produced by PLD (pathway 3). As depicted in Fig. 4, PA also serves as a second messenger signal for numerous important pathways including mTOR (Foster et al. 2014; Foster 2007). mTOR activation leads to accelerated cell growth, and its suppression leads to cell cycle arrest in G_1 (Saqcena et al. 2013; Fingar et al. 2004). mTOR also senses the presence of glutamine and essential amino acids that are crucial for the synthesis (S) phase of the cell cycle (Saqcena et al. 2013). The accessibility of PA to interact with mTOR positively correlates with cells' abilities to make phospholipids to synthesize new membranes during cell division. Elevated PLD activity leads to increased activation of mammalian target of rapamycin (mTOR), a survival signal often hyperactivated in cancer cells in response to nutrition deprivation (Chen et al. 2003, 2005) and subdues the tumor suppressors p53 and protein phosphatase 2A (Hui et al. 2004).

1.3 Surmounting Numbers of Reports Implicate the Role of PA in Cell Migration and Invasion

Efficient migration and/or invasion require the coordinated cytoskeletal reorganization including the formation of lamellipodia, filopodia, and membrane blebs and

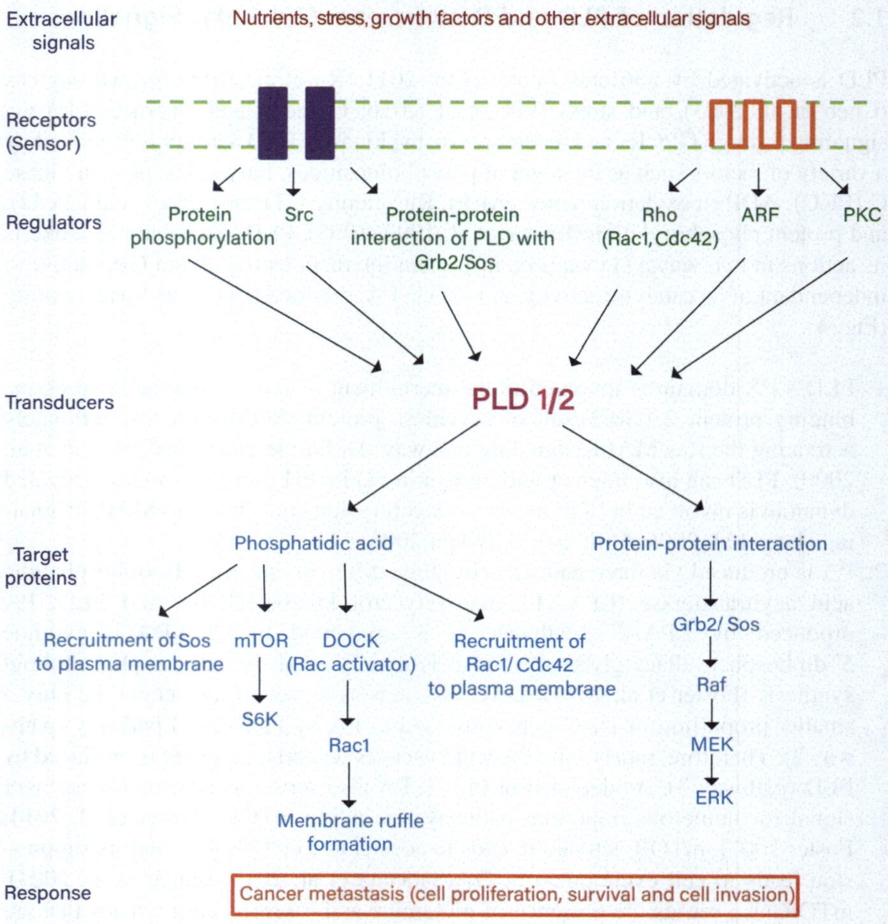

Fig. 4 Probable molecular signaling of classical PLD isoforms. G-protein-coupled receptors and/or tyrosine kinases act upstream of PLD and activate it by phosphorylation of specific targeted residues. Phosphoinositides and small GTPases also act on PLD2 signaling pathways. All of these upstream actions ultimately control PLD2's ability to interact with other protein partners via protein-protein interactions and modulate its lipase and GEF activities, which affect downstream outcomes such as chemotaxis and cell invasion

cell-cell and cell-extracellular matrix adhesions disruption, and these structures are tightly regulated by multiple signaling mechanisms. In particular, members of the Rho family of small GTPases, Rac1 and Cdc42, are known to promote actin polymerization at the leading edge and are involved in lamellipodia (Rac1) and filopodia (Cdc42) production. PA either recruits these small GTPases to the plasma membrane where they are in close proximity to their activators (guanine exchange factors, GEFs) or directly activates them. One study reported activation of Rac and

DOCK (dedicator of cytokinesis, a Rac GEF) by PA produced by PLD, which then increased membrane ruffle formation (Sanematsu et al. 2013). In a separate report, PA produced from PLD2 was shown to be sufficient to recruit son of sevenless (Sos) to the plasma membrane in a PLD2-dependent and Grb2-independent manner, which is important for Ras activity (Zhao et al. 2007) (Fig. 4). Moreover, Chae et al. (2008) proposed that PLD-generated PA modulates Rac1 downstream signaling by targeting it to the plasma membrane through its C-terminal polybasic motif (Chae et al. 2008). Overall, PA is likely involved in cell invasion through Rho family small GTPases-mediated cytoskeletal alterations.

According to a model by Zheng et al. (2006), cells inside the developing tumor mass were subjected to hypoxia and nutrient/growth factor deprivation. These stressed cells responded by elevating total PLD protein levels and survived presumably by gaining the ability to migrate via WASP signaling and to proliferate by Raf/MEK/ERK pathway activation (Zheng et al. 2006).

2 Chemical and Biological (Small Molecule) Inhibitors of PLD

Several natural products including resveratrol, quercetin, caffeic acid phenylether ester, calphostin C (PKC inhibitor), and marine fungal metabolite (SCH420789) have been shown to be PLD inhibitors but are relatively nonspecific (Park et al. 2013a; Park and do Min 2011; Puar et al. 2000; Sciorra et al. 2001; Tou and Urbizo 2001). Quercetin and caffeic acid phenylether ester inhibit transactivation, thereby interfering with PLD activation, and were found to inhibit cell invasion and proliferation for glioblastoma cells (Park et al. 2013a; Park and do Min 2011). Triptolide, another natural product, and rebamipide both suppress PLD1 and PLD2 activity in cancer cell lines (Arakawa et al. 1998; Qiu and Kao 2003). However the specificity of these compounds toward PLD is subjected to debate since the effect of triptolide on MDA-MB-231 breast cancer cell proliferation was attributed to its ability to inhibit the transcription factors NFκβ, NFAT, and p53 (Kang et al. 2009).

Primary alcohols like 1-butanol have also been used to block PLD activity, as they nonspecifically complete with water as a nucleophile; however, it is difficult to achieve complete inhibition using this approach (Motes et al. 2005). In 2007, Monovich et al. at Novartis identified halopemide, a dopamine blocker which was already approved as a psychotropic agent, and 14 analogs, as PLD2 inhibitors (Table 1), out of which 5-fluoro 2-indolyl des-chlorohalopemide (FIPI; Su et al. 2009) was shown to be the most potent ($IC_{50} = 0.02$ μM) (Monovich et al. 2007). FIPI is a direct inhibitor of PLD activity and is not known to interfere with any other signaling pathway or change the levels of PIP_2 (Fig. 5). FIPI-mediated inhibition of PLD impedes cytoskeleton reorganization, cell invasion, and metastasis (Su et al. 2009; Nishikimi et al. 2009). FIPI and another analog *N*-[2-(4-oxo-1-phenyl-1,3,8-triazaspiro (Ponting and Kerr 1996; Sung et al. 1997) dec-8-yl)ethyl]-2-naphthalenecarboxamide (NPOT, designed by Brown and colleagues in 2009 [Scott et al. 2009]) inhibit primary tumor growth in xenotransplanted mice (Henkels

Table 1 Chemical inhibitors of phospholipase D isoforms

IUPAC name and abbrev. name	Isoform specificity	Chemical structure
FIPI (5-fluoro-2-indolyl des-chlorohalopemide) (Frohman 2015; Sanematsu et al. 2013; Su et al. 2009; Nishikimi et al. 2009; Chen et al. 2012; Stegner et al. 2013; Elvers et al. 2010; Ali et al. 2013) *N*-[2-[4-(2,3-Dihydro-2-oxo-1H-benzimidazol-1-yl)-1-piperidinyl]ethy]-5-fluoro-1H-indole-2-carboxamide	Dual (PLD1/ PLD2)	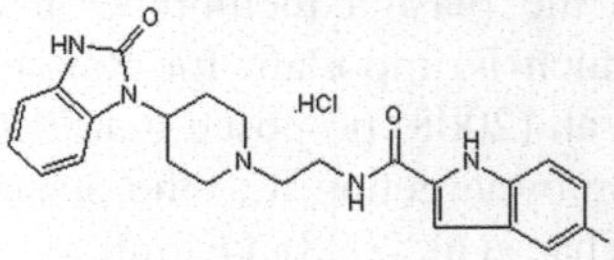
VU0155056 (Scott et al. 2009; Chaves-Moreira et al. 2017) *N*-(2-{4-[2-oxo-2,3-dihydro-1H-benzo(d) imidazol-1-yl]piperidin-1-yl}ethyl)-2-naphthamide	Dual (PLD1/ PLD2)	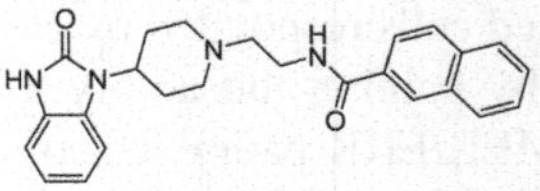
VU0155069 (NBOD/CAY10593) (Scott et al. 2009; Lewis et al. 2009; Lavieri et al. 2009; Sulzmaier et al. 2012) *N*-[2-[4-(5-chloro-2,3-dihydro-2-oxo-1H-benzimidazol-1-yl)-1-piperidinyl]-1-methylethyl]-2-naphthalenecarboxamide	PLD1	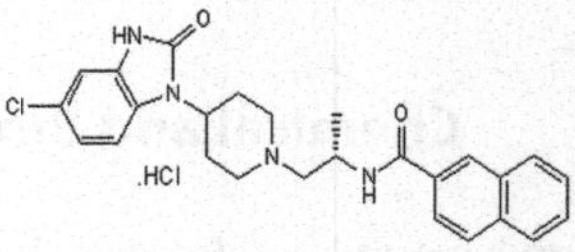
VU0359595 (RBPC/ML-270) (Lewis et al. 2009; Bruntz et al. 2014; Han et al. 2011) (1R,2R)-*N*-([S]-1-{4-[5-bromo-2-oxo-2,3-dihydro-1H-benzo(d)imidazol-1-yl] piperidin-1-yl}propan-2-yl)-phenyl cyclopropanecarboxamide	PLD1	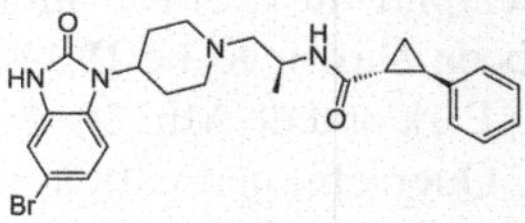
VU0364739 (NFOT) (Lavieri et al. 2009, 2010; Basiouni et al. 2013; Henkels et al. 2013; Jiang et al. 2016) *N*-[2-[1-(3-Fluorophenyl)-4-oxo-1,3,8-triazaspiro [4.5]decan-8-yl]ethyl]-2-naphthalene carboxamide	PLD2	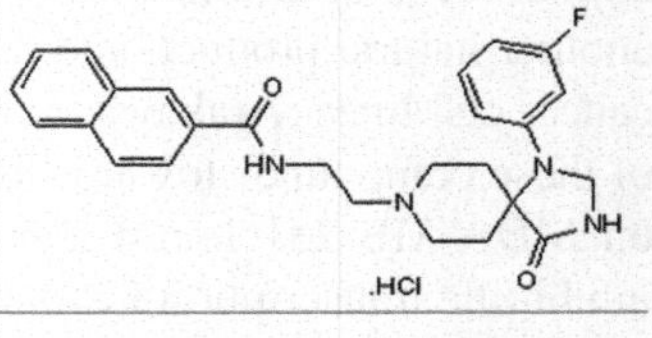
VU0155072-2 (NPOT/CAY10594) (Henkels et al. 2016; Lewis et al. 2009; Ganesan et al. 2015) *N*-[2-(4-oxo-1-phenyl-1,3,8-triazaspiro[4,5] dec-8-yl)ethyl]-2-naphthalenecarboxamide	PLD2	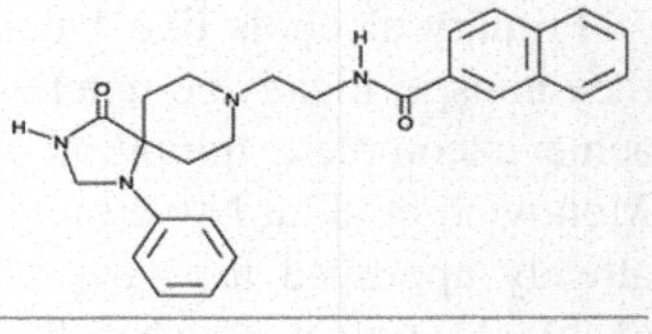
ML298 (O'Reilly et al. 2013) 3,4-Difluoro-*N*-[2-[1-(3-fluorophenyl)-4-oxo-1,3,8-triazaspiro[4.5]dec-8-yl]ethyl]-benzamide	PLD2	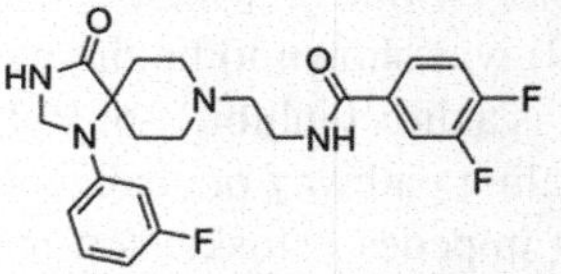

(continued)

Table 1 (continued)

IUPAC name and abbrev. name	Isoform specificity	Chemical structure
ML299 (O'Reilly et al. 2013) 4-bromo-*N*-[(1S)-2-[1-(3-fluorophenyl)-4-oxo-1,3,8-triazaspiro[4.5]dec-8-yl]-1-methylethyl]-benzamide	Dual (PLD1/ PLD2)	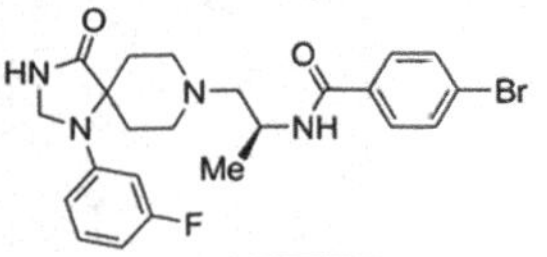
ML395 (O'Reilly et al. 2014)	PLD2	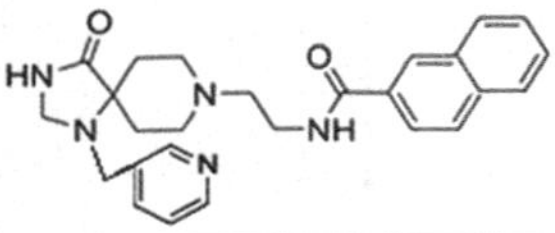

et al. 2016). Moreover, there was a significant reduction in infiltration of tumor-associated macrophages and neutrophils in the tumor microenvironment.

A second-generation, PLD2-selective inhibitor, VU0364739 reduced virus replication in A549 cells infected with influenza virus. Despite the isoform PLD selectivity, five different off-targets were identified for VU0364739, highlighting the need for better molecules. Third-generation improved PLD inhibitors include ML298, ML299, and ML395. For instance, compared to VU0364739, ML395 displayed almost no cell toxicity in A549 cells (O'Reilly et al. 2014). Moreover, ML395 was shown to be more effective in reducing viral load in A549 cells infected with influenza virus (H1N1, H3N2, H5N1, H7N9) in comparison to VU0364739. A separate study showed that the dual PLD1/PLD2 inhibitor ML299 and the PLD2-selective inhibitor ML298 both decreased cell invasion in U87-MG cells (O'Reilly et al. 2013). However, the third-generation inhibitors have yet to be employed in animal models of cancer, inflammation, and neurological disorders.

RNA interference can also be an effective way in inhibiting PLD isoforms. Many studies have reported using siRNA or shRNA to silence the PLD gene in various diseases, including breast cancer, lung cancer, ischemia, and stroke, which are discussed in the respective diseases in this chapter. MicroRNAs are noncoding RNA that can regulate gene expression through argonaute-based mRNA cleavage and translational repression (Bartel 2009). Studies have identified miR-203 to be specific to the PLD2 gene. A study reporting specificity of miR-203 to PLD2 showed downregulation of PLD2 expression miR-203 mimics transfection (Chen et al. 2014). Data from our lab shows higher basal expression of miR-203, 887, 3619, and miR 182 in low-aggressive breast cancer cells that possess low PLD2 levels (MCF-7), while the expression of these microRNAs was drastically lower in highly aggressive breast cancer cells with high PLD2 expression (MDA-MB-231) (Fite et al. 2016).

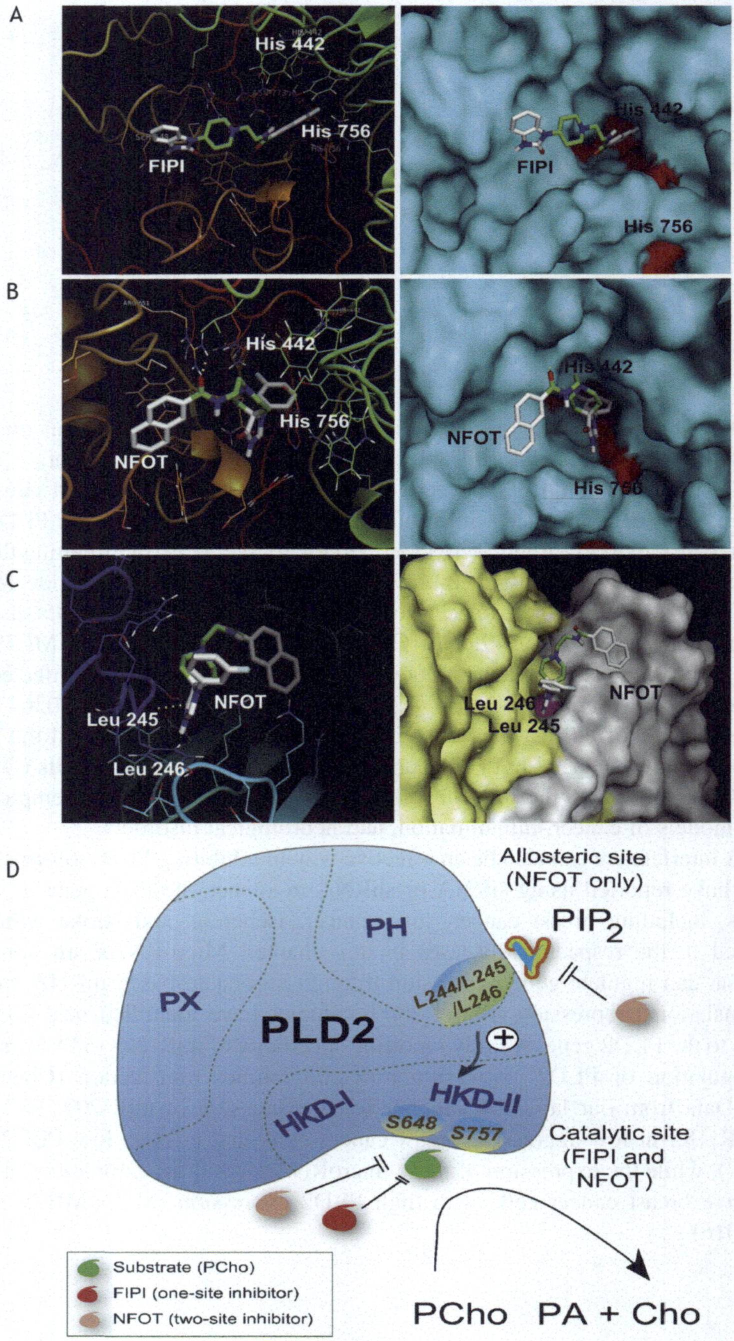

Fig. 5 Inhibitor binding sites on PLD2 and schematic representation of the mechanism of action of FIPI and NFOT. (**a**) Ribbon and surface models showing binding of FIPI to the active site. (**b**)

3 Pathological Role of PLD in Diseases and Therapeutic Potential of PLD Inhibitors

3.1 PLD in Cancer

PLD1 and PLD2 play an important role in maintaining the integrity of cellular membranes. PA produced by PLD activates important signaling pathways such as G-protein-coupled receptors, receptor tyrosine kinases, PI3K-Akt, mTOR, and Wnt/β-catenin and thus influence numerous cellular functions including cytoskeletal rearrangement, membrane trafficking, cell migration, invasion, and proliferation (Gomez-Cambronero 2014b). The role of PLD1/2 in these signaling events also makes them integral to cancer cell metastasis (Chen et al. 2012; Henkels et al. 2013; Knoepp et al. 2008; Uchida et al. 1997). Additionally, PLD1/2 transmit cellular signals that suppress apoptosis and contribute to cancer cell survival (Hui et al. 2004; Gomez-Cambronero 2014b; Cho et al. 2008). PLD1/2 are upregulated in human cancer, especially KRAS-driven cancers (colorectal cancer, pancreatic cancer, and non-small cell lung cancer) (Zheng et al. 2006; Garcia et al. 2008; Shi et al. 2007). Augmented PLD expression and enzymatic activity have also been reported in several other cancers, including breast cancer, liver cancer, prostate cancer, and gastric cancer (Uchida et al. 1997, 1999; Yamada et al. 2003; Levin et al. 1995).

3.2 PLD in Colorectal Cancer

The RB1/E2F pathway has been implicated in many cancers, including interacting with Wnt/β-catenin and PI3K-Akt in colorectal cancer cells to transcriptionally upregulate PLD1 and PLD2. In turn, PLD1 and PLD2 promote β-catenin-TCF-4 complex formation, further activating Wnt signaling, cell growth, and cell invasion (Kang and Min 2010). PLD1 ablation in $Apc^{min/+}$ mice increased apoptosis significantly, which was independent of p53 but correlated with miR-192/4465-mediated RB1 downregulation. PLD1 inactivation similarly suppressed PI3K/Akt-TopBP1 and Wnt/b-catenin signaling due to increased expression of PI3K-repressed E2F1. Similar results were obtained by pharmacologically targeting PLD1 using VU0155069.

Moreover, PLD1 overexpression decreased apoptosis in a colorectal cancer cell line (Kang et al. 2017) and high levels of PLD1 and RB1 along with decreased E2F1 correlated with lower survival rates in colorectal cancer patients (Kang et al. 2015a).

Fig. 5 (continued) Ribbon and surface models showing binding of NFOT to the active site in PLD2. Colored in red are the histidine residues. (**c**) Ribbon and surface models showing binding of NFOT to an allosteric site in PLD2. Colored in purple are the hydrophobic residues. (**d**) FIPI (a dual, PLD1/PLD2 inhibitor) and NFOT (a PLD2-specific inhibitor) act at a site in the vicinity of the lipase catalytic site. In addition, NFOT is a competitive, allosteric inhibitor. As indicated in the schematic, the possible sites of action of NFOT are F244, L245, and L246 in the PH region (PIP2 binding site) and S757/S648 near the HKD region, while the site of action of FIPI is at S648

Studies like these support the idea that PLD1 promotes cell survival, self-renewal, and anti-apoptosis in colorectal cancer cells by regulating RB1 and β-catenin posttranscriptionally and by modulating E2F1 and Akt pathways (Kang et al. 2015a, 2017; Selvy et al. 2011). In a separate set of studies, PLD2 overexpression in tumor samples from colorectal carcinoma patients (Oshimoto et al. 2003) correlated with progression and survival (Saito et al. 2007). Finally, PLD2 inhibition promotes autophagy and death of HT29 and HCT116 colorectal cancer cells, suggesting that PLD2 could be an effective target for cancer therapy (Hwang et al. 2014).

3.3 PLD in Breast Cancer

PLD1 mRNA levels are elevated in patients with basal-like breast tumors but not in those with ER-negative breast cancer (Gozgit et al. 2007). MDA-MB-231 cells, which have high PLD1 expression, show low phospho-Akt signals and elevated mTOR signaling (Chen et al. 2005). PLD activity may also upregulate PLD1 levels in breast cancer cells: PA induces Ras-ERK/PI3K-NFκβ signaling, which increases NFκβ binding to the PLD1 promoter and PLD1 expression. Inhibiting PLD1 in this setting decreased expression of EGF-induced matrix metalloproteinases (MMP) and decreased cell invasion (Kang et al. 2011).

PLD2 has also been linked to breast cancer cell invasion and tumor growth. SCID mice xenotransplanted with PLD2-silenced MDA-MB-231 cells exhibited a delayed onset of tumor growth and reduced tumor size (Henkels et al. 2013). Moreover, MCF-7 cells overexpressing PLD2 exhibited highly aggressive characteristics including larger tumors, faster growth, and metastasis. Chemical inhibition of PLD2 by FIPI and NOPT in SCID xenotransplanted mice reduced tumor growth and metastasis, supporting the proposal of PLD2 as a target for breast cancer therapy. The molecular mechanism behind PLD-mediated actin polymerization and cell invasion is thought to involve WASp, Grb2, and Rac2.

3.4 PLD in Lung Cancer

An in vitro study in BEAS-2B cells showed that expression of PLD1 increases in response to cigarette smoke, which correlates with increased IL-6 expression, a key event in COPD, cancer, and atherosclerosis. G_i protein, phospholipase C, protein kinase C, and p38MAPK are involved in the PLD1 and IL-6 upregulation (Koo and Han 2016). A noncoding RNA in the INK4 locus is upregulated in response to PLD inhibition in H460 lung cancer cells; upon INK4 silencing, apoptosis was decreased (Kang et al. 2015b), which may explain how elevated PLD expression promotes survival by inhibiting apoptosis and autophagy (i.e., through suppression of the INK4 ncRNA).

3.5 PLD in Other Cancers

Increased PLD1 and PLD2 expression levels were reported in high-grade serous carcinoma in 59 peritoneal and 14 pleural effusions, 28 ovarian tumors, and 24 solid tumor patient samples. The high levels of PLD1 and PLD2 in these patient samples were also confirmed by immunohistochemistry of ovarian tumors and effusions (Harel-Dassa et al. 2017). Increased expression of active PLD2 protein in EL4 lymphoma cells increased cell proliferation, adhesion, and cell invasion and ultimately contributed to lymphoma cell metastasis (Knoepp et al. 2008). Moreover, inhibiting PLD activity by FIPI led to a significant decrease in metastasis and growth of melanoma tumors in mice (Chen et al. 2012). The same study identified by histological examination that PLD inhibition by FIPI decreases microvessels in tumors by 79%.

4 PLD in Inflammation and Immune System Disorders

Aberrant PLD expression and activity is implicated in inflammation (Iyer et al. 2004, 2006; Mancini and Ciervo 2015; Park et al. 2013b; Schonberger et al. 2014). PLD is upregulated during many inflammatory conditions, such as atherosclerosis, infectious diseases, autoimmune disease, and ischemia/reperfusion injury (I/RI). PLD is important for the phagocytic activity of macrophages, which is crucial for innate immune functions as well as for inflammation and resolution (Ali et al. 2013; Gomez-Cambronero 2014b; Iyer et al. 2004, 2006; Gomez-Cambronero et al. 2007). PLD1 and PLD2 act at different stages of the phagocytic process (Corrotte et al. 2006) through the production of PA at the phagocytic cup (Kassas et al. 2012, 2017) and regulation of WASp function (Kantonen et al. 2011). PLD/PA also play a role in leukocyte adhesion (Gobel et al. 2014; Speranza et al. 2014). A potential role of PLD in atherogenesis downstream of oxidized LDL (ox-LDL) has also been proposed (Gomez-Munoz et al. 2000; Natarajan et al. 1995). Recently, our lab demonstrated that PLD2 in cooperation with CD36 interacts with actin, Grb2, and WASP to phagocytose Agg-Ox-LDL, leading to the transformation of macrophages into foam cells, one of the key steps in atherogenesis (Ganesan et al. 2018). Earlier studies from our lab showed increased infiltration of tumor-associated macrophages in secondary tumors, with an increase in PLD levels in these TAMs and tumor-associated neutrophils (TANs) (Henkels et al. 2016).

PLD is also actively involved in pro-inflammatory cytokine recruitment, reactive oxygen species (ROS) generation, endothelial dysfunction, chemotaxis, and cell migration (Koch et al. 2009; Usatyuk et al. 2009, 2013). PLD1 plays a crucial role in pro-inflammatory cytokine IL-1β-mediated activation of synoviocyte and chronic inflammatory arthritis (Park et al. 2013b). Moreover, PLD2$^{-/-}$ mice produce less pro-inflammatory cytokines in a sepsis model (Lee et al. 2015). PLD1 is a major mediator of peritonitis via TNF-α activation (Sethu et al. 2010) and is a peripheral blood marker for pancreatitis (Bluth et al. 2008).

During ischemia, depletion of ATP and high intracellular Ca2+ results in damage of the electron transport chain and elevated mitochondrial reactive oxygen species (ROS) synthesis; once oxygen is restored, cell death and release of harmful ROS into the circulation are further elevated (Murphy and Steenbergen 2008). Studies using PLD knockout (KO) mice or chemical inhibitors have reported that suppressing PLD is "protective" during ischemic stroke (Stegner et al. 2013), hypertension (Olala et al. 2013), thrombosis (Noh et al. 2010; Thielmann et al. 2012), and myocardial infarction (Elvers et al. 2010). Mice having chemical-induced injury in carotid arteries or mesenterial arterioles showed reduced thrombus formation and infarct progression upon treatment with FIPI, a dual PLD inhibitor. The authors showed that the underlying mechanism involves decreased α-granule release and integrin activation in platelets. A study also reported that FIPI-induced PLD inhibition decreased mercury and oxidant-induced cytotoxicity in mouse aortic epithelial cells (Secor et al. 2011).

Finally, PLD2 has been reported to negatively regulate blood pressure through the production of the vasodilator nitrous oxide (NO) via eNOS (Nelson et al. 2017). Mice lacking PLD2 develop hypertension and display long-term effects of it in their vasculature.

5 PLD in Neurological Disorders

5.1 Alzheimer's Disease (AD)

PLD1 is upregulated in mitochondrial fraction of AD brains and interacts with amyloid precursor protein (APP) for its processing (Jin et al. 2006). Overexpressed PLD1 has been shown to interact with presenilin 1, which is a subunit of γ secretase complex (Cai et al. 2006). γ secretase is an intramembrane protease that cleaves APP and notch. Ablation of PLD2 ameliorated cognitive defects in a high amyloid β plaque-expressing AD mouse model (SwAPP transgenic mice) (Oliveira et al. 2010) conferring synaptic protection. Intense accumulation of PLD3 is found in neuritic plaques in Alzheimer's (Satoh et al. 2014). As cited earlier, rare variants in PLD3 have been linked to AD (Cruchaga et al. 2014), but this remains controversial (Cacace et al. 2015).

5.2 Stroke

PLD KO mice are protected from thrombotic brain ischemia (Elvers et al. 2010); PLD inhibition via FIPI provides similar benefits when the mice are dosed prior to the ischemic insult (Stegner et al. 2013). Mechanistically, PLD1 signaling is important for activation of the αIIbβ3 integrin that drives platelet activation and thrombus formation. These findings suggest that a PLD inhibitor could be therapeutically useful in thrombotic events (also aortic thrombosis and pulmonary embolisms) if one with a quick enough onset of activation can be developed. The current inhibitors would be best employed for individuals at high risk of future events or with thrombotic ischemic events in evolution (Frohman 2015).

5.3 Multiple Sclerosis and Related Conditions

Phospholipase D has been thought to be a promising target for several neurological disorders since its discovery in the rat brain in 1973. Increased PLD activity activates macrophages in inflammatory conditions, including in the CNS, thereby contributing to neuroinflammatory conditions such as experimental autoimmune encephalomyelitis (EAE) (Ahn et al. 2001). EAE is a model for studying brain inflammation that best represents a multiple sclerosis-like condition. PLD1 is also upregulated in EAE lesions in rat models (Ahn et al. 2001). PLD1-mediated lymphocyte migration through the blood-brain barrier may underlie PLD1's role in CNS autoimmune conditions; PLD1 KO mice exhibit decreased lymphocyte migration and interaction with ICAM and VCAM and thus decreased adhesion. These results suggest that PLD1 inhibition might be beneficial in multiple sclerosis.

5.4 Parkinson's Disease

There are contrasting views about PLD being involved in Parkinson's disease. One study showed in 2002 that α-synuclein, a protein implicated in Alzheimer's and Parkinson's pathophysiology, interacts with and inhibits PLD in HEK 293 cells (Ahn et al. 2002). But another group found that α-synuclein does not inhibit PLD, using HEK 293, HeLa, and PC12 cells as well as cell-free assays (Rappley et al. 2009). Subsequent reports have suggested that PLD1 regulates clearance of α-synuclein (Bae et al. 2014) and that α-synuclein modulates PLD1 expression (Conde et al. 2018), further highlighting the interconnection between PLD1 and α-synuclein.

5.5 Neurite Growth

Overexpression of PLD1 and PLD2 in mouse brains results in hippocampal mossy fiber outgrowth. Physiologically, PLD1 expression is more prominent in neurons, whereas PLD2 is expressed more strongly in astrocytes (Zhang et al. 2004). Neurite outgrowth is also increased by PDGF-induced PLD activation for hippocampal stem cells (Sung et al. 2001). Inhibition of PLD activity by ethanol in cerebellar granule cells suppresses neurite outgrowth that can be rescued by PLD2 overexpression (Watanabe et al. 2004). PLD1 or PLD2 KO mice exhibit reduced neurite outgrowth and delayed neuronal development (Ammar et al. 2013). PLD1 overexpression is also observed in spinal cord injury rat models, suggesting that PLD1 inhibition might be used in the treatment of spinal cord injury (Jung et al. 2003).

6 PLD in Viral Diseases

Influenza virus infection of alveolar basal epithelial cells (A549) activates PLD, and inhibition of the PLD activation using the PLD2 inhibitor VU0364739 blocked the increase in PLD activity upon influenza virus challenge in A549 cells reduces viral entry (Oguin et al. 2014). Mice challenged with a 4,000 EID_{50} viral load and treated with VU0364739 three times a day for 3 days and showed significantly decreased viral replication and an increased survival rate. ML395, which is more selective toward PLD2, has been shown to have similar antiviral action (O'Reilly et al. 2014).

T cell proliferation after its activation and reprogramming requires large amounts of deoxyribonucleotide triphosphates (dNTPs) (Korin and Zack 1999; Pan et al. 2013). Addition of dNTPs to resting T cells significantly increases human immunodeficiency virus (HIV) integration in the host genome (Plesa et al. 2007). The ability of dNTP treatment of CD4+ to promote HIV replication was significantly reduced upon VU0359595 application, suggesting that PLD activity is required for optimal viral replication (Taylor et al. 2015) and suggesting a possible therapeutic potential in the management of HIV.

7 Future Prospects: Possible Pharmacological Approaches for Inflammation and Cancer Involving PLD as a Target

PLD has an "entourage" of protein partners in signaling (ROCK, SOS, GRB2, WASP, S6K); these partners and its product PA may form a target platform for discovering new "players" in understanding the underlying pathophysiology in many diseases. Based on all of the pre-existing cellular, preclinical, and clinical data, it is important to find out the diseases for which PLD is a key contributor to pathogenesis. For designing and successfully screening small molecule and chemical inhibitors of PLD, a detailed pharmacological evaluation of each molecule is needed. All the chemical compounds known to inhibit PLD in vitro and in vivo should be investigated for their efficacy, safety, pharmacokinetic-pharmacodynamic profile, and toxicological profile before they can be presented as a therapeutic intervention in clinical trials and marketed. For example, in the specific case of PLD and breast cancer, the best hope for treating advanced and metastatic breast cancer is to understand the molecular biology of tumor progression and metastasis and to identify the molecules and/or signaling pathways related to PLD that confer cancer cell aggressiveness, thereby developing effective targeted therapeutic drugs. For example, FIPI, a widely used PLD inhibitor (a derivative of halopemide, originally approved as a drug in psychiatric disorders), has been used in cancer cells in vitro and in in vivo models for breast cancer and pulmonary metastases. It has a great efficacy (100% reduction in enzyme activity at 100 nM) but limited solubility, hampering (for now) its use in clinical trials.

References

Ahn M et al (2001) Increased expression of phospholipase D1 in the spinal cords of rats with experimental autoimmune encephalomyelitis. Neurosci Lett 316(2):95–98

Ahn B-H et al (2002) α-Synuclein interacts with phospholipase D isozymes and inhibits pervanadate-induced phospholipase D activation in human embryonic kidney-293 cells. J Biol Chem 277(14):12334–12342

Ali WH et al (2013) Deficiencies of the lipid-signaling enzymes phospholipase D1 and D2 alter cytoskeletal organization, macrophage phagocytosis, and cytokine-stimulated neutrophil recruitment. PLoS One 8(1):e55325

Ammar MR et al (2013) The Coffin-Lowry syndrome-associated protein RSK2 regulates neurite outgrowth through phosphorylation of phospholipase D1 (PLD1) and synthesis of phosphatidic acid. J Neurosci 33(50):19470–19479

Arakawa T et al (1998) Rebamipide: overview of its mechanisms of action and efficacy in mucosal protection and ulcer healing. Dig Dis Sci 43(9 Suppl):5s–13s

Bae EJ et al (2014) Phospholipase D1 regulates autophagic flux and clearance of alpha-synuclein aggregates. Cell Death Differ 21(7):1132–1141

Bartel DP (2009) MicroRNAs: target recognition and regulatory functions. Cell 136(2):215–233

Basiouni S, Fuhrmann H, Schumann J (2013) The influence of polyunsaturated fatty acids on the phospholipase d isoforms trafficking and activity in mast cells. Int J Mol Sci 14(5):9005–9017

Bluth M et al (2008) Use of gene expression profiles in cells of peripheral blood to identify new molecular markers of acute pancreatitis. Arch Surg 143(3):227–233

Brown HA et al (1993) ADP-ribosylation factor, a small GTP-dependent regulatory protein, stimulates phospholipase D activity. Cell 75(6):1137–1144

Brown HA et al (1995) Partial purification and characterization of Arf-sensitive phospholipase D from porcine brain. J Biol Chem 270(25):14935–14943

Bruntz RC et al (2014) Phospholipase D2 mediates survival signaling through direct regulation of Akt in glioblastoma cells. J Biol Chem 289(2):600–616

Cacace R et al (2015) Rare variants in PLD3 do not affect risk for early-onset Alzheimer disease in a European consortium cohort. Hum Mutat 36(12):1226–1235

Cai D et al (2006) Presenilin-1 uses phospholipase D1 as a negative regulator of beta-amyloid formation. Proc Natl Acad Sci U S A 103(6):1941–1946

Chae YC et al (2008) Phospholipase D activity regulates integrin-mediated cell spreading and migration by inducing GTP-Rac translocation to the plasma membrane. Mol Biol Cell 19(7):3111–3123

Chaves-Moreira D et al (2017) Potential implications for designing drugs against the Brown spider venom phospholipase-D. J Cell Biochem 118(4):726–738

Chen Y, Zheng Y, Foster DA (2003) Phospholipase D confers rapamycin resistance in human breast cancer cells. Oncogene 22(25):3937–3942

Chen Y, Rodrik V, Foster DA (2005) Alternative phospholipase D/mTOR survival signal in human breast cancer cells. Oncogene 24(4):672–679

Chen Q et al (2012) Key roles for the lipid signaling enzyme phospholipase D1 in the tumor microenvironment during tumor angiogenesis and metastasis. Sci Signal 5(249):ra79

Chen Z et al (2014) MicroRNA-203 inhibits the proliferation and invasion of U251 glioblastoma cells by directly targeting PLD2. Mol Med Rep 9(2):503–508

Cho JH et al (2008) Overexpression of phospholipase D suppresses taxotere-induced cell death in stomach cancer cells. Biochim Biophys Acta 1783(5):912–923

Choi SY et al (2006) A common lipid links Mfn-mediated mitochondrial fusion and SNARE-regulated exocytosis. Nat Cell Biol 8(11):1255–1262

Colley WC et al (1997) Phospholipase D2, a distinct phospholipase D isoform with novel regulatory properties that provokes cytoskeletal reorganization. Curr Biol 7(3):191–201

Conde MA et al (2018) Phospholipase D1 downregulation by alpha-synuclein: implications for neurodegeneration in Parkinson's disease. Biochim Biophys Acta Mol Cell Biol Lipids 1863 (6):639–650
Corrotte M et al (2006) Dynamics and function of phospholipase D and phosphatidic acid during phagocytosis. Traffic 7(3):365–377
Cruchaga C et al (2014) Rare coding variants in the phospholipase D3 gene confer risk for Alzheimer's disease. Nature 505(7484):550–554
Di Fulvio M et al (2006) The elucidation of novel SH2 binding sites on PLD2. Oncogene 25 (21):3032–3040
Du G et al (2003) Regulation of phospholipase D1 subcellular cycling through coordination of multiple membrane association motifs. J Cell Biol 162(2):305–315
Du GW et al (2004) Phospholipase D2 localizes to the plasma membrane and regulates angiotensin II receptor endocytosis. Mol Biol Cell 15(3):1024–1030
Elvers M et al (2010) Impaired alpha(IIb)beta(3) integrin activation and shear-dependent thrombus formation in mice lacking phospholipase D1. Sci Signal 3(103):ra1
Fingar DC et al (2004) mTOR controls cell cycle progression through its cell growth effectors S6K1 and 4E-BP1/eukaryotic translation initiation factor 4E. Mol Cell Biol 24(1):200–216
Fite K, Elkhadragy L, Gomez-Cambronero J (2016) A repertoire of MicroRNAs regulates cancer cell starvation by targeting phospholipase D in a feedback loop that operates maximally in cancer cells. Mol Cell Biol 36(7):1078–1089
Foster DA (2007) Regulation of mTOR by phosphatidic acid? Cancer Res 67(1):1–4
Foster DA et al (2014) Phospholipase D and the maintenance of phosphatidic acid levels for regulation of mammalian target of rapamycin (mTOR). J Biol Chem 289(33):22583–22588
Frohman MA (2015) The phospholipase D superfamily as therapeutic targets. Trends Pharmacol Sci 36(3):137–144
Ganesan R et al (2015) Two sites of action for PLD2 inhibitors: the enzyme catalytic center and an allosteric, phosphoinositide biding pocket. Biochim Biophys Acta 1851(3):261–272
Ganesan R et al (2018) Oxidized LDL phagocytosis during foam cell formation in atherosclerotic plaques relies on a PLD2-CD36 functional interdependence. J Leukoc Biol 103(5):867–883
Gao Q, Frohman MA (2012) Roles for the lipid-signaling enzyme MitoPLD in mitochondrial dynamics, piRNA biogenesis, and spermatogenesis. BMB Rep 45(1):7–13
Garcia A et al (2008) Honokiol suppresses survival signals mediated by Ras-dependent phospholipase D activity in human cancer cells. Clin Cancer Res 14(13):4267–4274
Gavin AL et al (2018) PLD3 and PLD4 are single-stranded acid exonucleases that regulate endosomal nucleic-acid sensing. Nat Immunol 19(9):942–953
Gobel K et al (2014) Phospholipase D1 mediates lymphocyte adhesion and migration in experimental autoimmune encephalomyelitis. Eur J Immunol 44(8):2295–2305
Gomez-Cambronero J (2014a) Phosphatidic acid, phospholipase D and tumorigenesis. Adv Biol Regul 54:197–206
Gomez-Cambronero J (2014b) Phospholipase D in cell signaling: from a myriad of cell functions to cancer growth and metastasis. J Biol Chem 289(33):22557–22566
Gomez-Cambronero J, di Fulvio M, Knapek K (2007) Understanding phospholipase D (PLD) using leukocytes: PLD involvement in cell adhesion and chemotaxis. J Leukoc Biol 82(2):272–281
Gomez-Munoz A, Martens JS, Steinbrecher UP (2000) Stimulation of phospholipase D activity by oxidized LDL in mouse peritoneal macrophages. Arterioscler Thromb Vasc Biol 20(1):135–143
Gottlin EB et al (1998) Catalytic mechanism of the phospholipase D superfamily proceeds via a covalent phosphohistidine intermediate. Proc Natl Acad Sci U S A 95(16):9202–9207
Gozgit JM et al (2007) PLD1 is overexpressed in an ER-negative MCF-7 cell line variant and a subset of phospho-Akt-negative breast carcinomas. Br J Cancer 97(6):809–817
Hammond SM et al (1995) Human ADP-ribosylation factor-activated phosphatidylcholine-specific phospholipase D defines a new and highly conserved gene family. J Biol Chem 270 (50):29640–29643

Hammond SM et al (1997) Characterization of two alternately spliced forms of phospholipase D1. Activation of the purified enzymes by phosphatidylinositol 4,5-bisphosphate, ADP-ribosylation factor, and Rho family monomeric GTP-binding proteins and protein kinase C-alpha. J Biol Chem 272:3860–3868. 1997(0021–9258 (Print))

Han X et al (2011) beta-1,3-Glucan-induced host phospholipase D activation is involved in Aspergillus fumigatus internalization into type II human pneumocyte A549 cells. PLoS One 6(7):e21468

Harel-Dassa K et al (2017) Phospholipase D messenger RNA expression and clinical role in high-grade serous carcinoma. Hum Pathol 62:115–121

Henkels KM et al (2013) Phospholipase D (PLD) drives cell invasion, tumor growth and metastasis in a human breast cancer xenograph model. Oncogene 32(49):5551–5562

Henkels KM, Muppani NR, Gomez-Cambronero J (2016) PLD-specific small-molecule inhibitors decrease tumor-associated macrophages and neutrophils infiltration in breast tumors and lung and liver metastases. PLoS One 11(11):e0166553

Hodgkin MN et al (2000a) Phospholipase D regulation and localisation is dependent upon a phosphatidylinositol 4,5-biphosphate-specific PH domain. Curr Biol 10:43–46. (0960–9822 (Print))

Hodgkin MN et al (2000b) Phospholipase D regulation and localisation is dependent upon a phosphatidylinositol 4,5-bisphosphate-specific PH domain. Curr Biol 10(1):43–46

Huang H et al (2011) piRNA-associated germline nuage formation and spermatogenesis require MitoPLD profusogenic mitochondrial-surface lipid signaling. Dev Cell 20(3):376–387

Hui L et al (2004) Phospholipase D elevates the level of MDM2 and suppresses DNA damage-induced increases in p53. Mol Cell Biol 24(13):5677–5686

Hwang WC et al (2014) Inhibition of phospholipase D2 induces autophagy in colorectal cancer cells. Exp Mol Med 46(12):e124–e124

Iyer SS et al (2004) Phospholipases D1 and D2 coordinately regulate macrophage phagocytosis. J Immunol 173(4):2615–2623

Iyer SS et al (2006) Phospholipase D1 regulates phagocyte adhesion. J Immunol 176(6):3686–3696

Jiang Y et al (2016) Phosphatidic acid produced by RalA-activated PLD2 stimulates caveolae-mediated endocytosis and trafficking in endothelial cells. J Biol Chem 291(39):20729–20738

Jin J-K et al (2006) Phospholipase D1 is up-regulated in the mitochondrial fraction from the brains of Alzheimer's disease patients. Neurosci Lett 407(3):263–267

Jung K et al (2003) Upregulation of phospholipase D1 in the spinal cords of rats with clip compression injury. Neurosci Lett 336(2):126–130

Jung S et al (2014) A nonsense mutation in PLD4 is associated with a zinc deficiency-like syndrome in Fleckvieh cattle. BMC Genomics 15:623

Kang DW, Min DS (2010) Positive feedback regulation between phospholipase D and Wnt signaling promotes Wnt-driven anchorage-independent growth of colorectal cancer cells. PLoS One 5(8):e12109

Kang DW et al (2009) Triptolide-induced suppression of phospholipase D expression inhibits proliferation of MDA-MB-231 breast cancer cells. Exp Mol Med 41(9):678

Kang DW et al (2011) Autoregulation of phospholipase D activity is coupled to selective induction of phospholipase D1 expression to promote invasion of breast cancer cells. Int J Cancer 128 (4):805–816

Kang DW et al (2015a) Targeting phospholipase D1 attenuates intestinal tumorigenesis by controlling β-catenin signaling in cancer-initiating cells. J Exp Med 212(8):1219–1237

Kang YH, Kim D, Jin EJ (2015b) Down-regulation of phospholipase D stimulates death of lung cancer cells involving up-regulation of the long ncRNA ANRIL. Anticancer Res 35 (5):2795–2803

Kang DW et al (2017) Phospholipase D1 acts through Akt/TopBP1 and RB1 to regulate the E2F1-dependent apoptotic program in cancer cells. Cancer Res 77(1):142–152

Kantonen S et al (2011) A novel phospholipase D2-Grb2-WASp heterotrimer regulates leukocyte phagocytosis in a two-step mechanism. Mol Cell Biol 31(22):4524–4537

Kassas N et al (2012) Genetically encoded probes for phosphatidic acid. Methods Cell Biol 108:445–459

Kassas N et al (2017) Comparative characterization of phosphatidic acid sensors and their localization during frustrated phagocytosis. J Biol Chem 292(10):4266–4279

Katayama K et al (1998) Cloning, differential regulation and tissue distribution of alternatively spliced isoforms of ADP-ribosylation-factor-dependent phospholipase D from rat liver. Biochem J 329:647–652

Knoepp SM et al (2008) Effects of active and inactive phospholipase D2 on signal transduction, adhesion, migration, invasion, and metastasis in EL4 lymphoma cells. Mol Pharmacol 74 (3):574–584

Koch T et al (2009) Mu-opioid receptor-stimulated synthesis of reactive oxygen species is mediated via phospholipase D2. J Neurochem 110(4):1288–1296

Koo JB, Han J-S (2016) Cigarette smoke extract-induced interleukin-6 expression is regulated by phospholipase D1 in human bronchial epithelial cells. J Toxicol Sci 41(1):77–89

Korin YD, Zack JA (1999) Nonproductive human immunodeficiency virus type 1 infection in nucleoside-treated G0 lymphocytes. J Virol 73(8):6526–6532

Lavieri R et al (2009) Design and synthesis of isoform-selective phospholipase D (PLD) inhibitors. Part II. Identification of the 1,3,8-triazaspiro[4,5]decan-4-one privileged structure that engenders PLD2 selectivity. Bioorg Med Chem Lett 19(8):2240–2243

Lavieri RR et al (2010) Design, synthesis, and biological evaluation of halogenated N-(2-(4-oxo-1-phenyl-1, 3, 8-triazaspiro [4.5] decan-8-yl) ethyl) benzamides: discovery of an isoform-selective small molecule phospholipase D2 inhibitor. J Med Chem 53(18):6706–6719

Lee JS et al (2005) Phosphatidylinositol (3,4,5)-trisphosphate specifically interacts with the phox homology domain of phospholipase D1 and stimulates its activity. J Cell Sci 118 (19):4405–4413

Lee CS et al (2006) The phox homology domain of phospholipase D activates dynamin GTPase activity and accelerates EGFR endocytosis. Nat Cell Biol 8(5):477–484

Lee SK et al (2015) Phospholipase D2 drives mortality in sepsis by inhibiting neutrophil extracellular trap formation and down-regulating CXCR2. J Exp Med 212(9):1381–1390

Leiros I, McSweeney S, Hough E (2004) The reaction mechanism of phospholipase D from Streptomyces sp strain PMF. Snapshots along the reaction pathway reveal a pentacoordinate reaction intermediate and an unexpected final product. J Mol Biol 339(4):805–820

Lerchner A et al (2006) Probing conserved amino acids in phospholipase D (*Brassica oleracea var. capitata*) for their importance in hydrolysis and transphosphatidylation activity. Protein Eng Des Sel 19(10):443–452

Levin WJ et al (1995) Expression patterns of immediate early transcription factors in human non-small cell lung cancer. The Lung Cancer Study Group. Oncogene 11(7):1261–1269

Lewis JA et al (2009) Design and synthesis of isoform-selective phospholipase D (PLD) inhibitors. Part I: impact of alternative halogenated privileged structures for PLD1 specificity. Bioorg Med Chem Lett 19(7):1916–1920

Li G, Lin F, Xue HW (2007) Genome-wide analysis of the phospholipase D family in Oryza sativa and functional characterization of PLD beta 1 in seed germination. Cell Res 17(10):881–894

Mancini F, Ciervo A (2015) Enzymatic characterization of Chlamydophila pneumoniae phospholipase D. New Microbiol 38(1):59–66

Monovich L et al (2007) Optimization of halopemide for phospholipase D2 inhibition. Bioorg Med Chem Lett 17(8):2310–2311

Motes CM et al (2005) Differential effects of two phospholipase D inhibitors, 1-butanol and N-acylethanolamine, on in vivo cytoskeletal organization and Arabidopsis seedling growth. Protoplasma 226(3–4):109–123

Murphy E, Steenbergen C (2008) Mechanisms underlying acute protection from cardiac ischemia-reperfusion injury. Physiol Rev 88(2):581–609

Natarajan V et al (1995) Oxidized low density lipoprotein-mediated activation of phospholipase D in smooth muscle cells: a possible role in cell proliferation and atherogenesis. J Lipid Res 36(9):2005–2016
Nelson RK et al (2017) Phospholipase D2 loss results in increased blood pressure via inhibition of the endothelial nitric oxide synthase pathway. Sci Rep 7(1):9112
Nishikimi A et al (2009) Sequential regulation of DOCK2 dynamics by two phospholipids during neutrophil chemotaxis. Science 324(5925):384–387
Noh JY et al (2010) Procoagulant and prothrombotic activation of human erythrocytes by phosphatidic acid. Am J Phys Heart Circ Phys 299(2):H347–H355
Nureki O (2014) Is zucchini a phosphodiesterase or a ribonuclease? Biom J 37(6):369–374
O'Reilly MC et al (2013) Development of dual PLD1/2 and PLD2 selective inhibitors from a common 1,3,8-Triazaspiro[4.5]decane core: discovery of ML298 and ML299 that decrease invasive migration in U87-MG glioblastoma cells. J Med Chem 56(6):2695–2699
Oguin TH et al (2014) Phospholipase D facilitates efficient entry of influenza virus, allowing escape from innate immune inhibition. J Biol Chem 289(37):25405–25417
Olala LO et al (2013) A role for phospholipase D in angiotensin II-induced protein kinase D activation in adrenal glomerulosa cell models. Mol Cell Endocrinol 366(1):31–37
Oliveira TG et al (2010) Phospholipase D2 ablation ameliorates Alzheimer's disease-linked synaptic dysfunction and cognitive deficits. J Neurosci 30(49):16419–16428
O'Reilly MC et al (2014) Discovery of a highly selective PLD2 inhibitor (ML395): a new probe with improved physiochemical properties and broad-Spectrum antiviral activity against influenza strains. ChemMedChem 9(12):2633–2637
Orth JD, McNiven MA (2006) Get off my back! Rapid receptor internalization through circular dorsal ruffles. Cancer Res 66(23):11094–11096
Oshimoto H et al (2003) Increased activity and expression of phospholipase D2 in human colorectal cancer. Oncol Res 14(1):31–37
Osisami M, Ali W, Frohman MA (2012) A role for phospholipase D3 in myotube formation. PLoS One 7(3):e33341
Otani Y et al (2011) PLD4 is involved in phagocytosis of microglia: expression and localization changes of PLD4 are correlated with activation state of microglia. PLoS One 6(11):e27544
Pan X et al (2013) Restrictions to HIV-1 replication in resting CD4+ T lymphocytes. Cell Res 23(7):876–885
Park MH, do Min S (2011) Quercetin-induced downregulation of phospholipase D1 inhibits proliferation and invasion in U87 glioma cells. Biochem Biophys Res Commun 412(4):710–715
Park SH et al (1998a) Assignment of human PLD1 to human chromosome band 3q26 by fluorescence in situ hybridization. Cytogenet Cell Genet 82(3–4):224–224
Park SH et al (1998b) Assignment of human PLD2 to chromosome band 17p13.1 by fluorescence in situ hybridization. Cytogenet Cell Genet 82(3–4):225
Park MH et al (2013a) Caffeic acid phenethyl ester downregulates phospholipase D1 via direct binding and inhibition of NFκB transactivation. Biochem Biophys Res Commun 442(1–2):1–7
Park DW et al (2013b) TLR2 stimulates ABCA1 expression via PKC-eta and PLD2 pathway. Biochem Biophys Res Commun 430(3):933–937
Plesa G et al (2007) Addition of deoxynucleosides enhances human immunodeficiency virus type 1 integration and 2LTR formation in resting CD4+ T cells. J Virol 81(24):13938–13942
Ponting CP, Kerr ID (1996) A novel family of phospholipase D homologues that includes phospholipid synthases and putative endonucleases: identification of duplicated repeats and potential active site residues. Protein Sci 5(5):914–922
Puar MS et al (2000) Sch 420789. A novel fungal metabolite with phospholipase D inhibitory activity. J Antibiot 53(8):837–838
Qiu D, Kao PN (2003) Immunosuppressive and anti-inflammatory mechanisms of triptolide, the principal active diterpenoid from the Chinese medicinal herb Tripterygium wilfordii Hook. F. Drugs R D 4(1):1–18

Rappley I et al (2009) Evidence that α-synuclein does not inhibit phospholipase D. Biochemistry 48(5):1077–1083

Redina OE, Frohman MA (1998a) Genomic analysis of murine phospholipase D1 and comparison to phospholipase D2 reveals an unusual difference in gene size. Gene 222(1):53–60

Redina OE, Frohman MA (1998b) Organization and alternative splicing of the murine phospholipase D2 gene. Biochem J 331(Pt 3):845–851

Saito M et al (2007) Expression of phospholipase D2 in human colorectal carcinoma. Oncol Rep 18:1329–1334

Sanematsu F et al (2013) Phosphatidic acid-dependent recruitment and function of the Rac activator DOCK1 during dorsal ruffle formation. J Biol Chem 288(12):8092–8100

Saqcena M et al (2013) Amino acids and mTOR mediate distinct metabolic checkpoints in mammalian G1 cell cycle. PLoS One 8(8):e74157

Saqib KM, Wakelam MJ (1997) Differential expression of human phospholipase D genes. Biochem Soc Trans 25(4):S586

Satoh J-i et al (2014) PLD3 is accumulated on neuritic plaques in Alzheimer's disease brains. Alzheimer's Res Ther 6(5–8):70

Schonberger T et al (2014) Pivotal role of phospholipase D1 in tumor necrosis factor-alpha-mediated inflammation and scar formation after myocardial ischemia and reperfusion in mice. Am J Pathol 184(9):2450–2464

Sciorra VA et al (1999) Identification of a phosphoinositide binding motif that mediates activation of mammalian and yeast phospholipase D isoenzymes. EMBO J 18(21):5911–5921

Sciorra VA, Hammond SM, Morris AJ (2001) Potent direct inhibition of mammalian phospholipase D isoenzymes by calphostin-c. Biochemistry 40(8):2640–2646

Sciorra VA et al (2002) Dual role for phosphoinositides in regulation of yeast and mammalian phospholipase D enzymes. J Cell Biol 159(6):1039–1049

Scott SA et al (2009) Design of isoform-selective phospholipase D inhibitors that modulate cancer cell invasiveness. Nat Chem Biol 5(2):108–117

Secor JD et al (2011) Novel lipid-soluble thiol-redox antioxidant and heavy metal chelator, N,N-bis (2-mercaptoethyl)isophthalamide (NBMI) and phospholipase D-specific inhibitor, 5-fluoro-2-indolyl des-chlorohalopemide (FIPI) attenuate mercury-induced lipid signaling leading to protection against cytotoxicity in aortic endothelial cells. Int J Toxicol 30(6):619–638

Selvy PE et al (2011) Phospholipase D: enzymology, functionality, and chemical modulation. Chem Rev 111(10):6064–6119

Sethu S, Pushparaj PN, Melendez AJ (2010) Phospholipase D1 mediates TNFalpha-induced inflammation in a murine model of TNFalpha-induced peritonitis. PLoS One 5(5):e10506

Shi M et al (2007) Phospholipase D provides a survival signal in human cancer cells with activated H-Ras or K-Ras. Cancer Lett 258(2):268–275

Sorkin A et al (2000) Interaction of EGF receptor and grb2 in living cells visualized by fluorescence resonance energy transfer (FRET) microscopy. Curr Biol 10(21):1395–1398

Speranza F et al (2014) The molecular basis of leukocyte adhesion involving phosphatidic acid and phospholipase D. J Biol Chem 289(42):28885–28897

Stahelin RV et al (2004) Mechanism of membrane binding of the phospholipase D1 PX domain. J Biol Chem 279(52):54918–54926

Steed PM et al (1998) Characterization of human PLD2 and the analysis of PLD isoform splice variants. FASEB J 12(13):1309–1317

Stegner D et al (2013) Pharmacological inhibition of phospholipase D protects mice from occlusive Thrombus formation and ischemic stroke-brief report. Arterioscler Thromb Vasc Biol 33 (9):2212–2217

Su W et al (2009) 5-Fluoro-2-indolyl des-chlorohalopemide (FIPI), a phospholipase D pharmacological inhibitor that alters cell spreading and inhibits chemotaxis. Mol Pharmacol 75 (3):437–446

Sugars JM et al (1999) Fatty acylation of phospholipase D1 on cysteine residues 240 and 241 determines localization on intracellular membranes. J Biol Chem 274(42):30023–30027

Sulzmaier FJ et al (2012) PEA-15 potentiates H-Ras-mediated epithelial cell transformation through phospholipase D. Oncogene 31(30):3547–3560

Sung TC et al (1997) Mutagenesis of phospholipase D defines a superfamily including a trans-Golgi viral protein required for poxvirus pathogenicity. EMBO J 16(15):4519–4530

Sung TC et al (1999) Structural analysis of human phospholipase D1. J Biol Chem 274 (6):3659–3666

Sung JY et al (2001) Differential activation of phospholipases by mitogenic EGF and neurogenic PDGF in immortalized hippocampal stem cell lines: activation of phospholipase C and D during neuronal differentiation. J Neurochem 78(5):1044–1053

Taylor HE et al (2015) Phospholipase D1 couples CD4+ T cell activation to c-Myc-dependent deoxyribonucleotide Pool expansion and HIV-1 replication. PLoS Pathog 11(5):e1004864

Terao C et al (2013) PLD4 as a novel susceptibility gene for systemic sclerosis in a Japanese population. Arthritis Rheum 65(2):472–480

Thielmann I et al (2012) Redundant functions of phospholipases D1 and D2 in platelet alpha-granule release. J Thromb Haemost 10(11):2361–2372

Tou J-S, Urbizo C (2001) Resveratrol inhibits the formation of phosphatidic acid and diglyceride in chemotactic peptide- or phorbol ester-stimulated human neutrophils. Cell Signal 13(3):191–197

Uchida N et al (1997) Increased phospholipase D activity in human breast cancer. J Cancer Res Clin Oncol 123(5):280–285

Uchida N, Okamura S, Kuwano H (1999) Phospholipase D activity in human gastric carcinoma. Anticancer Res 19(1B):671–675

Usatyuk PV et al (2009) Phospholipase D-mediated activation of IQGAP1 through Rac1 regulates hyperoxia-induced p47phox translocation and reactive oxygen species generation in lung endothelial cells. J Biol Chem 284(22):15339–15352

Usatyuk PV et al (2013) Phospholipase D signaling mediates reactive oxygen species-induced lung endothelial barrier dysfunction. Pulm Circ 3(1):108–115

Watanabe H et al (2004) Phospholipase D2 functions as a downstream signaling molecule of MAP kinase pathway in L1-stimulated neurite outgrowth of cerebellar granule neurons. J Neurochem 89(1):142–151

Xie Z, Ho WT, Exton JH (2001) Requirements and effects of palmitoylation of rat PLD1. J Biol Chem 276(12):9383–9391

Xu LM et al (2011) Phospholipase D mediates nutrient input to mammalian target of rapamycin complex 1 (mTORC1). J Biol Chem 286(29):25477–25486

Yamada Y et al (2003) Association of a polymorphism of the phospholipase D2 gene with the prevalence of colorectal cancer. J Mol Med 81(2):126–131

Yoon MS et al (2011) Class III PI-3-kinase activates phospholipase D in an amino acid-sensing mTORC1 pathway. J Cell Biol 195(3):435–447

Yoshikawa F et al (2010) Phospholipase D family member 4, a transmembrane glycoprotein with no phospholipase D activity, expression in spleen and early postnatal microglia. PLoS One 5(11):e13932

Zeniou-Meyer M et al (2008) The Coffin-Lowry syndrome-associated protein RSK2 is implicated in calcium-regulated exocytosis through the regulation of PLD1. Proc Natl Acad Sci U S A 105(24):8434–8439

Zhang Y et al (2004) Increased expression of two phospholipase D isoforms during experimentally induced hippocampal mossy fiber outgrowth. Glia 46(1):74–83

Zhao C et al (2007) Phospholipase D2-generated phosphatidic acid couples EGFR stimulation to Ras activation by Sos. Nat Cell Biol 9(6):707

Zheng Y et al (2006) Phospholipase D couples survival and migration signals in stress response of human cancer cells. J Biol Chem 281(23):15862–15868

Role of Phospholipase D-Derived Phosphatidic Acid in Regulated Exocytosis and Neurological Disease

Emeline Tanguy, Qili Wang, and Nicolas Vitale

Contents

Abstract

Lipids play a vital role in numerous cellular functions starting from a structural role as major constituents of membranes to acting as signaling intracellular or extracellular entities. Accordingly, it has been known for decades that lipids, especially those coming from diet, are important to maintain normal physiological functions and good health. On the other side, the exact molecular nature of these beneficial or deleterious lipids, as well as their precise mode of action, is only starting to be unraveled. This recent improvement in our knowledge is largely resulting from novel pharmacological, molecular, cellular, and genetic tools to study lipids in vitro and in vivo. Among these important lipids, phosphatidic acid plays a unique and central role in a great variety of cellular functions. This review will focus on the proposed functions of phosphatidic acid

E. Tanguy · Q. Wang
Institut des Neurosciences Cellulaires et Intégratives, CNRS UPR 3212 and Université de Strasbourg, Strasbourg, France

N. Vitale (✉)
Institut des Neurosciences Cellulaires et Intégratives, CNRS UPR 3212 and Université de Strasbourg, Strasbourg, France

INSERM, Paris, Cedex 13, France
e-mail: vitalen@inci-cnrs.unistra.fr

J. Gomez-Cambronero, M. A. Frohman (eds.), *Lipid Signaling in Human Diseases*, Handbook of Experimental Pharmacology 259, https://doi.org/10.1007/164_2018_180

generated by phospholipase D in the last steps of regulated exocytosis with a specific emphasis on hormonal and neurotransmitter release and its potential impact on different neurological diseases.

Keywords
Exocytosis · Lipid · Neuroendocrine · Neuron · Phosphatidic acid · Phospholipase D

1 Introduction

Complex organisms have evolved through their capacity to maintain global homeostasis. This is usually achieved by numerous cellular processes, of which some require cells to get information from distant cells/organs. Hence, a specific mechanism called regulated exocytosis allows cells to tightly control the release of informative molecules in the extracellular space before they are transported to the target cells/organs. Over the last three decades, considerable insight in this process has been gained through the study of neurotransmitter and hormonal release from neurons and neuroendocrine cells, respectively. As such, the chromaffin cell model, largely described in this review, has been very valuable to delineate the different steps of exocytosis (Bader et al. 2002). The regulated secretory pathway begins in the Golgi apparatus with the formation of specific vesicular structures called synaptic vesicles or dense-core secretory granules that are progressively filled with neurotransmitters, hormones, or neuropeptides to be secreted. After their biogenesis, these secretory vesicles are matured during their transport toward specific regions at the cell periphery, where their journey ends by the fusion with the plasma membrane and vesicular content release into the extracellular space, generally following a rise in cytosolic calcium (Burgess and Kelly 1987). This final stage of the secretory process, known as regulated exocytosis, implies successive docking and the priming of mature granules before merging of vesicular and plasma membranes to enable partial or total release of the secretory vesicle content.

It has been proposed that depending on physiological demand, at least three distinct modes of release co-exist: (1) the so-called "kiss-and-run" mode, when small molecules such as hormones and neurotransmitters are released through a narrow fusion pore, while larger molecules such as neuropeptides are retained in the vesicle; (2) vesicle cavity capture (cavicapture), in which dilation of the fusion pore permits partial release of large molecules but the omega shape of the fusing granule is maintained before closure; and (3) full collapse, wherein the vesicles flatten out in the plane of the plasma membrane, losing their round shape and completely emptying their contents (Taraska et al. 2003; Fulop and Smith 2006; van Kempen et al. 2011). It must be noted that the physiological importance of these different modes of secretion remains to be established and the molecular mechanisms that control the transition between these different modes identified.

Most studies on calcium-regulated exocytosis have focused on the minimal molecular machinery, which involves the formation of a tripartite soluble *N*-ethylmaleimide-sensitive factor attachment protein receptor (SNARE) complex between vesicular and plasma membrane proteins (Jahn and Fasshauer 2012). However, since exocytosis ends by the fusion of two membrane compartments, it is likely that lipids also play a leading role (Tanguy et al. 2016). In the following sections, we review observations detailing the functional roles performed during exocytosis by the simplest glycerophospholipid naturally existing in all-living organisms, phosphatidic acid (PA), and consequently its potential implication in neurological disease. Indeed, although it constitutes only a minor fraction of the total cell lipids, PA has attracted considerable attention for being both a lipid second messenger and a modulator of membrane shape.

2 The Different Sources of Phosphatidic Acid

The pleiotropic functions of PA are the direct consequence of its very simple chemical structure, consisting of two acyl chains linked by ester bonds to glycerol, whose remaining hydroxyl group is esterified with a phosphomonoester group. Hence, the small phosphate headgroup of PA provides a cone-shaped structure generating flexibility and negative curvatures in the context of a lipid bilayer. In addition, the negatively charged phosphomonoester headgroup of PA can carry one or two negative charges, depending on pH and surrounding lipids, and thus can assist in the recruitment of positively charged molecules to membrane surfaces.

There are four major routes of cellular PA production in mammals. Structural PA is synthesized through two acylation reactions: the glycerol 3-phosphate (G-3-P) pathway and the dihydroxyacetone phosphate (DHAP) pathway leading to lysoPA (LPA), a mono-acylated form of PA (Fig. 1a). LPA is subsequently transformed in a second acylation step into PA (Vance and Vance 2004) (Fig. 1a). PA generated from these de novo pathways is a key intermediate in the synthesis of all triacylglycerols and glycerophospholipids, as it is rapidly converted by phosphatidic acid phosphohydrolase (PAP) to diacylglycerol (DAG), which represents a major source for the biosynthesis of these lipids (Vance and Goldfine 2002) (Fig. 1a). Furthermore, PA can be degraded by CDP-DAG synthetase into CDP-diacylglycerol, which is directly used as substrate for the synthesis of phosphatidylinositol (PI), phosphatidylglycerol (PG), and cardiolipin (CL) (Fig. 1a). Finally, the many isoforms of phospholipase A (PLA) can deacylate PA into LPA (Fig. 1a). Three alternative biosynthetic pathways use distinct lipid precursors to produce what is called "signaling" PA. The first pathway involves the phosphorylation of DAG using ATP as a phosphate source by DAG kinase (DGK) to produce PA (Fig. 1a). Ten isoforms of mammalian DGK (α, β, γ, δ, η, k, ε, ζ, ι, and θ) have been cloned, characterized, and classified in five subtypes sharing a conserved catalytic domain and at least two cysteine-rich domains (Topham 2006). The second pathway involves acylation of LPA by specific lysoPA acyltransferases (LPAAT) to generate PA (Jenkins and Frohman 2005) (Fig. 1a). Six human LPAAT isoforms have been cloned and

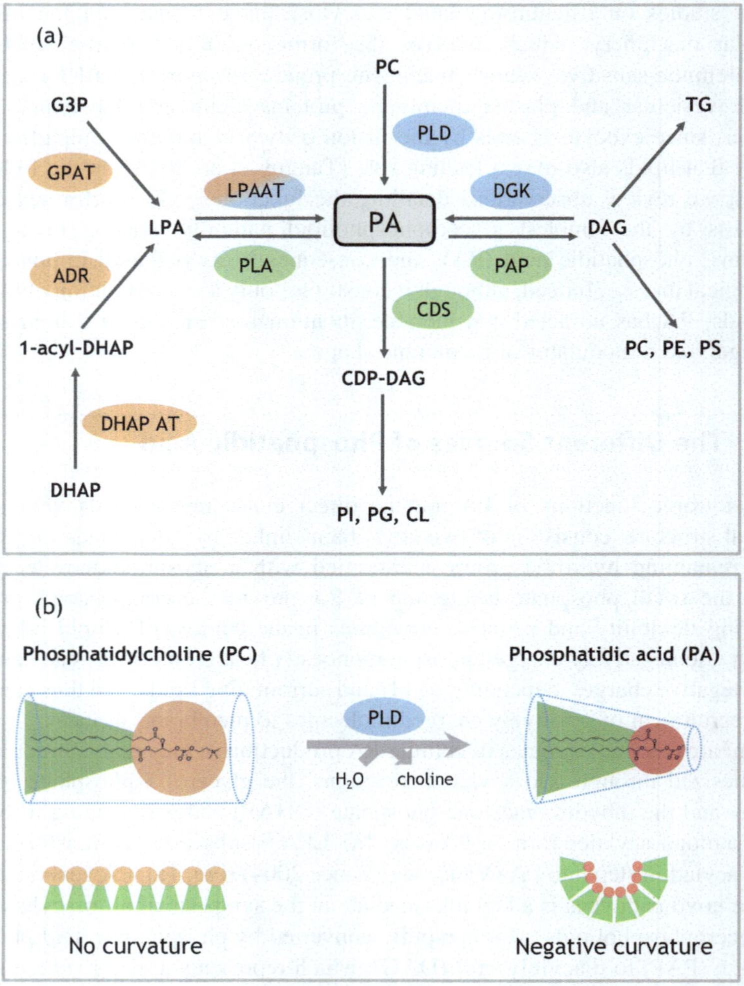

Fig. 1 PA synthesis modifies membrane topology. (**a**) Biosynthetic pathways of structural and signaling PA. PA is a central phospholipid for biosynthetic and signaling reactions. Enzymes in orange denote biosynthetic reactions that lead to structural PA synthesis, whereas enzymes involved in formation of signaling pools of PA are shown in blue. Enzymes involved in PA catabolism are shown in green. (**b**) Phosphatidylcholine hydrolysis by PLD and modification in lipid geometry. The cylindrical PC is transformed into conical PA by enzymatic PLD activity. The accumulation of cone-shaped PA creates regions of negative membrane curvature. Of note, PA exists in a single or a double negative charge mode depending on the local pH environment

characterized (Leung 2001), but more proteins displaying LPAAT activities have been recently identified. For instance, the protein RIBEYE in synaptic ribbon possesses LPAAT activity, providing PA for ultra-fast synaptic release (Schwarz et al. 2011). The third pathway involves phospholipase D (PLD), which catalyzes the hydrolysis of the distal phosphodiester bond in phosphatidylcholine (PC) to form PA and choline (Fig. 1a). Six isoforms of PLDs have been identified based on sequence homology, but PLD1 and PLD2 are the major isoforms characterized, while thus far no direct PLD activity per se has been demonstrated for PLD3-5 (Frohman 2015). The complexity and diversity of PLD, DGK, and LPAAT families suggest that they are involved in various specific cellular functions and are probably not redundant. In general, signaling PA generated from these enzymes is implicated in multiple cell functions such as cytoskeleton organization, cell survival and proliferation, and membrane and vesicle trafficking (Nelson and Frohman 2015). Intriguingly PC to PA conversion by PLD transforms a cylindrical phospholipid into a conical one (Fig. 1b). Furthermore PA has been shown to produce negative membrane curvature through X-ray diffraction studies (Kooijman et al. 2005). Since biophysical models have proposed that intermediates of the membrane fusion reaction require such cone- or inverted cone-shaped lipid, a direct role of PA as a fusogenic lipid has been proposed (Vitale 2010).

3 A Fusogenic Role of PLD-Generated Phosphatidic Acid in Membrane Fusion

The first elements in favor of a role for PA in regulated exocytosis came from experiments showing a correlation between PLD activation and secretory activity in HL60 cells (Xie et al. 1991; Stutchfield and Cockcroft 1993). Furthermore 1-Butanol, an inhibitor of PA accumulation through the PLD pathway, also strongly affects exocytosis in a number of different cell types (Xie et al. 1991; Stutchfield and Cockcroft 1993; Caumont et al. 1998; Choi et al. 2002). Later, molecular tools established that PLD1 is a key isoform responsible for PA synthesis during catecholamine and insulin secretion (Vitale et al. 2001; Hughes et al. 2004; Huang et al. 2005; Waselle et al. 2005). Accordingly, capacitance recordings from chromaffin cells injected with a dominant-negative form of PLD1 or expressing PLD1 siRNA indicated that PLD1 controls the number of fusion-competent secretory granules docked at the plasma membrane as well as the kinetics of individual fusion events (Vitale et al. 2001; Zeniou-Meyer et al. 2007). Using similar tools, PLD1-generated PA was also reported to contribute actively to the regulated secretion of von Willebrand factor from endothelial cells (Disse et al. 2009). Phagocytosis is another important physiological process that depends on exocytosis of intracellular vesicles. Indeed macrophages engulf and degrade pathogens after generation of extensive plasma membrane protrusions, coming in part from different intracellular membrane compartments. This highly regulated process requires PLD2 activity at the plasma membrane for PA synthesis at the phagocytotic cup, as well as PLD1 activation required for the fusion of intracellular PLD1-positive vesicles with the plasma membrane (Corrotte et al. 2006). Another documented role for PA in secretion relates to the induction of neutrophil exocytosis of azurophilic granules by anti-neutrophil cytoplasmic antibodies (Williams et al. 2007). In apicomplexan parasites, such as *Toxoplasma gondii* and *Plasmodium* spp., specialized organelles termed micronemes release their contents including adhesins, perforins, and proteases in a PA-dependent manner, critically contributing to invasion and egress from infected cells (Bullen et al. 2016). Sperm acrosome exocytosis also appears to be regulated by PA (Lopez et al. 2012). It must be noted, however, that in the latter case, it is rather DGK-produced PA that is important than PLD-synthesized PA. Nevertheless these results strongly support the notion that PLD-generated PA plays an important role in the last stages of exocytosis but that other sources can also provide PA for efficient secretion.

Many observations support the notion that lipids, in addition to localizing essential components of the exocytotic machinery, also directly contribute to the fusion reaction. The most widely accepted model for membrane fusion involves a combination of protein and lipid elements at the fusion site. It entails the merging of cis-contacting monolayers, leading to the formation of a specific negatively curved lipid structure called the stalk (Chernomordik and Kozlov 2008). The stalk in this case results from the merging of the inner leaflet of the plasma membrane with the outer leaflet of the vesicle prior to fusion pore formation. Cone-shaped lipids, such as PA, have been proposed to facilitate fusion through their intrinsic negative curvatures when accumulated in the inner (cis) leaflets of the contacting bilayers (Fig. 1b). Indeed the property of PA to generate non-bilayer hexagonal II phase membrane domains, particularly in the presence of calcium ions, is well documented (Jouhet 2013). This is important for exocytosis where vesicles have a large positive curvature and the formation of non-bilayer phases may help to lower the energy needed for fusion (Kozlovsky et al. 2002).

In addition to changing membrane topology, PA is unique among anionic lipids because of its small and highly charged headgroup very close to the glycerol backbone. PA tends to form microdomains through intermolecular hydrogen bonding (Boggs 1987; Demel et al. 1992). A partial reduction in charge (e.g., upon divalent cation interaction) reduces electrostatic repulsion between the PA headgroups and increases attractive hydrogen-bonding interactions, possibly resulting in fluid-fluid immiscibility and the formation of PA-enriched microdomains (Garidel et al. 1997). These highly charged microdomains may induce conformational changes in associated proteins (Iversen et al. 2015) and serve as membrane insertion sites for numerous proteins important for exocytosis that tend to accumulate at regions of membrane curvature (Jung et al. 2010; Martens 2010). More directly, PA has been proposed to contribute to many biological processes through its ability to interact with the positively charged domains of numerous proteins (Jenkins and Frohman 2005). PA can also directly serve as source for other lipids, such as DAG, that play positive function in exocytosis. Finally PA stimulates PI kinase to produce PtdIns(4,5)P_2, another key lipid needed for exocytosis (Jones et al. 2000). In fact, it is likely that PA is a critical lipid in any given physiological event through a combination of these functions (Fig. 2).

The biophysical properties of PA also imply that it should rapidly disperse within planar membranes. One possible explanation for the accumulation of PA at the exocytotic site is the occurrence of a PA-binding site that prevents PA diffusion. Such binding of PA to a protein with a highly basic motif has been reported for the

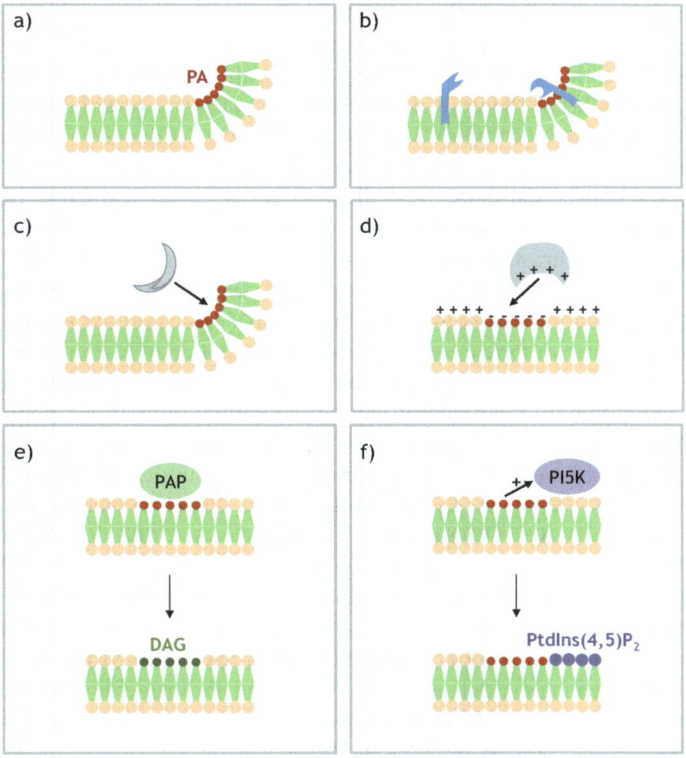

Fig. 2 Model of how PA drives signaling events. (**a**) Local accumulation of PA generates negative membrane curvature or (**b**) membrane-dependent enzymatic activity such as for interfacial activation of lipases. (**c**) Specific curvature-sensing proteins are recruited to PA-induced membrane curved domains. (**d**) Clusters of PA create local negatively charged regions that recruit PA effectors containing positively charged domains. (**e**) PA-phosphatases (PAP) convert PA into DAG, another signaling lipid. (**f**) PA potentiates the activity of PI4P5-kinase, producing PtdIns $(4,5)P_2$, another key signaling lipid

plasma membrane-associated SNARE protein syntaxin-1 (Lam et al. 2008) and for NSF (Jang et al. 2013). A mutation in the polybasic juxtamembrane region of syntaxin-1, which prevents binding to acidic phospholipids such as PA, strongly affects the exocytotic response of chromaffin and PC12 cells, suggesting that PA-binding may be required for the function of syntaxin-1 (Lam et al. 2008). Furthermore, the X-ray structure of this polybasic region of syntaxin-1 confirms that it is important for SNARE complex assembly and that a lipid such as PA may stabilize its orientation (Stein et al. 2009). This idea is further underscored by the observation that cone-shaped lipids that promote negative membrane curvature purify with active zone SNARE proteins (Lewis et al. 2014). Finally the strongest evidence for a direct role of PA in membrane fusion derives from in vitro reconstituted assays that revealed that PA present in a t-SNARE-containing membrane promoted fusion with a v-SNARE-containing membrane (Vicogne et al. 2006) and studies involving a liposomal flotation assay for fusion with purified yeast vacuolar SNARE chaperones Sec17p/Sec18p and the multifunctional HOPS complex with the Sec1-Munc18 family. In the latter assay, PA was one of the lipids shown to be critical for SNARE complex assembly and fusion (Mima and Wickner 2009).

Intracellular PA levels are tightly controlled, i.e., PA is maintained at very low levels under resting conditions. Visualization of the local formation of PA has necessitated the design of a novel PA-specific sensor derived from the yeast homologue of SNAP25. Ultrastructural analysis revealed PA accumulation near docking sites at the plasma membrane during exocytosis in chromaffin cells (Zeniou-Meyer et al. 2007). Supporting the notion that the intrinsic curvature of PA in the inner leaflet of the plasma membrane contributes to the regulation of fusion pore formation and/or expansion, extracellular application of the inverted cone-shaped lipid lysophosphatidylcholine (LPC) partially rescued secretion from PLD1-depleted cells (Zeniou-Meyer et al. 2007). Interestingly, low levels of PA before exocytosis are probably maintained, since the major source of PA during exocytosis is low-level basal activity PLD1 (Vitale et al. 2001; Hughes et al. 2004). In fact, a complex node of GTPases including Arf6 (Vitale et al. 2002; Béglé et al. 2009), Ral A (Vitale et al. 2005), and Rac1 (Momboisse et al. 2009) and their own regulators (Audebert et al. 2004; Meyer et al. 2006), but also the kinase RSK2, involved in X-linked mental retardation (Zeniou-Meyer et al. 2008), and PtdIns(4,5)P_2 itself (Du et al. 2003), appear altogether to control PLD1 activation for efficient exocytosis in chromaffin cells. Similarly regulators such as Arf6, RalA, and PtdIns(4,5)P_2 have also been identified in the activation of PLD as required for insulin secretion (Grodnitzky et al. 2007; Ljubicic et al. 2009; Waselle et al. 2005).

In conclusion the local buildup of fusogenic lipids such as PA together with other key lipids such as PtdIns(4,5)P_2, DAG, and cholesterol presumably at the neck or near the fusion pore may synergize by changing membrane curvature, together with SNARE-mediated membrane apposition and destabilization, to promote fusion pore formation and/or regulate its stability. The recent development of isoform-specific inhibitors will most likely prove to be useful to define more precisely steps controlled by PLD-generated PA. In addition, the precise localization of these different fusogenic lipids during the short-lived fusion pore formation, expansion, and closure is still unknown and needs important improvement in high-resolution imaging techniques and lipid probes to be adequately addressed. It must be also noted that the contribution of PA in early steps of the secretory pathway have not been as well investigated (Gasman and Vitale 2017). For instance, recent findings suggest that PLD-generated PA mostly affects docking and priming in sea urchin egg fusion (Rogasevskaia and Coorssen 2015) and as well is involved in early steps of sperm acrosomal exocytosis (Lopez et al. 2012).

4 A Role for PLD-Generated PA in Neurological Diseases?

Numerous lipids have been shown to be involved in pre- and post-synaptic functions and neurological diseases (Lauwers et al. 2016). PLD1 largely localizes to neurons in the central nervous system but is also present in oligodendrocytes, while PLD2 is largely found in astrocytes (Kim et al. 2010; Rohrbough and Broadie 2005; Zhang et al. 2004). However, the expression of PLD isoforms in the brain has been relatively controversial in regard to the cell type, isoform expression, and pattern of expression throughout development (Klein 2005). In fact, only a few recent papers have reported the time course of PLD1 expression in maturing neuronal cell cultures, with optimal expression at DIV5-6, then decreasing by more than 50% (Zhu et al. 2012) or 80% (Ammar et al. 2015). It is likely that the relative uncertainty of the PLD isoform expression pattern relies from the limited quality of the anti-PLD antibodies available and from the different types of neuronal culture used in these studies. To date, the strongest evidence that PLD1 may be involved in neurotransmission comes from experiments where injection of catalytically inactive PLD1 protein into presynaptic cholinergic neurons in the buccal ganglion of *Aplysia californica* led to a fast and dose-dependent inhibition of acetylcholine release, suggesting that a rapid exchange of inactive dominant-negative PLD1 for wild-type PLD1 causes a dramatic decrease in the amount of exocytosis (Humeau et al. 2001). These results support the notion that PLD1 generates PA-rich microdomains that recruit or activate proteins required for synaptic vesicle fusion with the plasma membrane (Humeau et al. 2009). These PA-rich domains might also physically bend the membrane to promote mixing of the lipids in the plasma and vesicle membranes during fusion as described previously. Since null mutations in RSK2, a kinase that regulates PLD1 activity, are responsible for the symptoms of the Coffin Lowry Syndrome disease, it has been proposed that alteration of PLD1 activation could explain the intellectual disabilities of patients through at least partially inhibiting neurotransmitter exocytosis (Zeniou-Meyer et al. 2008, 2010). Conversely, PLD2 has been implicated in the modulation of glutamate transporter function (Mateos et al. 2012) and the internalization of mGluR (Bhattacharya et al. 2004), both of which could potentially affect synaptic activity. Alteration of the DAG-PA balance could also be responsible for some of the cellular and behavioral symptoms observed in a mouse model of fragile X disease (Tabet et al. 2016a, b).

In the presence of low amounts of ethanol, PLD produces phosphatidylethanol at the expense of PA. So although ethanol does not inhibit PLD activity per se, it has long been used as disruptor of signaling pathways that involve PLD activation (Frohman 2015). As indicated above, PA is a lipid second messenger in its own right, with several downstream targets that relate to cell proliferation. Ethanol, on the other hand, has long been known to suppress proliferation of brain cells, especially astrocytes in vitro and in vivo. Astrocytes are more sensitive than neurons to ethanol, at least concerning proliferation. Thus, the inhibition of astroglial proliferation by ethanol has been suggested to be responsible for some features of fetal alcohol syndrome. Children born from heavy-drinking pregnant women have characteristic facial features and reduced brain and body weights, with microcephaly indicating a delay in growth and maturation of the brain (Guerri and Renau-Piqueras 1997; Guizzetti et al. 1997). As numerous studies have validated the activation of PLD in the brain by mitogenic and growth factors, it is likely that PLD1/2-generated PA plays an important role in normal brain development and that alteration of these PLD activities is responsible for some of the brain developmental pathologies.

In addition to its effect on cell proliferation, PLD is also likely to play a role in neuronal development by promoting extension of neurites. PLD activity has been implicated in neurite outgrowth in various neuronal models for over two decades, but most of the original findings relied on the use of ethanol as a non-specific inhibitor of PA synthesis, and in most cases the PLD isoform involved was not identified (Klein 2005). Using a combination of knockout mice, a gene-silencing approach, and the recently described isoform-specific PLD inhibitors, it has more recently been demonstrated that PLD1 contributes to neurite outgrowth, dendrite branching, and spine development (Ammar et al. 2013). It is also worth mentioning that the GTPase RalB promotes neuronal branching through a pathway involving PLD (Lalli and Hall 2005). Conversely, however, using different methods to modulate protein levels and neuronal type, PLD1 has been described to negatively regulate dendritic branching in hippocampal neurons (Zhu et al. 2012). Interestingly, PLD1 was recently shown to participate in the BDNF signaling pathway in cortical neurons, supporting the notion of neuronal development regulation by PLD (Ammar et al. 2015).

The data discussed above implicate the PLD pathway in brain development, but PLD-generated PA has also been shown to be involved in neurodegeneration. Indeed, increased PLD activity has been found in Alzheimer brains postmortem (Kanfer et al. 1996), and other studies have noted that β-amyloid increases PLD expression and activity (Klein 2005). Moreover, synucleins, which are present in amyloid plaques in Alzheimer's disease and in Parkinson's disease, interact with and inhibit PLD (Jenco et al. 1998; Ahn et al. 2002; Payton et al. 2004). However, mass spectrometry analysis of Huntington's disease mouse brains reveals modification of the levels of few PA species (Vodicka et al. 2015). Of note, it was recently suggested that α-synuclein may cross-bridge vesicular SNARE and acidic phospholipids such as PA to facilitate SNARE-dependent vesicle docking, suggesting a possible link between these diseases and alteration of vesicular trafficking regulated by PLD (Lou et al. 2017). Furthermore both oxidative and antioxidative compounds have been reported to modulate PLD activity in neuronal and glial cells (Oh et al. 2000; Servitja et al. 2000; Kim et al. 2004a, b). Interestingly, PLD1 appears to regulate the intracellular trafficking of preselinin 1/γ-secretase (Liu et al. 2009), while the memory deficit in a transgenic model of Alzheimer disease was rescued when the PLD2 gene was ablated (Oliveira et al. 2010). In line with this finding, lipidomic analysis revealed that levels of several PA species were modified in this mouse model and in Alzheimer's disease brain patients (Oliveira et al. 2010). PLD activities were also investigated in acute neurodegeneration induced by brain ischemia. In vitro, acute hypoxia did not change PLD activity in hippocampal slices (Klein et al. 1993), but global ischemia in vivo diminished PLD activity in rat brain (Nishida et al. 1994). A massive increase in PLD1 expression was observed in reactive astrocytes from the hippocampus at 7 to 10 days after forebrain ischemia in vivo (Lee et al. 2000). Increased PLD expression apparently accompanies astrogliosis, repair, and remodeling of tissue after ischemia, and astrogliosis during inflammation could underlie increased PLD1 expression in scrapie-infected mouse brain (Jin et al. 2005) and in sciatic neurons during experimental autoimmune neuritis (Shin et al. 2002). Prenatal stress induces brain abnormalities of the offspring, with disruption of dendritic profiles, spine distribution, and adult neurogenesis, all of which can lead to pain hypersensitivity that is dependent on PLD1 signaling (Sun et al. 2013). Finally, compression injury of rat spinal cord (Jung et al. 2010), cryoinjury in rat cortex (Kim et al. 2004a), and kainate-induced seizures in rat hippocampus (Kim et al. 2004c) lead to increased PLD activity in astrocytes. Taken together, these pioneer studies contributed to the notion that PLD expression and activity accompany normal brain development and remodeling and that alterations of PLD-generated PA levels correlate and/or are directly responsible for different human neurological diseases. It is evident that understanding the exact role of PA in these pathologies remains the next challenge.

5 Conclusion

The last two decades have seen generation of substantial evidence that PA synthesized by different enzymatic pathways contributes to normal and pathological conditions. Among these strong indications is a direct contribution of PLD-generated PA in the last steps of regulated exocytosis, a key process that allows cells to release informative molecules such as hormones, neurotransmitters, and neuropeptides. Despite our increased understanding, the exact molecular steps affected and targets of PA action are still elusive. In addition, recent lipidomic analyses have revealed that, based on their fatty acid composition, three to four dozen distinct species of PA co-exist in most cells (Andreyev et al. 2010; Kassas et al. 2017; Oliveira et al. 2010). The function of each of these PA species, however, remains completely unknown. Therefore, the development of novel tools to further decipher the role of each PA species in regulated exocytosis, neurological diseases, and many other key cellular functions is now required. This is especially important as membrane-lipid therapies are expected to become new efficient treatments for many human pathologies (Escribá 2017).

References

Ahn BH, Rhim H, Kim SY, Sung YM, Lee MY, Choi JY, Wolozin B, Chang JS, Lee YH, Kwon TK, Chung KC, Yoon SH, Hahn SJ, Kim MS, Jo YH, Min DS (2002) alpha-Synuclein interacts with phospholipase D isozymes and inhibits pervanadate-induced phospholipase D activation in human embryonic kidney-293 cells. J Biol Chem 277(14):12334–12342

Ammar MR, Humeau Y, Hanauer A, Nieswandt B, Bader MF, Vitale N (2013) The Coffin-Lowry syndrome-associated protein RSK2 regulates neurite outgrowth through phosphorylation of phospholipase D1 (PLD1) and synthesis of phosphatidic acid. J Neurosci 33(50):19470–19479

Ammar MR, Thahouly T, Hanauer A, Stegner D, Nieswandt B, Vitale N (2015) PLD1 participates in BDNF-induced signalling in cortical neurons. Sci Rep 5:14778

Andreyev AY, Fahy E, Guan Z, Kelly S, Li X, McDonald JG, Milne S, Myers D, Park H, Ryan A, Thompson BM, Wang E, Zhao Y, Brown HA, Merrill AH, Raetz CR, Russell DW, Subramaniam S, Dennis EA (2010) Subcellular organelle lipidomics in TLR-4-activated macrophages. J Lipid Res 51(9):2785–2797

Audebert S, Navarro C, Nourry C, Chasserot-Golaz S, Lécine P, Bellaiche Y, Dupont JL, Premont RT, Sempéré C, Strub JM, Van Dorsselaer A, Vitale N, Borg JP (2004) Mammalian Scribble forms a tight complex with the betaPIX exchange factor. Curr Biol 14(11):987–995

Bader MF, Holz RW, Kumakura K, Vitale N (2002) Exocytosis: the chromaffin cell as a model system. Ann N Y Acad Sci 971:178–183

Béglé A, Tryoen-Tóth P, de Barry J, Bader MF, Vitale N (2009) ARF6 regulates the synthesis of fusogenic lipids for calcium-regulated exocytosis in neuroendocrine cells. J Biol Chem 284 (8):4836–4845

Bhattacharya M, Babwah AV, Godin C, Anborgh PH, Dale LB, Poulter MO, Ferguson SS (2004) Ral and phospholipase D2-dependent pathway for constitutive metabotropic glutamate receptor endocytosis. J Neurosci 24(40):8752–8761

Boggs JM (1987) Lipid intermolecular hydrogen bonding: influence on structural organization and membrane function. Biochim Biophys Acta 906(3):353–404

Bullen HE, Jia Y, Yamaryo-Botté Y, Bisio H, Zhang O, Jemelin NK, Marq JB, Carruthers V, Botté CY, Soldati-Favre D (2016) Phosphatidic acid-mediated signaling regulates microneme secretion in toxoplasma. Cell Host Microbe 19(3):349–360

Burgess TL, Kelly RB (1987) Constitutive and regulated secretion of proteins. Annu Rev Cell Biol 3:243–293

Caumont AS, Galas MC, Vitale N, Aunis D, Bader MF (1998) Regulated exocytosis in chromaffin cells. Translocation of ARF6 stimulates a plasma membrane-associated phospholipase D. J Biol Chem 273(3):1373–1379

Chernomordik LV, Kozlov MM (2008) Mechanics of membrane fusion. Nat Struct Mol Biol 15(7):675–683

Choi WS, Kim YM, Combs C, Frohman MA, Beaven MA (2002) Phospholipases D1and D2 regulate different phases of exocytosis in mast cells. J Immunol 168(11):5682–5689

Corrotte M, Chasserot-Golaz S, Huang P, Du G, Ktistakis NT, Frohman MA, Vitale N, Bader MF, Grant NJ (2006) Dynamics and function of phospholipase D and phosphatidic acid during phagocytosis. Traffic 7(3):365–377

Demel RA, Yin CC, Lin BZ, Hauser H (1992) Monolayer characteristics and thermal behaviour of phosphatidic acids. Chem Phys Lipids 60:209–223

Disse J, Vitale N, Bader MF, Gerke V (2009) Phospholipase D1 is specifically required for regulated secretion of von Willebrand factor from endothelial cells. Blood 113:973–980

Du G, Altshuller YM, Vitale N, Huang P, Chasserot-Golaz S, Morris AJ, Bader MF, Frohman MA (2003) Regulation of phospholipase D1 subcellular cycling through coordination of multiple membrane association motifs. J Cell Biol 162(2):305–315

Escribá PV (2017) Membrane-lipid therapy: a historical perspective of membrane-targeted therapies – from lipid bilayer structure to the pathophysiological regulation of cells. Biochim Biophys Acta 1859(9 PtB):1493–1506

Frohman MA (2015) The phospholipase D superfamily as therapeutic targets. Trends Pharmacol Sci 36(3):137–144

Fulop T, Smith C (2006) Physiological stimulation regulates the exocytic mode through calcium activation of protein kinase C in mouse chromaffin cells. Biochem J 399(1):111–119

Garidel P, Johann C, Blume A (1997) Nonideal mixing and phase separation in phosphatidylcholine-phosphatidic acid mixtures as a function of acyl chain length and pH. Biophys J 72(5):2196–2210

Gasman S, Vitale N (2017) Lipid remodelling in neuroendocrine secretion. Biol Cell 109 (11):381–390

Grodnitzky JA, Syed N, Kimber MJ, Day TA, Donaldson JG, Hsu WH (2007) Somatostatin receptors signal through EFA6A-ARF6 to activate phospholipase D in clonal beta-cells. J Biol Chem 282(18):13410–13418

Guerri C, Renau-Piqueras J (1997) Alcohol, astroglia, and brain development. Mol Neurobiol 15 (1):65–81

Guizzetti M, Catlin M, Costa LG (1997) The effects of ethanol on glial cell proliferation: relevanceto the fetal alcohol syndrome. Front Biosci 2:e93–e98

Huang P, Altshuller YM, Hou JC, Pessin JE, Frohman MA (2005) Insulin-stimulated plasma membrane fusion of Glut4 glucose transporter-containing vesicles is regulated by phospholipase D1. Mol Biol Cell 16(6):2614–2623

Hughes WE, Elgundi Z, Huang P, Frohman MA, Biden TJ (2004) Phospholipase D1 regulates secretagogue-stimulated insulin release in pancreatic p-cells. J Biol Chem 279:27534–27541

Humeau Y, Vitale N, Chasserot-Golaz S, Dupont JL, Du G, Frohman MA, Bader MF, Poulain B (2001) A role for phospholipase D1 in neurotransmitter release. Proc Natl Acad Sci U S A 98 (26):15300–15305

Humeau Y, Gambino F, Chelly J, Vitale N (2009) X-linked mental retardation: focus on synaptic function and plasticity. J Neurochem 109(1):1–14

Iversen L, Mathiasen S, Larsen JB, Stamou D (2015) Membrane curvature bends the laws of physicsand chemistry. Nat Chem Biol 11(11):822–825

Jahn R, Fasshauer D (2012) Molecular machines governing exocytosis of synaptic vesicles. Nature 490(7419):201–207

Jang HJ, Yang YR, Kim JK, Choi JH, Seo YK, Lee YH, Lee JE, Ryu SH, Suh PG (2013) Phospholipase C-γ1 involved in brain disorders. Adv Biol Regul 53(1):51–62

Jenco JM, Rawlingson A, Daniels B, Morris AJ (1998) Regulation of phospholipase D2: selective inhibition of mammalian phospholipase D isoenzymes by alpha- and beta-synucleins. Biochemistry 37(14):4901–4909

Jenkins GM, Frohman MA (2005) Phospholipase D: a lipid centric review. Cell Mol Life Sci 62 (19–20):2305–2316

Jin JK, Kim NH, Min DS, Kim JI, Choi JK, Jeong BH, Choi SI, Choi EK, Carp RI, Kim YS (2005) Increased expression of phospholipase D1 in the brains of scrapie-infected mice. J Neurochem 92(3):452–461

Jones DH, Morris JB, Morgan CP, Kondo H, Irvine RF, Cockcroft S (2000) Type I phosphatidylinositol 4-phosphate 5-kinase directly interacts with ADP-ribosylation factor 1 and is responsible for phosphatidylinositol 4,5-bisphosphate synthesis in the golgi compartment. J Biol Chem 275(18):13962–13966

Jouhet J (2013) Importance of the hexagonal lipid phase in biological membrane organization. Front Plant Sci 4:494

Jung AG, Labarrera C, Jansen AM, Qvortrup K, Wild K, Kjaerulff O (2010) A mutational analysis of the endophilin-A N-BAR domain performed in living flies. PLoS One 5:e9492

Kanfer JN, Singh IN, Pettegrew JW, McCartney DG, Sorrentino G (1996) Phospholipid metabolism in Alzheimer's disease and in a human cholinergic cell. J Lipid Mediat Cell Signal 14 (1–3):361–363

Kassas N, Tanguy E, Thahouly T, Fouillen L, Heintz D, Chasserot-Golaz S, Bader MF, Grant NJ, Vitale N (2017) Comparative characterization of phosphatidic acid sensors and their localization during frustrated phagocytosis. J Biol Chem 292(10):4266–4279

Kim J, Min G, Bae YS, Min DS (2004a) Phospholipase D is involved in oxidative stress-induced migration of vascular smooth muscle cells via tyrosine phosphorylation and protein kinase C. Exp Mol Med 36(2):103–109

Kim SY, Ahn BH, Min KJ, Lee YH, Joe EH, Min DS (2004b) Phospholipase D isozymes mediate epigallocatechin gallate-induced cyclooxygenase-2 expression in astrocyte cells. J Biol Chem 279(37):38125–38133

Kim SY, Min DS, Choi JS, Choi YS, Park HJ, Sung KW, Kim J, Lee MY (2004c) Differential expression of phospholipase D isozymes in the hippocampus following kainic acid-induced seizures. J Neuropathol Exp Neurol 63:812–820

Kim M, Moon C, Kim H, Shin MK, Min do S, Shin T (2010) Developmental levels of phospholipase D isozymes in the brain of developing rats. Acta Histochem 112(1):81–91

Klein J (2005) Functions and pathophysiological roles of phospholipase D in the brain. J Neurochem 94(6):1473–1487

Klein J, Holler T, Cappel E, Köppen A, Löffelholz K (1993) Release of choline from rat brain under hypoxia: contribution from phospholipase A2 but not from phospholipase D. Brain Res 630 (1–2):337–340

Kooijman EE, Chupin V, Fuller NL, Kozlov MM, de Kruijff B, Burger KN, Rand PR (2005) Spontaneous curvature of phosphatidic acid and lysophosphatidic acid. Biochemistry 44 (6):2097–2102

Kozlovsky Y, Chernomordik LV, Kozlov MM (2002) Lipid intermediates in membrane fusion: formation, structure, and decay of hemifusion diaphragm. Biophys J 83(5):2634–2651

Lalli G, Hall A (2005) Ral GTPases regulate neurite branching through GAP-43 and the exocyst complex. J Cell Biol 171(5):857–869

Lam IP, Siu FK, Chu JY, Chow BK (2008) Multiple actions of secretin in the human body. Int Rev Cytol 265:159–190

Lauwers E, Goodchild R, Verstreken P (2016) Membrane lipids in presynaptic function and disease. Neuron 90(1):11–25

Lee MY, Kim SY, Min DS, Choi YS, Shin SL, Chun MH, Lee SB, Kim MS, Jo YH (2000) Upregulation of phospholipase D in astrocytes in response to transient forebrain ischemia. Glia 30(3):311–317

Leung DW (2001) The structure and functions of human lysophosphatidic acid acyltransferases. Front Biosci 6(1):D944–D953

Lewis KT, Maddipati KR, Taatjes DJ, Jena BP (2014) Neuronal porosome lipidome. J Cell MolMed 18(10):1927–1937

Liu Y, Zhang YW, Wang X, Zhang H, You X, Liao FF, Xu H (2009) Intracellular trafficking of presenilin 1 is regulated by beta-amyloid precursor protein and phospholipase D1. J Biol Chem 284(18):12145–12152

Ljubicic S, Bezzi P, Vitale N, Regazzi R (2009) The GTPase RalA regulates different steps of the secretory process in pancreatic beta-cells. PLoS One 4(11):e7770

Lopez JA, Brennan AJ, Whisstock JC, Voskoboinik I, Trapani JA (2012) Protecting a serial killer: pathways for perforin trafficking and self-defence ensure sequential target cell death. Trends Immunol 33(8):406–412

Lou X, Kim J, Hawk BJ, Shin YK (2017) α-Synuclein may cross-bridge v-SNARE and acidic phospholipids to facilitate SNARE-dependent vesicle docking. Biochem J 474(12):2039–2049

Martens S (2010) Role of C2 domain proteins during synaptic vesicle exocytosis. Biochem Soc Trans 38:213–216

Mateos MV, Giusto NM, Salvador GA (2012) Distinctive roles of PLD signaling elicited by oxidative stress in synaptic endings from adult and aged rats. Biochim Biophys Acta 1823 (12):2136–2148

Meyer MZ, Déliot N, Chasserot-Golaz S, Premont RT, Bader MF, Vitale N (2006) Regulation of neuroendocrine exocytosis by the ARF6 GTPase-activating protein GIT1. J Biol Chem 281 (12):7919–7926

Mima J, Wickner W (2009) Phosphoinositides and SNARE chaperones synergistically assemble and remodel SNARE complexes for membrane fusion. Proc Natl Acad Sci U S A 106 (38):16191–16196

Momboisse F, Lonchamp E, Calco V, Ceridono M, Vitale N, Bader MF, Gasman S (2009) betaPIX-activated Rac1 stimulates the activation of phospholipase D, which is associated with exocytosis in neuroendocrine cells. J Cell Sci 122(Pt 6):798–806

Nelson RK, Frohman MA (2015) Physiological and pathophysiological roles for phospholipase D. J Lipid Res 56(12):2229–2237

Nishida A, Emoto K, Shimizu M, Uozumi T, Yamawaki S (1994) Brain ischemia decreases phosphatidylcholine-phospholipase D but not phosphatidylinositol-phospholipase C in rats. Stroke 25(6):1247–1251

Oh SO, Hong JH, Kim YR, Yoo HS, Lee SH, Lim K, Hwang BD, Exton JH, Park SK (2000) Regulation of phospholipase D2 by H(2)O(2) in PC12 cells. J Neurochem 75(6):2445–2454
Oliveira TG, Chan RB, Tian H, Laredo M, Shui G, Staniszewski A, Zhang H, Wang L, Kim TW, Duff KE, Wenk MR, Arancio O, Di Paolo G (2010) Phospholipase d2 ablation ameliorates Alzheimer's disease-linked synaptic dysfunction and cognitive deficits. J Neurosci 30 (49):16419–16428
Payton JE, Perrin RJ, Woods WS, George JM (2004) Structural determinants of PLD2 inhibition by alpha-synuclein. J Mol Biol 337(4):1001–1009
Rogasevskaia TP, Coorssen JR (2015) The role of phospholipase D in regulated exocytosis. J Biol Chem 290(48):28683–28696
Rohrbough J, Broadie K (2005) Lipid regulation of the synaptic vesicle cycle. Nat Rev Neurosci 6 (2):139–150
Schwarz K, Natarajan S, Kassas N, Vitale N, Schmitz F (2011) The synaptic ribbon is a site of phosphatidic acid generation in ribbon synapses. J Neurosci 31(44):15996–16011
Servitja JM, Masgrau R, Pardo R, Sarri E, Picatoste F (2000) Effects of oxidative stress on phospholipid signaling in rat cultured astrocytes and brain slices. J Neurochem 75(2):788–794
Shin EY, Ma EK, Kim CK, Kwak SJ, Kim EG (2002) Src/ERK but not phospholipase D is involved in keratinocyte growth factor-stimulated secretion of matrix metalloprotease-9 and urokinase-type plasminogen activator in SNU-16 human stomach cancer cell. J Cancer Res Clin Oncol 128 (11):596–602
Stein A, Weber G, Wahl MC, Jahn R (2009) Helical extension of the neuronal SNARE complex into the membrane. Nature 460:525–528
Stutchfield J, Cockcroft S (1993) Correlation between secretion and phospholipase D activation in differentiated HL60 cells. Biochem J 293(Pt3):649–655
Sun H, Xia M, Shahane SA, Jadhav A, Austin CP, Huang R (2013) Are hERG channel blockers also phospholipidosis inducers? Bioorg Med Chem Lett 23(16):4587–4590
Tabet R, Moutin E, Becker JA, Heintz D, Fouillen L, Flatter E, Krężel W, Alunni V, Koebel P, Dembélé D, Tassone F, Bardoni B, Mandel JL, Vitale N, Muller D, Le Merrer J, Moine H (2016a) Fragile X Mental Retardation Protein (FMRP) controls diacylglycerol kinase activity in neurons. Proc Natl Acad Sci U S A 113:E3619–E3628
Tabet R, Vitale N, Moine H (2016b) Fragile X syndrome: are signaling lipids the missing culprits? Biochimie 130:188–194
Tanguy E, Carmon O, Wang Q, Jeandel L, Chasserot-Golaz S, Montero-Hadjadje M, Vitale N (2016) Lipids implicated in the journey of a secretory granule: from biogenesis to fusion. J Neurochem 137(6):904–912
Taraska JW, Perrais D, Ohara-Imaizumi M, Nagamatsu S, Almers W (2003) Secretory granules are recaptured largely intact after stimulated exocytosis in cultured endocrine cells. Proc Natl Acad Sci U S A 100(4):2070–2075. Epub 21 Jan 2003
Topham MK (2006) Signaling roles of diacylglycerol kinases. J Cell Biochem 97(3):474–484 Review
van Kempen GT, vanderLeest HT, van den Berg RJ, Eilers P, Westerink RH (2011) Three distinct modes of exocytosis revealed by amperometry in neuroendocrine cells. Biophys J 100 (4):968–977
Vance DE, Goldfine H (2002) Konrad Bloch – a pioneer in cholesterol and fatty acid biosynthesis. Biochem Biophys Res Commun 292(5):1117–1127
Vance JE, Vance DE (2004) Phospholipid biosynthesis in mammalian cells. Biochem Cell Biol 82 (1):113–128
Vicogne J, VollenweiderD SJR, Huang P, Frohman MA, Pessin JE (2006) Asymmetric phospholipid distribution drives in vitro reconstituted SNARE-dependent membrane fusion. Proc Natl Acad Sci U S A 103:14761–14766
Vitale N (2010) Synthesis of fusogenic lipids through activation of phospholipase D1 by GTPases and the kinase RSK2 is required for calcium-regulated exocytosis in neuroendocrine cells. Biochem Soc Trans 38(Pt 1):167–171

Vitale N, Caumont AS, Chasserot-Golaz S, Du G, Wu S, Sciorra VA, Morris AJ, Frohman MA, Bader MF (2001) Phospholipase D1: a key factor for the exocytotic machinery in neuroendocrine cells. EMBO J 20(10):2424–2434

Vitale N, Chasserot-Golaz S, Bader MF (2002) Regulated secretion in chromaffin cells: an essential role for ARF6-regulated phospholipase D in the late stages of exocytosis. Ann N Y Acad Sci 971:193–200

Vitale N, Mawet J, Camonis J, Regazzi R, Bader MF, Chasserot-Golaz S (2005) The small GTPase RalA controls exocytosis of large dense core secretory granules by interacting with ARF6-dependent phospholipase D1. J Biol Chem 280(33):29921–29928

Vodicka P, Mo S, Tousley A, Green KM, Sapp E, Iuliano M, Sadri-Vakili G, Shaffer SA, Aronin N, DiFiglia M, Kegel-Gleason KB (2015) Mass spectrometry analysis of wild-type and knock-in Q140/Q140 Huntington's disease mouse brains reveals changes in glycerophospholipids including alterations in phosphatidic acid and lyso-phosphatidic acid. J Huntingtons Dis 4(2):187–201

Waselle L, Gerona RR, Vitale N, Martin TF, Bader MF, Regazzi R (2005) Role of phosphoinositide signaling in the control of insulin exocytosis. Mol Endocrinol 19(12):3097–3106. Epub 4 Aug 2005

Williams JM, Pettitt TR, Powell W, Grove J, Savage CO, Wakelam MJ et al (2007) Antineutrophil cytoplasm antibody-stimulated neutrophil adhesion depends on diacylglycerol kinase-catalyzed phosphatidic acid formation. J Am Soc Nephrol 18(4):1112–1120

Xie MS, Jacobs LS, Dubyak GR (1991) Activation of phospholipase D and primary granule secretion by P2-purinergic- and chemotactic peptide-receptor agaonists is induced during granulocyte differenciation of HL-60 cells. J Clin Invest 88:45–54

Zeniou-Meyer M, Zabari N, Ashery U, Chasserot-Golaz S, Haeberlé AM, Demais V, Bailly Y, Gottfried I, Nakanishi H, Neiman AM, Du G, Frohman MA, Bader MF, Vitale N (2007) Phospholipase D1 production of phosphatidic acid at the plasma membrane promotes exocytosis of large dense-core granules at a late stage. J Biol Chem 282(30):21746–21757

Zeniou-Meyer M, Liu Y, Béglé A, Olanich ME, Hanauer A, Becherer U, Rettig J, Bader MF, Vitale N (2008) The Coffin-Lowry syndrome-associated protein RSK2 is implicated in calcium-regulated exocytosis through the regulation of PLD1. Proc Natl Acad Sci U S A 105 (24):8434–8439

Zeniou-Meyer M, Gambino F, Ammar MR, Humeau Y, Vitale N (2010) The Coffin-Lowry syndrome-associated protein RSK2 and neurosecretion. Cell Mol Neurobiol 30(8):1401–1406

Zhang Y, Huang P, Du G, Kanaho Y, Frohman MA, Tsirka SE (2004) Increased expression of two phospholipase D isoforms during experimentally induced hippocampal mossy fiber outgrowth. Glia 46(1):74–83

Zhu YB, Kang K, Zhang Y, Qi C, Li G, Yin DM, Wang Y (2012) PLD1 negatively regulates dendritic branching. J Neurosci 32(23):7960–7969

Part III

Lipid Kinases and Novel Regulatory Pathways

Diacylglycerol Kinase Malfunction in Human Disease and the Search for Specific Inhibitors

Isabel Merida, Javier Arranz-Nicolás, Pedro Torres-Ayuso, and Antonia Ávila-Flores

Contents

Abstract

The diacylglycerol kinases (DGKs) are master regulator kinases that control the switch from diacylglycerol (DAG) to phosphatidic acid (PA), two lipids with important structural and signaling properties. Mammalian DGKs distribute into five subfamilies that regulate local availability of DAG and PA pools in a tissue- and subcellular-restricted manner. Pharmacological manipulation of DGK activity holds great promise, given the critical contribution of specific DGK subtypes to the control of membrane structure, signaling complexes, and cell-cell communication. The latest advances in the DGK field have unveiled the differential

I. Merida (✉) · J. Arranz-Nicolás · A. Ávila-Flores
Department of Immunology and Oncology, National Center of Biotechnology (CNB-CSIC), Madrid, Spain
e-mail: imerida@cnb.csic.es

P. Torres-Ayuso
Laboratory of Cell and Developmental Signaling, National Cancer Institute (NCI-NIH), Frederick, MD, USA

J. Gomez-Cambronero, M. A. Frohman (eds.), *Lipid Signaling in Human Diseases*, Handbook of Experimental Pharmacology 259, https://doi.org/10.1007/164_2019_221

contribution of selected isoforms to human disease. Defects in the expression/activity of individual DGK isoforms contribute substantially to cognitive impairment, mental disorders, insulin resistance, and vascular pathologies. Abnormal DGK overexpression, on the other hand, confers the acquisition of malignant traits including invasion, chemotherapy resistance, and inhibition of immune attack on tumors. Translation of these findings into therapeutic approaches will require development of methods to pharmacologically modulate DGK functions. In particular, inhibitors that target the DGKα isoform hold particular promise in the fight against cancer, on their own or in combination with immune-targeting therapies.

Keywords

Cancer immunotherapy · Cognitive impairment · Diabetes · Protein kinase C · RasGRP · Src

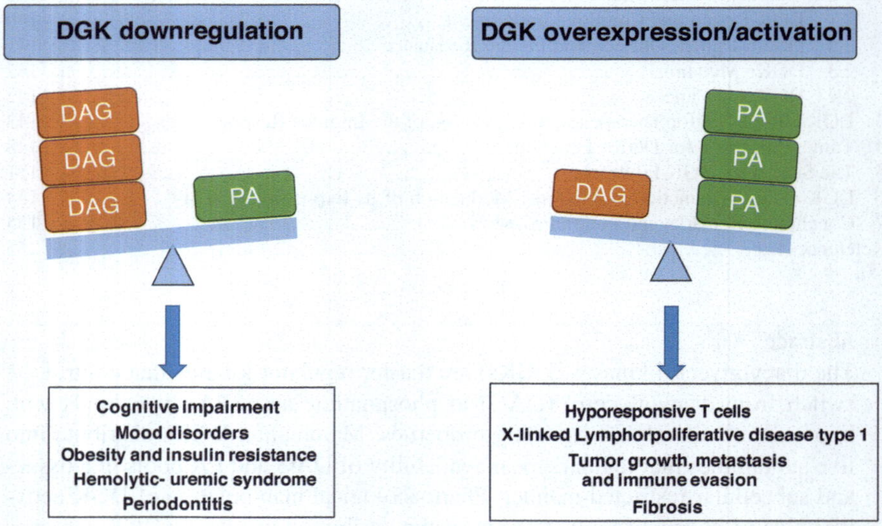

General model of DGK contribution to human disease. The DGK family of lipid kinases regulates the conversion of DAG into PA, two lipids that govern a variety of cellular processes. Deregulation of the DAG/PA homeostasis that results from DGK malfunction is associated with multiple human diseases. (**a**) Deficiency of selected DGK isoforms results in an excess of DAG that impairs synaptic transmission, favors insulin resistance, and triggers abnormal platelet or neutrophil activation. (**b**) Upregulation of DGK isoforms limits T and NK cytotoxic function and contributes to oncogenic transformation

1 Introduction

Diacylglycerol kinase (DGK) activity was first described, in the classical studies by Hokin and Hokin, as the limiting step that transforms the lipid diacylglycerol (DAG) into phosphatidic acid (PA), the precursor of phosphatidylinositol (PI) in the PI cycle (Hokin and Hokin 1959). Today we know that this enzyme activity is exerted by an extended family of lipid kinases that control numerous aspects of cell function. DGK-mediated transformation of DAG into PA regulates the abundance of two basic structural components of membranes. These two lipids have specific properties that modulate membrane fission and fusion and are also the precursors of other, more complex lipids (Carrasco and Merida 2007). In addition to their structural role, DAG and PA generated at the membrane create hot spots that facilitate localization and activation of many signaling proteins (Almena and Merida 2011; Stace and Ktistakis 2006).

DAG binds to proteins bearing the protein kinase C (PKC)-homology 1 (C1) domain, a conserved Zn^{2+}-containing region present in tandem with all members of the classical and novel PKC and the protein kinase D (PKD) families (Hurley et al. 1997). Studies with the DAG analog phorbol esters led to the characterization of specific residues required for DAG interaction that characterized the typical C1 domain. Proteins with typical C1 domains are candidates for DAG-dependent recruitment to the membrane. In addition to the classical and novel PKC and PDK, there are five additional families of C1 domain-containing proteins that include chimaerins, some DGK members, Ras guanine-releasing proteins (RasGRP), mammalian uncoordinated 13 (Munc13), and myotonic dystrophy kinase-related Cdc42-binding kinase (MRCK) families. Except for members of the Munc13 family, which have scaffolding functions, the rest of the DAG-receptor families range from lipid and protein kinases to modulators of small GTPases. The non-kinase receptors of DAG have uncovered new and strategic function of DAG in the regulation of Ras activation or Rac-mediated functions (Kazanietz 2002).

Albeit less characterized due to the lack of a recognizable binding domain, the negatively charged headgroup of PA facilitates membrane localization of proteins through nonspecific electrostatic interactions with patches of positively charged amino acids such as lysine and arginine (Shin and Loewen 2011). Electrostatic-based interactions of these two residues with PA increase the negative charge of the lipid via a mechanism termed the electrostatic/hydrogen bond switch (Kooijman et al. 2007). This ability converts PA into a sensor that directs pH-dependent membrane binding of target proteins (Young et al. 2010). Polybasic stretches that recognize PA have been identified in the rapamycin-binding domain of the mammalian target of rapamycin (mTOR) (Fang et al. 2001) and in the DEP (dishevelled, Egl-10, and pleckstrin) domain of Epac1 (Consonni et al. 2012) and dishevelled (Dsh) proteins (Simons et al. 2009).

DGKs are conserved from yeast to mammals, with specialization increasing with organism complexity (Merida et al. 2008). Yeast expresses a single DGK enzyme, whereas mammals express ten isozymes, some with splicing variants. All mammalian DGKs share a catalytic domain that contains the so-called common domain, whose features are conserved with the catalytic region of ceramide and sphingosine kinases (Labesse et al. 2002), and an accessory domain unique to the DGK family. The catalytic domain bears a highly conserved G-G-D-G motif that participates in ATP binding. Despite the interest in this enzyme family, there are no reports of successful eukaryotic DGK crystallization. Advances have been made by analyzing structures of related prokaryotic proteins. In this regard, studies based on the structure of the *Staphylococcus aureus* DgkB have identified several residues important for catalysis and substrate recognition in the membrane-binding region (Miller et al. 2008).

DGK family members contain additional characteristic domains that define different regulatory mechanisms (Fig. 1). Type I DGKs (α, β, and γ) have two EF-hand motifs characteristic of Ca^{2+}-regulated proteins, whereas type II DGKs (δ, η, and κ) have a PH (pleckstrin homology) and SAM (sterile alpha motif) domains as well as a large insert in the catalytic domain not present in other subtypes. Type III DGKε is the smallest, as it lacks regulatory domains. It is also the only DGK with specificity for a given DAG species, as it only phosphorylates 1-stearoyl-2-arachidonoyl glycerol (Epand et al. 2016). Type IV DGKζ and DGKι have a sequence homologous to the MARCKS (myristoylated alanine-rich C-kinase substrate) phosphorylation site that overlaps with a NLS (nuclear localization signal) and four ankyrin repeats. Type IV DGKs, as well as DGKη2 and DGKκ, contain a C-terminal sequence that binds proteins with a PDZ (postsynaptic density protein-95/disc large/zona occludens-1) domain. The sole type V member, DGKθ, has a PH-like domain that overlaps with a Ras-associating domain. All DGKs have two C1 domains except for DGKθ, which has three. Except for the first C1 domains of DGKβ and DGKγ, however, the C1 regions in DGK family members lack the key residues that define a canonical DAG-binding C1 domain (Hurley et al. 1997). These regions nonetheless contribute to membrane binding either through lipid-based interactions as described for DGKα and the lipid products of the PI3K (phosphoinositide 3-kinase) (Cipres et al. 2001) or through protein interaction as shown for DGKζ and β-arrestin (Nelson et al. 2007).

Conservation of at least one of the five isotypes in nonmammalian organisms such as *Drosophila* suggests nonredundant function for each DGK subtype (Merida et al. 2008). The activation of specific DGK isoforms based on their regulatory modules confers the ability to regulate restricted pools of DAG and PA. The nervous and immune synapses are two prominent sites at which DAG and PA serve as organizing centers that regulate the trafficking, interaction, and signaling properties of many proteins (Carrasco and Merida 2007; Dotti et al. 2014; Dustin and Choudhuri 2016). Not surprisingly, most DGK isoforms are abundantly expressed in the central nervous system (CNS) and in hematopoietic cells. The elevated representation of specific DGK isoforms in these two systems provides numerous mechanisms for the control of the two lipids that facilitate cell plasticity (Almena and Merida 2011) (Fig. 2a, b).

Cancer cells also need to form highly organized structures for their migration and invasion (Woodham and Machesky 2014) (Fig. 2c). As cancer progresses, cells

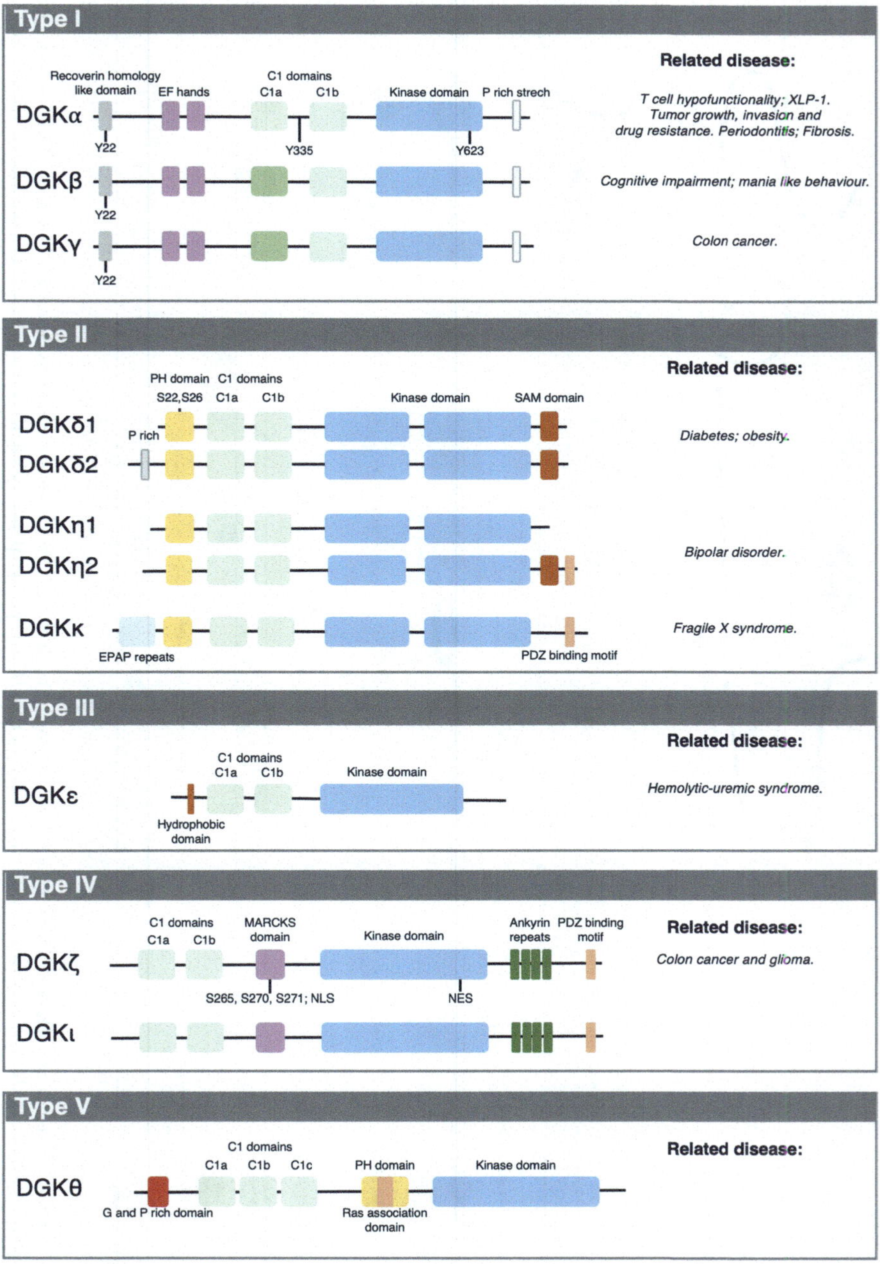

Fig. 1 The DGK family of proteins. Cartoon showing the mammalian DGK family of enzymes distributed into five subtypes according to the presence of specific regulatory domains. DGK regulatory domains and related human diseases are indicated. *Y* tyrosine, *P* proline, *G* glycine, *PH* pleckstrin homology, *SAM* sterile α-motif, *PDZ* postsynaptic density protein-95/disc large/zona occludens-1, *EPAP* glutamine-proline-alanine-proline repeats, *MARCKS* myristoylated alanine-rich C-kinase substrate, *NES* nuclear exporting sequence, *NLS* nuclear localization sequence

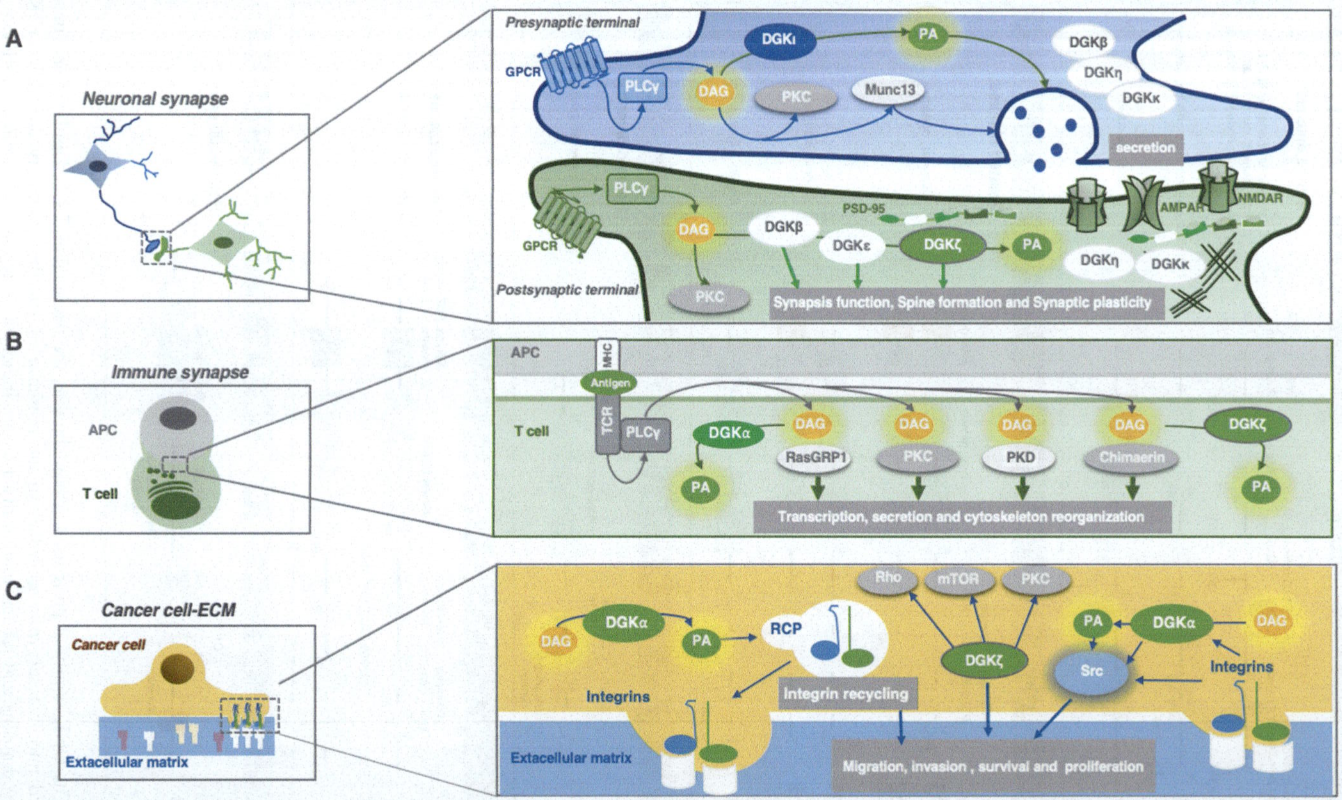

Fig. 2 DGKs contribute to local modulation of DAG and PA levels during cell-cell and cell-ECM contact. Functions described for selected DGK isoforms in highly polarized cell systems. (**a**) Neuronal synapse. DGKs are critical for controlling synaptic plasticity. DGKι controls secretion at presynaptic sites, whereas

Fig. 2 (continued) DGKζ controls spine formation. Additional DGK isoforms, including β, η, ε, and κ, also control synaptic transmission and neuronal function. (**b**) Immune synapse. DGKα and ζ activation downstream of the T cell receptor (TCR) regulates activation of DAG-regulated signaling proteins that control transcription, secretion, and cytoskeleton reorganization. DGK-derived PA may have additional targets that also help shape T cell responses. (**c**) Tumor extracellular matrix (ECM). In mesenchymal tumor cells, DGKα-dependent regulation of Src kinase sustains integrin-dependent regulation of migration, invasion, and survival signals. DGKα-mediated PA generation also controls integrin recycling. DGKζ contributes to the maintenance of multiple oncogenic functions including lipid metabolism and invasion

acquire the ability to undergo dynamic and reversible transition between differentiated epithelial and non-differentiated mesenchymal phenotypes (Tam and Weinberg 2013). During epithelial-mesenchymal transition, carcinoma cells acquire new traits including motility and invasiveness. Changes in the local concentration of DAG and PA in restricted membrane areas (such as synaptic spines, helper or cytotoxic synapses, and/or invadopodia) generate asymmetric membrane regions essential to regulate cell functions.

2 DGK Malfunction and Human Disease

2.1 DGK Deficit and Cognitive Impairment

Dynamic changes in the lipid composition of dendritic spines at excitatory synapses underlie memory and learning processes. The control of DAG and PA by the DGK family in the brain is a key feature of DGK physiology (Shirai and Saito 2014; Lee et al. 2016) (Fig. 2a). Studies in genetically deficient mice have demonstrated that several DGK isoforms affect brain function directly. *DGKB* was reported to be a learning-regulated gene (Hansell et al. 2015), and splice variant forms are differentially expressed in patients with mood disorder (Caricasole et al. 2002). DGKβ-deficient mice show impaired cognitive functions including spatial and long-term memories (Shirai et al. 2010) as well as hyperlocomotion, reduced anxiety, and attention-deficit behavior (Ishisaka and Hara 2014). Memory and emotional impairment in DGKβ-deficient mice can be rescued with the mood stabilizer lithium (Kakefuda et al. 2010), which suggests analysis of DGKβ expression as a biomarker in the selection of lithium-responsive bipolar patients (Mertens et al. 2015).

The DGKη isozyme is also expressed strongly in the CNS, and several genome-wide association studies on the etiology of bipolar disorders have reported DGKη mutations (Baum et al. 2008; Weber et al. 2011; Zeng et al. 2011). Enhanced DGKη mRNA expression is reported in some patients with bipolar disorders and schizophrenia (Moya et al. 2010). DGKη-deficient mice show mania-like behavior that includes hyperactivity, reduced anxiety, and diminished depression-like behavior. As in DGKβ-deficient mice, these symptoms are attenuated by lithium administration. The DGKβ expression pattern differs from that of DGKη, which implies that these isoforms regulate the mania phase in bipolar disorders via distinct mechanisms.

The type IV DGK isoforms (ζ and ι) are expressed abundantly in the brain although mouse studies demonstrate marked differences in their subcellular localization at neuronal synapses. DGKζ is targeted to excitatory synapses through direct interaction with the postsynaptic density protein-95 (PSD-95); when lacking, spine density is reduced (Kim et al. 2009). DGKι deficiency in mice does not visibly affect dendritic spines but causes a small increase in presynaptic release probability and a reduction in mGluRI-LTD (group 1 metabotropic glutamate receptor long-term depression) at neonatal stages (Yang et al. 2011).

One of the more interesting links between impaired DGK expression and abnormal brain function is the causal relationship reported between DGKκ deficiency and the fragile X syndrome (FXS) in a recent mouse study. Known as the most common form of inherited intellectual disability and a primary cause of autism, FXS arises from transcriptional inactivation of the gene *FMR1* (fragile X mental retardation gene 1) that encodes for FMRP (fragile X mental retardation protein), an RNA-binding protein (Hagerman et al. 2017). Very abundant in neurons, DGKκ has been identified as the main target for FMRP binding in these cells (Tabet et al. 2016). FXS correlates with increased DAG levels in human cerebellum suggesting that an excessive DAG signal directly links to FXS pathology. A model thus emerges for which, in healthy neurons, FMRP controls general translation in dendritic spines through DGKκ, which acts as a master switch of DAG and PA signals downstream of mGluRI. In FXS, DAG generated as the result of mGluRI activation is not transformed into PA, due to the lack of FMRP-dependent DGKκ translation. DAG signaling in the absence of PA leads to excess protein synthesis, amplified spine growth, and lack of spine stabilization. Reduction of DGKκ expression in the mouse brain recapitulates many of the alterations caused by FMRP loss (Tabet et al. 2016), which emphasizes the role of DGKκ in the control of synaptic plasticity. The identification of DGKκ as a main mRNA target of FMRP suggests research into DGKκ agonists as a promising therapy for FXS.

Genetic variants in the *DGKK* gene have been strongly associated with a high risk for hypospadias, a common congenital malformation of the male genitalia (van der Zanden et al. 2011). A study within a Swedish cohort of 9,262 males with hypospadia and their 4,936 brothers identified an increased risk for neurodevelopmental disorders in hypospadias-affected boys, with an increased risk for autism-related disorders in their brothers, suggesting a common genetic link between these two pathologies and DGKκ (Butwicka et al. 2015).

2.2 DGKδ Deficit, Obesity, and Insulin Resistance

The development of muscle insulin resistance in obese and diabetic patients is closely linked to an elevation of skeletal muscle DAG content that leads to PKC activation and serine phosphorylation of insulin receptor substrate 1 (IRS-1), limiting insulin-mediated functions (Szendroedi et al. 2014). A DGKδ expression deficit in skeletal muscle from type II diabetic patients is postulated as the cause of increased DAG accumulation, which contributes to the development of insulin resistance (Chibalin et al. 2008). In mice, DGKδ haploinsufficiency leads to a DAG increase in skeletal muscle, insulin resistance, and late-onset obesity (Jiang et al. 2016). DGKδ negative control of PKC is also necessary for proper activation of AMPK (AMP-activated kinase), an enzyme that controls lipid metabolism in muscle cells (Jiang et al. 2016). Although variations in the *DGKD* gene do not constitute a major genetic cause of type II diabetes, nine single-nucleotide polymorphisms (SNPs) have been described in the promoter and coding *DGKD* regions in type II diabetic families (Chibalin et al. 2008).

Studies of DGK expression in distinct insulin-sensitive tissues in lean and obese *ob/ob* mice have confirmed DGKδ alterations and also changes in other DGK isoforms (Manneras-Holm et al. 2015). DGKε deficiency preserves glucose tolerance and increases lipid metabolism (Manneras-Holm et al. 2017); DGKζ deficiency protects against peripheral insulin resistance and improves energy metabolism (Benziane et al. 2017); and DGKα, which appears dispensable for the regulation of whole-body insulin-mediated glucose utilization, modulates immune responses in white adipose tissue (Nascimento et al. 2017).

Diabetic nephropathy caused by hyperglycemia is one of the major diabetes complications and the leading cause of end-stage renal disease (Forbes and Cooper 2013). D-α-tocopherol (vitamin E) ameliorates diabetic nephropathy in wild-type mice but not in DGKα-deficient mice (Hayashi et al. 2017). These results agree with early findings showing vitamin E-specific activation of DGKα (Fukunaga-Takenaka et al. 2005) and suggest that DGKα activation might alleviate diabetic nephropathy in diabetic patients.

2.3 DGKε Mutations

The closest association between DGK mutations and human disease is seen in DGKε. Recessive loss-of-function DGKε mutations are associated with atypical hemolytic-uremic syndrome (aHUS), a disease characterized by vascular endothelial damage due to complement dysregulation (Lemaire et al. 2013). There is no obvious relationship between complement and DGKε, although complement deregulation influences the onset and severity of aHUS in carriers of DGKε mutations (Sanchez Chinchilla et al. 2014). The existence of a complement-independent mechanism leading to thrombotic angiopathy has clear therapeutic implications for children with this disease, who are normally treated with complement-blocking agents. *DGKE*-HUS typically manifests in the first year of life, although it is not limited exclusively to infancy, and viral triggers frequently precede HUS episodes (Azukaitis et al. 2017).

2.4 DGK and Cancer

Early observations demonstrating tumor-promoting actions of the DAG analog phorbol esters and the identification of PKC isoforms as high-affinity receptors for phorbol esters led to PKC being considered as an oncoprotein (Griner and Kazanietz 2007). As DGK negatively regulates PKC activation, one might predict that DGK malfunction would enhance tumor growth and survival. Several studies link DGK defects with tumor progression (Merida et al. 2017). Analysis of epigenetic silencing in colorectal cancer cell lines showed that *DGKG* methylation is positively associated with *KRAS* and *BRAF* mutations and with the CpG island methylator phenotype. *DGKG* methylation is also frequently detected in colorectal adenomas; this suggests that it is an early event in colorectal tumorigenesis (Kai et al. 2017). Diminished DGKα expression synergizes with oncogenic p53 and Ras mutations to promote cell transformation (McMurray et al. 2008). RNAseq and immunohistochemistry analyses show lower *DGKA* expression in gastric cancer (Kong et al.

2016), and *DGKA* expression is associated with improved survival in lung adenocarcinoma (Berrar et al. 2005).

A recent analysis of cancer-associated mutations in the PKC family challenged the contribution of PKC activation to cancer (Antal et al. 2015). This study revealed loss-of-function mutations in the majority of tumors analyzed, which suggests that for cancer therapy, PKC activity should be rescued and not inhibited (Newton and Brognard 2017). In keeping with a role for active PKC as tumor suppressors rather than oncoproteins, enhanced expression and/or activity of specific DGK isoforms has been linked to oncogenic transformation. DGKζ promotes invasiveness (Cai et al. 2014) and fosters the lipogenic metabolism and growth of colon cancer cells (Torres-Ayuso et al. 2015). DGKζ function is also necessary for growth and survival of gliomas (Diao et al. 2016).

Overexpression of the DGKα isoform in particular has a relevant function in cellular transformation, and several studies support the notion of tumors becoming addicted to this enzyme (Merida et al. 2017; Purow 2015). DGKα, which is absent in many healthy cells, such as hepatocytes, melanocytes, and neurons, is highly expressed and confers malignant properties in hepatocarcinoma (Takeishi et al. 2012), melanoma (Yanagisawa et al. 2007), and glioblastoma (Dominguez et al. 2013). Different from the other two type I DGKs, DGKα is preferentially expressed in the T cell lineage, where it controls T cell activation (Merida et al. 2017) (see the next section). Better characterization of the mechanisms that regulate DGKα expression in healthy T lymphocytes and in malignant cells, and of its effectors and partners, would increase our understanding of the complexity of the events that regulate tumor/T cell interactions.

3 DGKα Targeting for Therapeutic Manipulation of the Immune Response

Interest in DGK function in T lymphocytes was sparked by the purification and cloning of DGKα, as it showed a unique expression profile with abundance in thymus and mature T cells (Sakane et al. 1990). This tissue-specific distribution of DGKα suggested its participation in T cell-regulated functions. Several years later, experiments in human T cell lines confirmed that DGKα regulates DAG metabolism downstream of T cell receptor (TCR) triggering (Sanjuan et al. 2001). TCR-dependent activation of PLCγ generates Ca^{2+} and DAG at the immune synapse, which directly triggers activation of the GEF for Ras RasGRP1. This mechanism, which links the amount of DAG generated at the membrane with the intensity of Ras/ERK (extracellular-regulated kinase) signaling, provides a unique, tight technique to translate the affinity of the TCR for antigens into the intensity of the signals that ultimately define T cell activation (Figs. 2b and 3). Translocation to the synapse membrane of DGKα requires tyrosine phosphorylation of conserved residues and PLCγ-generated Ca^{2+} (Sanjuan et al. 2001; Merino et al. 2008). Membrane DGKα translocation is rapid, transient, and regulated by its own activity; the enzyme is retained at the membrane in the presence of inhibitors or when mutated to become

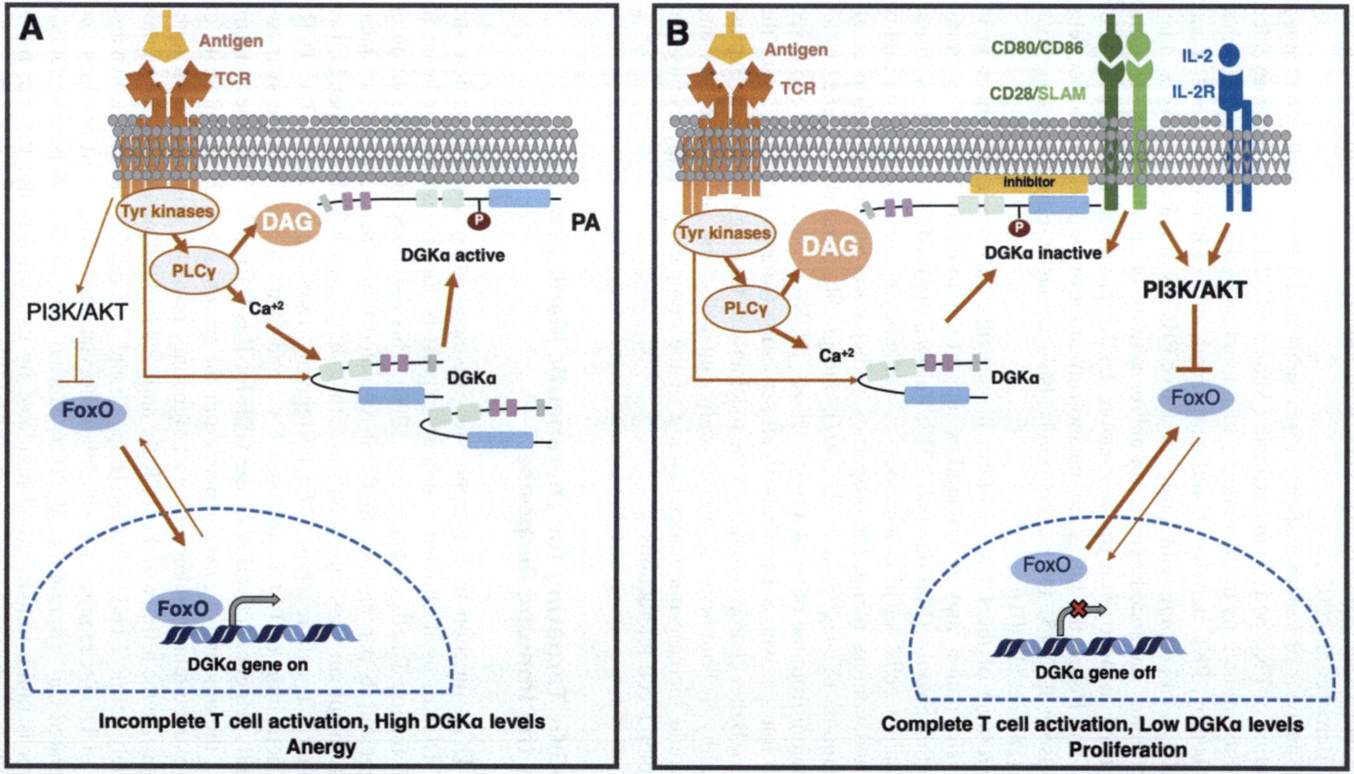

Fig. 3 Regulation of DGKα expression and activity in T cells. (**a**) TCR stimulation by cognate antigens triggers tyrosine kinase-dependent activation of PLCγ that generates DAG and inositol triphosphate-mediated Ca^{+2} elevation. Tyrosine phosphorylation and Ca^{+2} promote a conformational change in DGKα that exposes its membrane-binding domains, triggering localization to membranes where the enzyme phosphorylates DAG. Generation of PA at the membrane

Fig. 3 (continued) favors enzyme dissociation back to the cytosol. TCR signals provide weak activation of the PI3K/AKT pathway that is not sufficient to prevent the FoxO-dependent DGKα transcription that limits DAG activation of RasGRP1, activation of Ras, and IL-2 secretion, leading T cells into anergic, nonresponsive phenotypes. (**b**) Costimulatory signals such as those elicited by CD28 and/or SLAM promote initial DGKα inactivation that favors scaffolding functions at membranes. DGKα inhibition by costimulatory signals is reproduced by pharmacological DGK inhibitors that promote T cell activation. Costimulatory signals also promote strong activation of the PI3K/AKT pathway, inactivation of FoxO transcriptional activity, and repression of DGKα expression. Strong T cell stimulation leads to IL-2 production that also triggers PI3K/AKT activation, further repressing DGKα expression

inactive (Sanjuan et al. 2001). Mouse studies showed rapid DGKα translocation to the membrane in response to antigen recognition, with kinetics that mirrored those of RasGRP1 (Sanjuan et al. 2003). Experiments using dominant-negative and constitutive-active DGKα constructs confirmed a causal role in limiting RasGRP1 subcellular localization and consequent Ras activation. Costimulatory signals delivered by CD28 (Merino et al. 2008) or activation of the SLAM/SAP axis (signaling lymphocytic activation molecule-associated protein) (Baldanzi 2014) trigger DGKα inhibition, which sustains its membrane localization and facilitates RasGRP1-dependent Ras activation.

Studies in TCR transgenic mice demonstrated that DGKα expression, which is very high in resting cells, decreases rapidly following T cell activation (Sanjuan et al. 2003). The decrease in *Dgka* mRNA, which correlates with reduced protein expression and enzyme activity, ensures correct amplification of TCR signals. Incomplete activation of T cells leads to anergy, a condition characterized by defective Ras activation that limits interleukin 2 (IL-2) production and curbs T cell expansion (Valdor and Macian 2013). *Dgka* was identified as an anergy-induced gene, confirming a causal relationship between high DGKα expression and T cell tolerance (Macian et al. 2002). Studies in mouse models confirmed the correlation between DGKα abundance and T cell hypo-responses: its overexpression in T cells impairs T cell activation, whereas T cells from DGKα-deficient mice are anergy-resistant (Olenchock et al. 2006a; Zha et al. 2006).

Different from most of the genes that control T cell tolerance, early studies demonstrated that DGKα is not regulated by the Ca^{2+}-responsive transcription factor NFAT (nuclear factor of activated T cells) (Soto-Nieves et al. 2009). Analysis of the mouse *Dgka* gene revealed the presence of three binding sites for the forkhead box O (FoxO) transcription at the distal 5′ end region of the gene in a manner conserved in mammals (Martinez-Moreno et al. 2012) (Fig. 3). FoxO-mediated *Dgka* regulation directly links the regulation of enzyme abundance to the intensity of the signals received by T cells. FoxO phosphorylation and nuclear exclusion are regulated by the PI3K/AKT axis whose activation varies with the intensity of TCR signals and the presence of costimulation. TCR stimulation elicits PI3K activity through its p110δ catalytic isoform, leading to weak, transitory FoxO phosphorylation (Okkenhaug et al. 2002) that is insufficient to repress *DGKa* (Martinez-Moreno et al. 2012). Costimulatory signals delivered by CD28 or IL-2 result in the recruitment and activation of additional PI3K isoforms, enhancing FoxO phosphorylation (Garcon et al. 2008) and triggering *Dgka* repression (Fig. 3). The characterization of *Dgka* as a FoxO-regulated gene thus clarifies the causal relationship between incomplete TCR stimulation and anergy induction and also the capacity of IL-2 to rescue anergic cells.

Analysis of the 5′ upstream genomic region of the *Dgka* gene indicated the presence of binding sites for additional transcription factors (Martinez-Moreno et al. 2012). Some of these include p53, STAT, and Egr (early growth response) transcription factors, in accordance with microarray data (Merida et al. 2017). DGKα regulation by members of the Egr transcription factors has been confirmed in mouse (Zheng et al. 2013) and human (Weigel et al. 2016) studies. Analysis of the *Dgka* promoter also identified at least two alternative promoter regions that give rise to different transcripts. These variants include some that lack exon 10, and others with longer exons 13 and 21, that result in truncated proteins (Martinez-Moreno et al. 2012). Expression of a spliced DGKα variant that lacks exon 10 is found in the polymorphonuclear neutrophils (PMN) of localized aggressive periodontitis (LAP) patients (Batista et al. 2014). This is a rare syndrome characterized by abnormal neutrophil activation that leads to periodontal bone loss (Kantarci et al. 2003). Loss of exon 10 of *DGKA* results in expression of a truncated protein that lacks the catalytic domain but retains the ability to translocate to the membrane, acting as a dominant negative mutant. Overexpression of the truncated DGKα variant in HL60 cells promotes superoxide production, one of the causes of tissue damage in LAP (Batista et al. 2014).

DGKα-mediated DAG metabolism upon antigen recognition by T cells not only limits the activation of the Ras/ERK axis but also controls membrane trafficking and cytoskeletal reorganization at the immune synapse. An excess of DAG generation at the immune synapse as the result of DGKα deficiency impairs correct polarization of the MTOC (microtubule-organizing center) and polarized secretion (Alonso et al. 2011; Chauveau et al. 2014; Quann et al. 2009). In contrast, excessive DGKα activity prevents DAG-dependent recruitment of RasGRP1 and novel PKCs, reducing the stability of the immune synapse and T cell effector functions as described in X-linked lymphoproliferative disease (XLP-1) (Ruffo et al. 2016). This is a fatal primary immunodeficiency caused by germline mutations in the *SH2D1A* gene, which encodes the adaptor protein SAP. XLP-1-affected boys develop excessive lymphoproliferation after Epstein-Barr virus (EBV) infection characterized by massive accumulation of activated $CD8^+$ T cells that infiltrate and damage several organs (Veillette et al. 2013). It is suggested that the persistent DGKα activation that results from SAP absence prevents correct organization of DAG-regulated signals and facilitates resistance to AICD (activation-induced cell death).

In addition to DGKα, T lymphocytes also express DGKζ, although not with the strong tissue restriction observed for DGKα. DGKζ is expressed in the hematopoietic $CD34^+$ compartment, which includes dendritic ($BCCA4^+$), NK ($CD56^+$), and myeloid ($CD33^+$) cells, as well as in monocytes ($CD14^+$). BioGPS database analysis also shows strong expression of this gene in the brain (particularly in the amygdala and prefrontal cortex). This broader DGKζ expression correlates well with the multiple defects described in DGKζ-deficient mice, which range from abnormal dendritic spines (Kim et al. 2009) and impaired bone resorption (Iwazaki et al. 2017; Zamani et al. 2015) to reduced muscle hypertrophy (You et al. 2014).

As described for DGKα, DGKζ-deficient mice have anergy-resistant phenotypes and hyper-responsive T cells. DGKζ expression is upregulated in anergic cells through the control of Egr2 (Zheng et al. 2013), a transcription factor whose activity is promoted upon TCR engagement in an NFAT-dependent mechanism (Zheng et al. 2012). Double-deficient mice show impaired thymic development, confirming non-redundant functions for the two enzymes. Some excellent recent reviews summarize the multiple functions ascribed to DGKζ in the control of T cell responses (Chen et al. 2016; Singh and Kambayashi 2016; Merida et al. 2015). Similar to the findings described for T cells, DGKζ limits B cell antigen receptor-dependent activation of the Ras/ERK axis (Wheeler et al. 2013). In contrast to their hyperactive T cells, which enhance antiviral and antitumor responses, DGKζ-deficient mice have decreased mast cell functions characterized by impaired degranulation (Olenchock et al. 2006b). This phenomenon correlates with diminished PLCδ activity and decreased PKCβII recruitment to membranes. DGKζ-deficient mast cells, on the other hand, show enhanced IL-6 production, in accordance with higher activation of Ras/AKT/ERK pathways. The enhanced response of T cells as a result of DGKζ deficiency contrasts with the enhanced susceptibility of DGKζ-deficient mice to endotoxin-induced shock (Liu et al. 2007). This defect is attributed to the lack of PA needed for TLR (Toll-like receptor)-induced cytokine responses in dendritic cells and macrophages. In spite of its important contributions, no mutations are reported for DGKζ in humans.

4 Tumor Addiction for DGKα Functions

DGKα, whose expression is greatly restricted to the T cell lineage, is nonetheless associated with tumor progression. DGKα is not expressed in healthy liver, but hepatic tumors show high DGKα levels compared to untransformed neighboring tissue (Takeishi et al. 2012; Yanagisawa et al. 2007). DGKα expression is higher in metastases compared to the original tumor (Hao et al. 2004; Marchet et al. 2007). DGKα mediates numerous aspects of cancer cell progression including survival (Bacchiocchi et al. 2005; Dominguez et al. 2013; Takeishi et al. 2012; Torres-Ayuso et al. 2014; Yanagisawa et al. 2007), migration, and invasion (Baldanzi et al. 2008; Filigheddu et al. 2007; Rainero et al. 2012). These studies suggest that some tumors develop an "addiction" to DGKα-regulated pathways. The concept of "non-oncogenic addiction," first formulated by Solimini et al. (2007), is associated with a wide array of signaling enzymes that, although not inherently malignant, provide survival advantages to tumors. It usually relates to stress response mechanisms and contributes to drug resistance in many tumors. Targeting these pathways is a promising approach in cancer, since it provides a means of selectively targeting tumor cells while sparing untransformed tissues.

Studies using tumor cell culture in three-dimensional (3D) conditions reproduce DGKα upregulation and demonstrate that this enzyme is indispensable for growth and survival of highly metastatic tumors but not for non-transformed cells (Torres-Ayuso et al. 2014). DGKα silencing limits cell growth in 3D but not in 2D cell cultures, confirming that upregulation of this isoform contributes to tumor cell reprogramming. DGKα-silenced cells form smaller tumors when xenografted into immunocompromised mice (Torres-Ayuso et al. 2014). The higher DGKα expression observed in 3D-cultured colon and breast cancer cells correlates with enhanced activity of the tyrosine kinase Src, whereas DGKα silencing leads to Src inactivation. These studies complement the early identification of DGKα as a Src target (Baldanzi et al. 2008; Merino et al. 2008) and reveal mutual regulation of the two enzymes. A mechanistic link between these two enzymes helps to explain the addiction of highly metastatic, transformed tumors for DGKα. An increase in tyrosine signaling networks, specifically those of the Src family, is a characteristic of colon and breast cancers (Hochgrafe et al. 2010; Malek et al. 2002) and is critical in sustaining disorganized growth under 3D conditions (Arias-Romero et al. 2009).

This mutual DGKα/Src regulation agrees with the well-established mechanism of sequential activation of Src as a result of substrate interaction. The Src SH3 domain mediates target recognition through proline-rich sequences and target subsequent phosphorylation; this enforces interaction through the Src SH2 motif, which in turn promotes an open/active conformation of the kinase (Guarino 2010; Harrison 2003). DGKα interacts with Src through a proline stretch located at its C-terminal region that facilitates DGKα phosphorylation at Y335, which interacts with the SH2 motif (Baldanzi et al. 2008). The interaction of DGKα with Src is independent of PA production, but DGKα enzymatic activity is nonetheless necessary for Src activation (Torres-Ayuso et al. 2014). PA-dependent regulation of Src correlates with the presence of acidic lipid-binding motifs in the Src unique and SH3 domains (Perez et al. 2013). The contribution of the PA generated by DGKα to Src activation adds to other functions attributed to this pathway that also contribute to the survival and invasive properties of cancer cells. DGKα-derived PA promotes mobilization and membrane tethering of RCP (Rab-coupling protein), a modulator of Rab protein trafficking necessary for integrin recycling and cell migration (Rainero et al. 2012). DGKα-PA production is also suggested to activate phosphodiesterase activity, which controls cAMP levels and the expression of cAMP-responsive genes that are critical for cancer cell survival, including mTOR and HIF-1 (hypoxia-induced factor-1) (Dominguez et al. 2013). A DGKα-Src axis also mediates survival and proliferative signals downstream of the chimeric oncogenic kinase ALK (anaplastic lymphoma kinase) that is responsible for the hematopoietic malignancy known as ALCL (anaplastic large cell lymphoma) (Bacchiocchi et al. 2005).

DGKα upregulation in tumors is not restricted solely to malignant cells, but also occurs in the rest of the cells present in the tumor microenvironment; enhanced DGKα expression is found in renal tumor-infiltrating T and NK cells (Prinz et al. 2012, 2014). Similarly, enhanced expression of DGKα and DGKζ is found in chimeric antigen receptor-engineered T (CAR-T) cells when isolated from solid tumors (Riese et al. 2013). Overnight cultures of tumor-isolated CAR-T cells result in the rapid downregulation of DGKα/ζ expression (Riese et al. 2013), confirming that DGK upregulation, similar to that observed for epithelial tumor cells in 3D cultures (Torres-Ayuso et al. 2014), is triggered by the tumor microenvironment. The immunosuppressive, hypoxic tumor microenvironment thus promotes similar DGKα upregulation in tumors and infiltrating T cells, with contrasting consequences (Fig. 4). Whereas DGKα-dependent functions enhance tumor survival and metastasis, its upregulation in infiltrating T cells impedes cytotoxic functions. The control of DGKα expression in cancer thus emerges as one of the mechanisms that contributes to tumor immune evasion, suggesting that targeting this isoform could directly affect tumor survival, drug resistance, and immune escape mechanisms. The oncogenic addiction described for DGKα is not reported for other DGK isoforms, which suggests specific functions for this isoform. Analysis of DGKζ-deficient mice, on

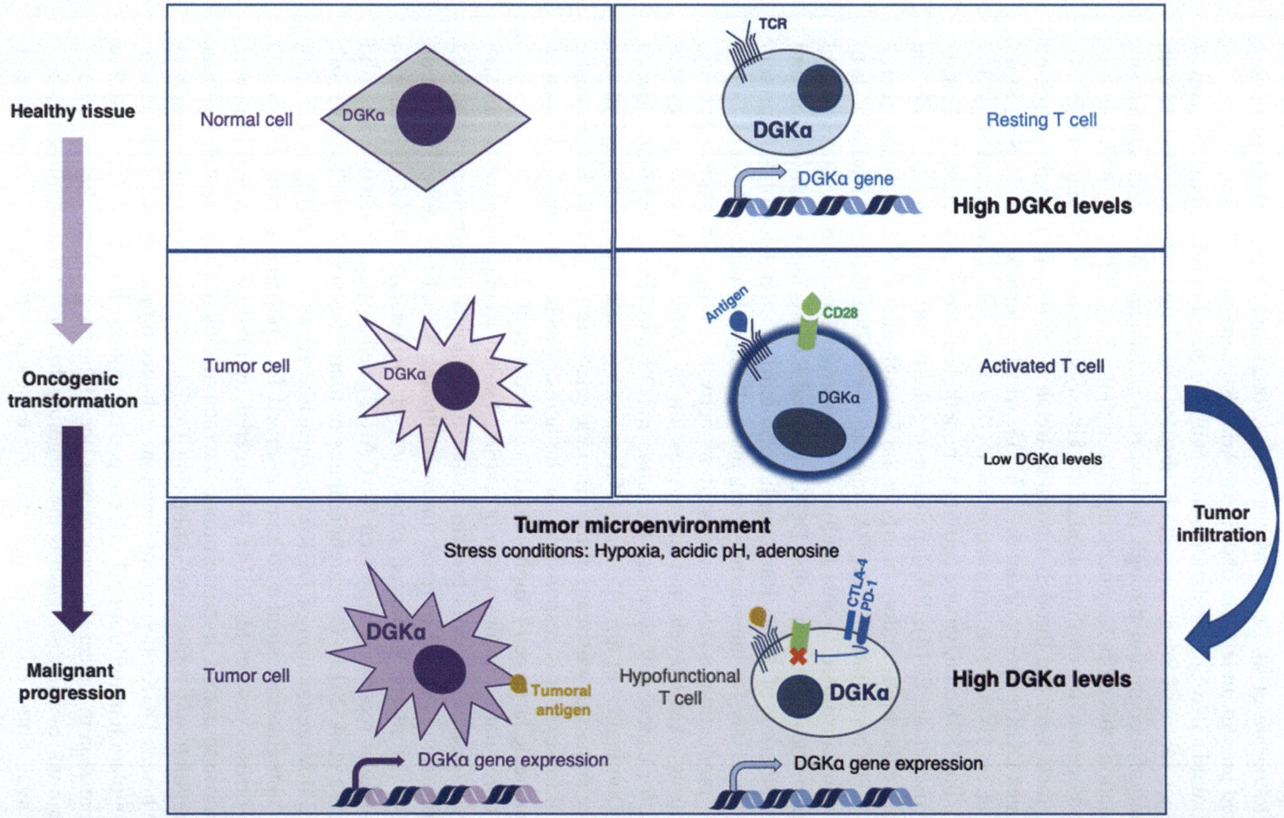

Fig. 4 High DGKα expression in tumors and tumor-infiltrating T cells. In healthy organs, DGKα is abundant in resting T lymphocytes. Expression of DGKα decreases in activated T lymphocytes and increases during oncogenic transformation. Stress conditions (hypoxia, low nutrient availability, acidic pH, etc.) enhance expression of DGKα in tumor cells and in tumor-infiltrating T cells. These became nonfunctional since TCR and costimulatory signals are blocked by the high expression of immune checkpoints, such as CTLA-4 and PD-1. This limits the T cell response to cancer cells, leading to tumor persistence

the other hand, confirms enhanced T cell (Andrada et al. 2017; Jing et al. 2017; Riese et al. 2013) as well as NK cell (Yang et al. 2016) antitumor functions. The wide expression of DGKζ nonetheless may limit the targeting of this isoform to foster immune tumor attack. The effectiveness of isoform-specific inhibitors vs. pan-DGK inhibitors, as well as the potential use of DGKα or DGKζ targeting combined with other checkpoint-blocking agents and/or anticancer therapies, will undoubtedly be the object of intense future study.

5 The Search for DGK Inhibitors

Recent discoveries have helped to clarify the functions of specific DGK isoforms and their potential as pharmacological targets, making DGK inhibition an important area for development of small molecule regulators of lipid-based responses. However, the development of DGK inhibitors has proved challenging. Early studies identified DAG lipid analogs such as dioctanoylethylene glycol and 1-monooleoylglycerol as DGK inhibitors in human platelets (Bishop et al. 1986). About the same time, a screen using isolated platelet membranes identified the synthetic small molecule R59022 as a DGK inhibitor (Chaffoy de Courcelles et al. 1985). The R59022 structural analog R59949 was subsequently reported to have an improved IC_{50} (Chaffoy de Courcelles et al. 1989), although head-to-head comparison later revealed a nearly identical IC_{50} of 3 μM (Rodriguez-Linares et al. 1991) (Fig. 5a). The two inhibitors show higher specificity for type I DGK isoforms, although they do not recognize the Ca^{2+}-binding motif common to this type of enzyme. Altered Mg/ATP binding in the presence of R59949 suggests recognition of an allosteric site adjacent to the active site (Jiang et al. 2000).

To date, R59022 and R59949 remain the best-characterized DGK inhibitors. Part of the problem when searching for DGK inhibitors is the optimization of robust systems for high-throughput screening. The conventional enzyme assay for DGK activity, which uses lipid substrates and radioactive ATP, is hard to adjust to screening formats. The use of a nonradioactive, high-throughput DGK assay for the screening of a 9,600-chemical library recently led to the identification of CU-3 as a selective DGKα inhibitor with an IC_{50} of 0.6 μM (Liu et al. 2016). CU-3 is not structurally similar to either R59949 or R59022 (Fig. 5a), and it acts as a competitive ATP inhibitor, probably through the 2-thioxo-1,3-thiazolidin-4-one ring. The reason for its selectivity for the type I DGK is not known. CU-3, as previously demonstrated for R59949 and R59022 (Dominguez et al. 2013; Torres-Ayuso et al. 2014), induces apoptosis in human cancer cells in vitro, supporting prior results for multiple tumor-derived cell lines.

Studies based on in vivo administration of DGK inhibitors are scarce. The therapeutic potential of R59022 as an antitumor agent has been demonstrated in vivo using SCID (severe combined immunodeficiency) mice implanted with U87 glioblastoma cells, in both orthotopic and subcutaneous models (Dominguez et al. 2013). After tumor establishment, mice receiving daily intraperitoneal injections of R59022 (2 mg/kg) for 23 consecutive days displayed significantly

A

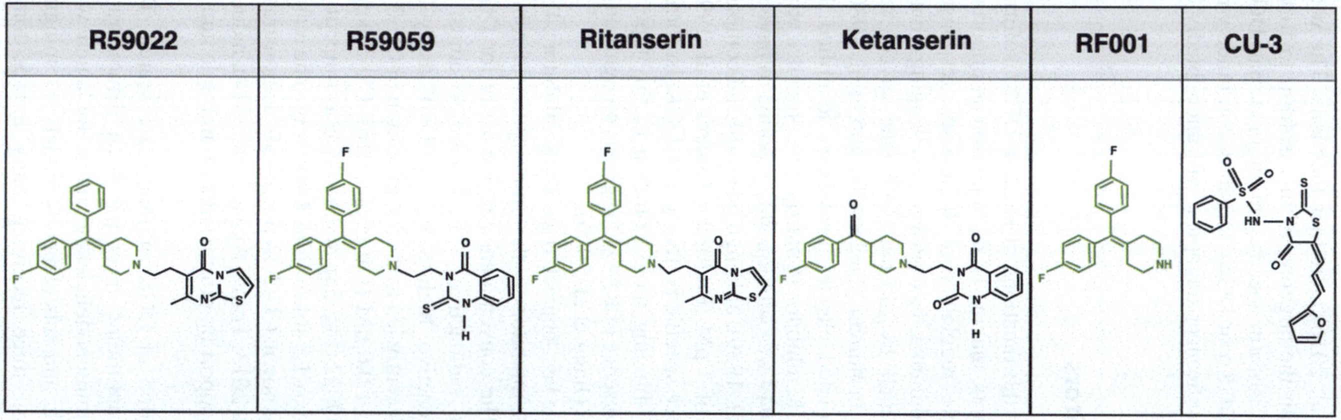

B

	R59022	R59059	Ritanserin	Ketanserin
DGKα	+	+	+	-
5-HT_{1B}	+++	+	+++	-
5-HT_{2A}	+++	+++	+++	+++
5-HT_{7A}	+++	+	+++	-

Fig. 5 The DGK inhibitor molecule R59022 and its related compounds. (**a**) Chemical structure of R59022 and structurally or functionally related molecules. R59022, R59059, and ritanserin share a conserved region (in green) that was recently identified as the minimal region necessary to target DGK activity and designated as RF001. The serotonin receptor (5-HTR) antagonist ketanserin only contains part of RF001 in agreement with its lack of function as a DGKα inhibitor. The similarity between the non-RF001 region of ketanserin (black) with the other molecules may explain targeting of 5-HTR by all of these molecules. CU-3 is not structurally related to the other molecules. (**b**) Summary of the effects of the indicated drugs against DGKα and the primary 5-HTR expressed in mouse T cells

increased survival compared to DMSO-injected controls. Tumors in R59022-treated mice showed reduced vascularity and increased apoptosis, in agreement with a role for DGKα-derived PA in angiogenesis (Baldanzi et al. 2004). Subcutaneous R59949 injection also reduces growth of xenografted colon cancer tumors when administered at a dose of 10 mg/kg every 48 h for 10 days (Torres-Ayuso et al. 2014).

R59022 has also been administered to *Sh2d1a*-deficient mice infected with lymphocytic choriomeningitis virus (LCMV) to evaluate the effects of DGKα inhibition in a model of FIM (fulminant infectious mononucleosis) similar to the disease observed in XLP-1 patients (Ruffo et al. 2016). LCMV-infected *Sh2d1a*-deficient mice receiving intraperitoneal injections of R59022 (2 mg/kg) twice a day showed significantly reduction of splenomegaly and decreased total lymphocyte counts in the spleen. Inhibitor treatment did not impair viral clearance in control LCMV-infected mice, suggesting that, as in the case of tumoral vs. non-transformed cells, inhibition only targets cells expressing aberrantly accumulated and/or activated DGKα.

These data offer proof of concept that DGKα could be a druggable target for reducing pathogenic accumulation of $CD8^+$ T cells in EBV-infected XLP-1 patients to prevent tumor-induced T and NK hypofunctional states and/or to treat highly transformed, chemotherapy-resistant forms of cancer. Translation of preclinical findings for clinical use will require development of new, clinical-grade-specific DGKα inhibitors. The pharmacokinetics studies indicate a short half-life for R59022 after a single intraperitoneal dose of 10 mg/kg, with peak concentration at 2 h and limited ability to cross the blood-brain barrier (Dominguez et al. 2013). In the search for better DGK inhibitors, it was recently noted that the R59022 structure is closely related to that of ritanserin, a well-known serotonin (5-HT) receptor (5-HTR) antagonist (Boroda et al. 2017). Ritanserin has a much longer half-life than R59022 and has been safely tested in humans, suggesting its repurposing as a DGKα inhibitor for cancer treatment. In vitro studies with purified DGKα confirmed that ritanserin inhibits enzyme activity at concentrations similar to those for R59022 (Boroda et al. 2017). DGKα targeting with ritanserin specially targets the mesenchymal subtype of glioblastoma and is synergistic with radiation and imatinib treatment that preferentially targets proneural glioblastoma (Olmez et al. 2018). The enhanced sensitivity to ritanserin of mesenchymal phenotypes is attributed to inhibition of geranylgeranyl transferase I.

The close structural similarity between ritanserin and R59022 suggests 5-HTR antagonizing properties for this DGKα inhibitor. Radioligand competition assays recently confirmed binding of R59022 and R59949 to all 5-HTR except 5-HTR3 (Boroda et al. 2017). Inhibition assays demonstrate antagonistic effects of both compounds for multiple 5-HTR, with the exception of R59949 for 5-HTR2C and 5-HTR7. The potential crosstalk between DGKα inhibitors and 5-HTR may be in conflict when modulating T cell responses. T cells synthesize and secrete 5-HT, which acts as costimulatory molecule through the 5-HTR2a and 5-HTR7 (Leon-Ponte et al. 2007). In agreement, ritanserin addition to primary mouse T cells impairs activation, an effect that is more pronounced in DGKα-deficient T cells (Arranz-Nicolás et al. 2018). The effect of ritanserin contrasts with the enhanced T cell activation induced by R59949 treatment (Arranz-Nicolás et al. 2018), suggesting that, when selecting DGKα inhibitors, particular care must be taken to avoid 5-HTR7 antagonistic functions (Fig. 5b). Evaluation of the pattern expression of distinct 5-HTR in the circulating T cells and those that are infiltrating tumors in humans will provide clues about the benefit of ritanserin repositioning as a DGKα inhibitor.

The characterization of ritanserin as a DGKα inhibitor has provided new clues about the contribution of the DGKα-C1 domains to catalytic function. Using ATP-acyl phosphate activity-based probes and chemical proteomics approaches, the site for inhibitor recognition in DGKα has been shown to encompass the catalytic domain and the C1 tandem domains (Franks et al. 2017). Fragment-based deconstruction studies have identified a hydrophobic region in ritanserin (RF001) (Fig. 5a) that recapitulates DGKα inhibition and retains binding to the C1 and catalytic DGKα domains. The nucleotide-like region common to R59022 and ritanserin competes not only for the ATP-binding site of DGKα but also for those of several protein kinases and ATPases and could be responsible for the off-target effects of ritanserin.

6 DGKα Gain of Function and Indirect Modulation of Its Expression/Activity

The DGK-deficient mouse phenotype, together with disease-linked alterations in DGK expression/activity, supports the concept of individual specialized functions for each DGK isoform. These functions are probably dictated by tissue restriction as well as by the distinct regulatory domains that couple DGK to specific activation pathways. In contrast to the restricted isoform-specific functions of most DGK family members, membrane targeting of inactive DGKα as the result of inhibitor treatment confers gain-of-function abilities on this isoform. T cell treatment with a DGKα inhibitor mimics costimulatory signals, in contrast with the reduced activation observed when this enzyme is deleted (Arranz-Nicolás et al. 2018). Inhibitor-mediated DGKα targeting to the T cell membrane also restores synapse localization of novel PKCs and triggers AICD in SAP-deficient cells (Ruffo et al. 2016). Whereas inhibitor-mediated DGKα targeting to membrane promotes DAG-dependent signals, relocalization of the active enzyme might alleviate pathological DAG overproduction. This is the case for vitamin E, which attenuates diabetic nephropathy and podocyte loss by promoting specific DGKα translocation to podocyte cell membranes (Hayashi et al. 2017). Deeper understanding of the mechanisms that control DGKα expression and activation could offer therapeutic approaches for a number of different diseases.

In addition to pharmacological inhibition, limiting DGKα expression might provide a therapeutic window. DGKα is regulated by FoxO transcription factors, whose targeting is being studied for treatment of various conditions that include predisposition to neoplasia, drug resistance in cancer, and/or prevention of ageing by maintenance of the hematopoietic stem cell niche (de Keizer 2017; Hornsveld et al. 2017). The use of FoxO-targeting drugs ranging from those that modulate the

PI3K/AKT axis (Monsalve and Olmos 2011) to those that block nuclear export such as selinexor (Abdul Razak et al. 2016; Farren et al. 2017) might allow modulation of DGKα gene expression in distinct contexts. In addition to FoxO-mediated regulation, DGKα expression by bromodomain and extraterminal domain (BET) proteins contributes to irradiation-induced fibrosis in a subset of breast cancer patients (Weigel et al. 2016). Targeting epigenetic modulation might thus offer additional possibilities for limiting DGKα expression in these situations. BET inhibitors block DGKα upregulation in fibrosis (Valinciute et al. 2017), having an anti-fibrotic effect that is similar to that seen for DGK inhibitors (Weigel et al. 2016). An agonist of the peroxisome proliferator-activated receptor γ (PPARγ), a transcription factor involved in diabetes development, is also reported to increase DGKα expression (Verrier et al. 2004). Analysis of the DGKα promoter shows multiple transcription factor binding sites (Martinez-Moreno et al. 2012), which suggests additional means for repressing or augmenting DGKα expression for therapeutic purposes.

7 Concluding Remarks and Future Prospects

Through their combined actions on membrane dynamics and protein activation, DAG and PA organize a large variety of cell processes. DGK function is essential for sustaining organization of distinct DAG and PA signaling nodes, as shown by the many alterations and pathologies associated with anomalous DGK activity. Manipulation of DGK function offers an opportunity for intervention in such different processes; this is encouraged by the promising effects observed in distinct experimental approaches that modulate their activity or expression. Translation of laboratory and preclinical findings to clinical use nonetheless will require the development of new, clinical-grade-specific DGKα inhibitors, as well as further characterization of the mechanisms that control the function and expression of DGK, of their targets, and of their effectors.

Acknowledgments JAN holds predoctoral FPI fellowships from the Spanish Ministry of Economy and Competitiveness (MINECO). This work was supported in part by grants from the MINECO/FEDER/UE (BFU2013-47640-P) and from the Madrid regional government (IMMUNOTHERCAM Consortium B2017/BMD-3733) to IM. We thank Catherine Mark for excellent editorial assistance.

References

Abdul Razak AR, Mau-Soerensen M, Gabrail NY, Gerecitano JF, Shields AF, Unger TJ, Saint-Martin JR, Carlson R, Landesman Y, McCauley D et al (2016) First-in-class, first-in-human phase I study of selinexor, a selective inhibitor of nuclear export, in patients with advanced solid tumors. J Clin Oncol 34:4142–4150

Almena M, Merida I (2011) Shaping up the membrane: diacylglycerol coordinates spatial orientation of signaling. Trends Biochem Sci 36:593–603

Alonso R, Mazzeo C, Rodriguez MC, Marsh M, Fraile-Ramos A, Calvo V, Avila-Flores A, Merida I, Izquierdo M (2011) Diacylglycerol kinase alpha regulates the formation and polarisation of mature multivesicular bodies involved in the secretion of Fas ligand-containing exosomes in T lymphocytes. Cell Death Differ 18:1161–1173

Andrada E, Liebana R, Merida I (2017) Diacylglycerol kinase zeta limits cytokine-dependent expansion of CD8(+) T cells with broad antitumor capacity. EBioMedicine 19:39–48

Antal CE, Hudson AM, Kang E, Zanca C, Wirth C, Stephenson NL, Trotter EW, Gallegos LL, Miller CJ, Furnari FB et al (2015) Cancer-associated protein kinase C mutations reveal kinase's role as tumor suppressor. Cell 160:489–502

Arias-Romero LE, Saha S, Villamar-Cruz O, Yip SC, Ethier SP, Zhang ZY, Chernoff J (2009) Activation of Src by protein tyrosine phosphatase 1B is required for ErbB2 transformation of human breast epithelial cells. Cancer Res 69:4582–4588

Arranz-Nicolás J, Ogando J, Soutar D, Arcos-Pérez R, Meraviglia-Crivelli D, Mañes S, Mérida I, Ávila-Flores A (2018) Diacylglycerol kinase α inactivation is an integral component of the costimulatory pathway that amplifies TCR signals. Cancer Immunol Immunother 67:965–980

Azukaitis K, Simkova E, Majid MA, Galiano M, Benz K, Amann K, Bockmeyer C, Gajjar R, Meyers KE, Cheong HI et al (2017) The phenotypic spectrum of nephropathies associated with mutations in diacylglycerol kinase epsilon. J Am Soc Nephrol 28:3066–3075

Bacchiocchi R, Baldanzi G, Carbonari D, Capomagi C, Colombo E, van Blitterswijk WJ, Graziani A, Fazioli F (2005) Activation of alpha-diacylglycerol kinase is critical for the mitogenic properties of anaplastic lymphoma kinase. Blood 106:2175–2182

Baldanzi G (2014) Inhibition of diacylglycerol kinases as a physiological way to promote diacylglycerol signaling. Adv Biol Regul 55:39–49

Baldanzi G, Mitola S, Cutrupi S, Filigheddu N, van Blitterswijk WJ, Sinigaglia F, Bussolino F, Graziani A (2004) Activation of diacylglycerol kinase alpha is required for VEGF-induced angiogenic signaling in vitro. Oncogene 23:4828–4838

Baldanzi G, Cutrupi S, Chianale F, Gnocchi V, Rainero E, Porporato P, Filigheddu N, van Blitterswijk WJ, Parolini O, Bussolino F et al (2008) Diacylglycerol kinase-alpha phosphorylation by Src on Y335 is required for activation, membrane recruitment and Hgf-induced cell motility. Oncogene 27:942–956

Batista EL Jr, Kantarci AI, Hasturk H, van Dyke TE (2014) Alternative splicing generates a diacylglycerol kinase alpha transcript that acts as a dominant-negative modulator of superoxide production in localized aggressive periodontitis. J Periodontol 85:934–943

Baum AE, Akula N, Cabanero M, Cardona I, Corona W, Klemens B, Schulze TG, Cichon S, Rietschel M, Nothen MM et al (2008) A genome-wide association study implicates diacylglycerol kinase eta (DGKH) and several other genes in the etiology of bipolar disorder. Mol Psychiatry 13:197–207

Benziane B, Borg ML, Tom RZ, Riedl I, Massart J, Bjornholm M, Gilbert M, Chibalin AV, Zierath JR (2017) DGKzeta deficiency protects against peripheral insulin resistance and improves energy metabolism. J Lipid Res 58:2324–2333

Berrar D, Sturgeon B, Bradbury I, Downes CS, Dubitzky W (2005) Survival trees for analyzing clinical outcome in lung adenocarcinomas based on gene expression profiles: identification of neogenin and diacylglycerol kinase alpha expression as critical factors. J Comput Biol 12:534–544

Bishop WR, Ganong BR, Bell RM (1986) Attenuation of sn-1,2-diacylglycerol second messengers by diacylglycerol kinase. Inhibition by diacylglycerol analogs in vitro and in human platelets. J Biol Chem 261:6993–7000

Boroda S, Niccum M, Raje V, Purow BW, Harris TE (2017) Dual activities of ritanserin and R59022 as DGKalpha inhibitors and serotonin receptor antagonists. Biochem Pharmacol 123:29–39

Butwicka A, Lichtenstein P, Landen M, Nordenvall AS, Nordenstrom A, Nordenskjold A, Frisen L (2015) Hypospadias and increased risk for neurodevelopmental disorders. J Child Psychol Psychiatry 56:155–161

Cai K, Mulatz K, Ard R, Nguyen T, Gee SH (2014) Increased diacylglycerol kinase zeta expression in human metastatic colon cancer cells augments Rho GTPase activity and contributes to enhanced invasion. BMC Cancer 14:208

Caricasole A, Bettini E, Sala C, Roncarati R, Kobayashi N, Caldara F, Goto K, Terstappen GC (2002) Molecular cloning and characterization of the human diacylglycerol kinase beta (DGKbeta) gene: alternative splicing generates DGKbeta isotypes with different properties. J Biol Chem 277:4790–4796

Carrasco S, Merida I (2007) Diacylglycerol, when simplicity becomes complex. Trends Biochem Sci 32:27–36

de Chaffoy de Courcelles DC, Roevens P, Van Belle H (1985) R 59 022, a diacylglycerol kinase inhibitor. Its effect on diacylglycerol and thrombin-induced C kinase activation in the intact platelet. J Biol Chem 260:15762–15770

de Chaffoy de Courcelles D, Roevens P, Van Belle H, Kennis L, Somers Y, de Clerck F (1989) The role of endogenously formed diacylglycerol in the propagation and termination of platelet activation. A biochemical and functional analysis using the novel diacylglycerol kinase inhibitor, R 59 949. J Biol Chem 264:3274–3285

Chauveau A, Le Floc'h A, Bantilan NS, Koretzky GA, Huse M (2014) Diacylglycerol kinase alpha establishes T cell polarity by shaping diacylglycerol accumulation at the immunological synapse. Sci Signal 7:ra82

Chen SS, Hu Z, Zhong XP (2016) Diacylglycerol kinases in T cell tolerance and effector function. Front Cell Dev Biol 4:130

Chibalin AV, Leng Y, Vieira E, Krook A, Bjornholm M, Long YC, Kotova O, Zhong Z, Sakane F, Steiler T et al (2008) Downregulation of diacylglycerol kinase delta contributes to hyperglycemia-induced insulin resistance. Cell 132:375–386

Cipres A, Carrasco S, Merida I (2001) Deletion of the acidic-rich domain of the IL-2Rbeta chain increases receptor-associated PI3K activity. FEBS Lett 500:99–104

Consonni SV, Gloerich M, Spanjaard E, Bos JL (2012) cAMP regulates DEP domain-mediated binding of the guanine nucleotide exchange factor Epac1 to phosphatidic acid at the plasma membrane. Proc Natl Acad Sci U S A 109:3814–3819

de Keizer PL (2017) The fountain of youth by targeting senescent cells? Trends Mol Med 23:6–17

Diao J, Wu C, Zhang J, Liu J, Zhang X, Hao P, Zhao S, Zhang Z (2016) Loss of diacylglycerol kinase-zeta inhibits cell proliferation and survival in human gliomas. Mol Neurobiol 53:5425–5435

Dominguez CL, Floyd DH, Xiao A, Mullins GR, Kefas BA, Xin W, Yacur MN, Abounader R, Lee JK, Wilson GM et al (2013) Diacylglycerol kinase alpha is a critical signaling node and novel therapeutic target in glioblastoma and other cancers. Cancer Discov 3:782–797

Dotti CG, Esteban JA, Ledesma MD (2014) Lipid dynamics at dendritic spines. Front Neuroanat 8:76

Dustin ML, Choudhuri K (2016) Signaling and polarized communication across the T cell immunological synapse. Annu Rev Cell Dev Biol 32:303–325

Epand RM, So V, Jennings W, Khadka B, Gupta RS, Lemaire M (2016) Diacylglycerol kinase-epsilon: properties and biological roles. Front Cell Dev Biol 4:112

Fang Y, Vilella-Bach M, Bachmann R, Flanigan A, Chen J (2001) Phosphatidic acid-mediated mitogenic activation of mTOR signaling. Science 294:1942–1945

Farren MR, Hennessey RC, Shakya R, Elnaggar O, Young G, Kendra K, Landesman Y, Elloul S, Crochiere M, Klebanov B et al (2017) The Exportin-1 inhibitor selinexor exerts superior antitumor activity when combined with T-cell checkpoint inhibitors. Mol Cancer Ther 16:417–427

Filigheddu N, Cutrupi S, Porporato PE, Riboni F, Baldanzi G, Chianale F, Fortina E, Piantanida P, De Bortoli M, Vacca G et al (2007) Diacylglycerol kinase is required for HGF-induced invasiveness and anchorage-independent growth of MDA-MB-231 breast cancer cells. Anticancer Res 27:1489–1492

Forbes JM, Cooper ME (2013) Mechanisms of diabetic complications. Physiol Rev 93:137–188

Franks CE, Campbell ST, Purow BW, Harris TE, Hsu KL (2017) The ligand binding landscape of diacylglycerol kinases. Cell Chem Biol 24:870–880 e875

Fukunaga-Takenaka R, Shirai Y, Yagi K, Adachi N, Sakai N, Merino E, Merida I, Saito N (2005) Importance of chroman ring and tyrosine phosphorylation in the subtype-specific translocation and activation of diacylglycerol kinase alpha by D-alpha-tocopherol. Genes Cells 10:311–319

Garcon F, Patton DT, Emery JL, Hirsch E, Rottapel R, Sasaki T, Okkenhaug K (2008) CD28 provides T-cell costimulation and enhances PI3K activity at the immune synapse independently of its capacity to interact with the p85/p110 heterodimer. Blood 111:1464–1471

Griner EM, Kazanietz MG (2007) Protein kinase C and other diacylglycerol effectors in cancer. Nat Rev Cancer 7:281–294

Guarino M (2010) Src signaling in cancer invasion. J Cell Physiol 223:14–26

Hagerman RJ, Berry-Kravis E, Hazlett HC, Bailey DB Jr, Moine H, Kooy RF, Tassone F, Gantois I, Sonenberg N, Mandel JL, Hagerman PJ (2017) Fragile X syndrome. Nat Rev Dis Primers 3:17065

Hansell NK, Halford GS, Andrews G, Shum DH, Harris SE, Davies G, Franic S, Christoforou A, Zietsch B, Painter J et al (2015) Genetic basis of a cognitive complexity metric. PLoS One 10: e0123886

Hao X, Sun B, Hu L, Lahdesmaki H, Dunmire V, Feng Y, Zhang SW, Wang H, Wu C, Wang H et al (2004) Differential gene and protein expression in primary breast malignancies and their lymph node metastases as revealed by combined cDNA microarray and tissue microarray analysis. Cancer 100:1110–1122

Harrison SC (2003) Variation on an Src-like theme. Cell 112:737–740

Hayashi D, Yagi K, Song C, Ueda S, Yamanoue M, Topham M, Suzaki T, Saito N, Emoto N, Shirai Y (2017) Diacylglycerol kinase alpha is involved in the vitamin E-induced amelioration of diabetic nephropathy in mice. Sci Rep 7:2597

Hochgrafe F, Zhang L, O'Toole SA, Browne BC, Pinese M, Porta Cubas A, Lehrbach GM, Croucher DR, Rickwood D, Boulghourjian A et al (2010) Tyrosine phosphorylation profiling reveals the signaling network characteristics of basal breast cancer cells. Cancer Res 70:9391–9401

Hokin LE, Hokin MR (1959) Diglyceride phosphokinase: an enzyme which catalyzes the synthesis of phosphatidic acid. Biochim Biophys Acta 31:285–287

Hornsveld M, Dansen TB, Derksen PW, Burgering BMT (2017) Re-evaluating the role of FOXOs in cancer. Semin Cancer Biol 50:90–100

Hurley JH, Newton AC, Parker PJ, Blumberg PM, Nishizuka Y (1997) Taxonomy and function of C1 protein kinase C homology domains. Protein Sci 6:477–480

Ishisaka M, Hara H (2014) The roles of diacylglycerol kinases in the central nervous system: review of genetic studies in mice. J Pharmacol Sci 124:336–343

Iwazaki K, Tanaka T, Hozumi Y, Okada M, Tsuchiya R, Iseki K, Topham MK, Kawamae K, Takagi M, Goto K (2017) DGKzeta downregulation enhances osteoclast differentiation and bone resorption activity under inflammatory conditions. J Cell Physiol 232:617–624

Jiang Y, Sakane F, Kanoh H, Walsh JP (2000) Selectivity of the diacylglycerol kinase inhibitor 3-[2-(4-[bis-(4-fluorophenyl)methylene]-1-piperidinyl)ethyl]-2, 3-dihydro-2-thioxo-4 (1H)quinazolinone (R59949) among diacylglycerol kinase subtypes. Biochem Pharmacol 59:763–772

Jiang LQ, de Castro Barbosa T, Massart J, Deshmukh AS, Lofgren L, Duque-Guimaraes DE, Ozilgen A, Osler ME, Chibalin AV, Zierath JR (2016) Diacylglycerol kinase-delta regulates AMPK signaling, lipid metabolism, and skeletal muscle energetics. Am J Physiol Endocrinol Metab 310:E51–E60

Jing W, Gershan JA, Holzhauer S, Weber J, Palen K, McOlash L, Pulakanti K, Wesley E, Rao S, Johnson BD, Riese MJ (2017) T cells deficient in diacylglycerol kinase zeta are resistant to PD-1 inhibition and help create persistent host immunity to leukemia. Cancer Res 77:5676–5686

Kai M, Yamamoto E, Sato A, Yamano HO, Niinuma T, Kitajima H, Harada T, Aoki H, Maruyama R, Toyota M et al (2017) Epigenetic silencing of diacylglycerol kinase gamma in colorectal cancer. Mol Carcinog 56:1743–1752

Kakefuda K, Oyagi A, Ishisaka M, Tsuruma K, Shimazawa M, Yokota K, Shirai Y, Horie K, Saito N, Takeda J, Hara H (2010) Diacylglycerol kinase beta knockout mice exhibit lithium-sensitive behavioral abnormalities. PLoS One 5:e13447

Kantarci A, Oyaizu K, van Dyke TE (2003) Neutrophil-mediated tissue injury in periodontal disease pathogenesis: findings from localized aggressive periodontitis. J Periodontol 74:66–75

Kazanietz MG (2002) Novel "nonkinase" phorbol ester receptors: the C1 domain connection. Mol Pharmacol 61:759–767

Kim K, Yang J, Zhong XP, Kim MH, Kim YS, Lee HW, Han S, Choi J, Han K, Seo J et al (2009) Synaptic removal of diacylglycerol by DGKzeta and PSD-95 regulates dendritic spine maintenance. EMBO J 28:1170–1179

Kong Y, Zheng Y, Jia Y, Li P, Wang Y (2016) Decreased LIPF expression is correlated with DGKA and predicts poor outcome of gastric cancer. Oncol Rep 36:1852–1860

Kooijman EE, Tieleman DP, Testerink C, Munnik T, Rijkers DT, Burger KN, de Kruijff B (2007) An electrostatic/hydrogen bond switch as the basis for the specific interaction of phosphatidic acid with proteins. J Biol Chem 282:11356–11364

Labesse G, Douguet D, Assairi L, Gilles AM (2002) Diacylglyceride kinases, sphingosine kinases and NAD kinases: distant relatives of 6-phosphofructokinases. Trends Biochem Sci 27:273–275

Lee D, Kim E, Tanaka-Yamamoto K (2016) Diacylglycerol kinases in the coordination of synaptic plasticity. Front Cell Dev Biol 4:92

Lemaire M, Fremeaux-Bacchi V, Schaefer F, Choi M, Tang WH, Le Quintrec M, Fakhouri F, Taque S, Nobili F, Martinez F et al (2013) Recessive mutations in DGKE cause atypical hemolytic-uremic syndrome. Nat Genet 45:531–536

Leon-Ponte M, Ahern GP, O'Connell PJ (2007) Serotonin provides an accessory signal to enhance T-cell activation by signaling through the 5-HT7 receptor. Blood 109:3139–3146

Liu CH, Machado FS, Guo R, Nichols KE, Burks AW, Aliberti JC, Zhong XP (2007) Diacylglycerol kinase zeta regulates microbial recognition and host resistance to toxoplasma gondii. J Exp Med 204:781–792

Liu K, Kunii N, Sakuma M, Yamaki A, Mizuno S, Sato M, Sakai H, Kado S, Kumagai K, Kojima H et al (2016) A novel diacylglycerol kinase alpha-selective inhibitor, CU-3, induces cancer cell apoptosis and enhances immune response. J Lipid Res 57:368–379

Macian F, Garcia-Cozar F, Im SH, Horton HF, Byrne MC, Rao A (2002) Transcriptional mechanisms underlying lymphocyte tolerance. Cell 109:719–731

Malek RL, Irby RB, Guo QM, Lee K, Wong S, He M, Tsai J, Frank B, Liu ET, Quackenbush J et al (2002) Identification of Src transformation fingerprint in human colon cancer. Oncogene 21:7256–7265

Manneras-Holm L, Kirchner H, Bjornholm M, Chibalin AV, Zierath JR (2015) mRNA expression of diacylglycerol kinase isoforms in insulin-sensitive tissues: effects of obesity and insulin resistance. Physiol Rep 3:e12372

Manneras-Holm L, Schonke M, Brozinick JT, Vetterli L, Bui HH, Sanders P, Nascimento EBM, Bjornholm M, Chibalin AV, Zierath JR (2017) Diacylglycerol kinase epsilon deficiency preserves glucose tolerance and modulates lipid metabolism in obese mice. J Lipid Res 58:907–915

Marchet A, Mocellin S, Belluco C, Ambrosi A, DeMarchi F, Mammano E, Digito M, Leon A, D'Arrigo A, Lise M, Nitti D (2007) Gene expression profile of primary gastric cancer: towards the prediction of lymph node status. Ann Surg Oncol 14:1058–1064

Martinez-Moreno M, Garcia-Lievana J, Soutar D, Torres-Ayuso P, Andrada E, Zhong XP, Koretzky GA, Merida I, Avila-Flores A (2012) FoxO-dependent regulation of diacylglycerol kinase alpha gene expression. Mol Cell Biol 32:4168–4180

McMurray HR, Sampson ER, Compitello G, Kinsey C, Newman L, Smith B, Chen SR, Klebanov L, Salzman P, Yakovlev A, Land H (2008) Synergistic response to oncogenic mutations defines gene class critical to cancer phenotype. Nature 453:1112–1116

Merida I, Avila-Flores A, Merino E (2008) Diacylglycerol kinases: at the hub of cell signalling. Biochem J 409:1–18

Merida I, Andrada E, Gharbi SI, Avila-Flores A (2015) Redundant and specialized roles for diacylglycerol kinases alpha and zeta in the control of T cell functions. Sci Signal 8:re6

Merida I, Torres-Ayuso P, Avila-Flores A, Arranz-Nicolas J, Andrada E, Tello-Lafoz M, Liebana R, Arcos R (2017) Diacylglycerol kinases in cancer. Adv Biol Regul 63:22–31

Merino E, Avila-Flores A, Shirai Y, Moraga I, Saito N, Merida I (2008) Lck-dependent tyrosine phosphorylation of diacylglycerol kinase alpha regulates its membrane association in T cells. J Immunol 180:5805–5815

Mertens J, Wang QW, Kim Y, Yu DX, Pham S, Yang B, Zheng Y, Diffenderfer KE, Zhang J, Soltani S et al (2015) Differential responses to lithium in hyperexcitable neurons from patients with bipolar disorder. Nature 527:95–99

Miller DJ, Jerga A, Rock CO, White SW (2008) Analysis of the *Staphylococcus aureus* DgkB structure reveals a common catalytic mechanism for the soluble diacylglycerol kinases. Structure 16:1036–1046

Monsalve M, Olmos Y (2011) The complex biology of FOXO. Curr Drug Targets 12:1322–1350

Moya PR, Murphy DL, McMahon FJ, Wendland JR (2010) Increased gene expression of diacylglycerol kinase eta in bipolar disorder. Int J Neuropsychopharmacol 13:1127–1128

Nascimento EBM, Manneras Holm L, Chibalin AV, Bjornholm M, Zierath JR (2017) Diacylglycerol kinase alpha deficiency alters inflammation markers in adipose tissue in response to high fat diet. J Lipid Res 59:273–282

Nelson CD, Perry SJ, Regier DS, Prescott SM, Topham MK, Lefkowitz RJ (2007) Targeting of diacylglycerol degradation to M1 muscarinic receptors by beta-arrestins. Science 315:663–666

Newton AC, Brognard J (2017) Reversing the paradigm: protein kinase C as a tumor suppressor. Trends Pharmacol Sci 38:438–447

Okkenhaug K, Bilancio A, Farjot G, Priddle H, Sancho S, Peskett E, Pearce W, Meek SE, Salpekar A, Waterfield MD et al (2002) Impaired B and T cell antigen receptor signaling in p110delta PI 3-kinase mutant mice. Science 297:1031–1034

Olenchock BA, Guo R, Carpenter JH, Jordan M, Topham MK, Koretzky GA, Zhong XP (2006a) Disruption of diacylglycerol metabolism impairs the induction of T cell anergy. Nat Immunol 7:1174–1181

Olenchock BA, Guo R, Silverman MA, Wu JN, Carpenter JH, Koretzky GA, Zhong XP (2006b) Impaired degranulation but enhanced cytokine production after Fc epsilonRI stimulation of diacylglycerol kinase zeta-deficient mast cells. J Exp Med 203:1471–1480

Olmez I, Love S, Xiao A, Manigat L, Randolph P, McKenna BD, Neal BP, Boroda S, Li M, Brenneman B et al (2018) Targeting the mesenchymal subtype in glioblastoma and other cancers via inhibition of diacylglycerol kinase alpha. Neuro-Oncology 20:192–202

Perez Y, Maffei M, Igea A, Amata I, Gairi M, Nebreda AR, Bernado P, Pons M (2013) Lipid binding by the unique and SH3 domains of c-Src suggests a new regulatory mechanism. Sci Rep 3:1295

Prinz PU, Mendler AN, Masouris I, Durner L, Oberneder R, Noessner E (2012) High DGK-alpha and disabled MAPK pathways cause dysfunction of human tumor-infiltrating CD8+ T cells that is reversible by pharmacologic intervention. J Immunol 188:5990–6000

Prinz PU, Mendler AN, Brech D, Masouris I, Oberneder R, Noessner E (2014) NK-cell dysfunction in human renal carcinoma reveals diacylglycerol kinase as key regulator and target for therapeutic intervention. Int J Cancer 135:1832–1841

Purow B (2015) Molecular pathways: targeting diacylglycerol kinase alpha in cancer. Clin Cancer Res 21:5008–5012

Quann EJ, Merino E, Furuta T, Huse M (2009) Localized diacylglycerol drives the polarization of the microtubule-organizing center in T cells. Nat Immunol 10:627–635

Rainero E, Caswell PT, Muller PA, Grindlay J, McCaffrey MW, Zhang Q, Wakelam MJ, Vousden KH, Graziani A, Norman JC (2012) Diacylglycerol kinase alpha controls RCP-dependent integrin trafficking to promote invasive migration. J Cell Biol 196:277–295

Riese MJ, Wang LC, Moon EK, Joshi RP, Ranganathan A, June CH, Koretzky GA, Albelda SM (2013) Enhanced effector responses in activated CD8+ T cells deficient in diacylglycerol kinases. Cancer Res 73:3566–3577

Rodriguez-Linares B, Walker T, Watson S (1991) The diacylglycerol kinase inhibitor, R59949, potentiates secretion but not increased phosphorylation of a 47 kDalton protein in human platelets. Biochem Pharmacol 41:835–838

Ruffo E, Malacarne V, Larsen SE, Das R, Patrussi L, Wulfing C, Biskup C, Kapnick SM, Verbist K, Tedrick P et al (2016) Inhibition of diacylglycerol kinase alpha restores restimulation-induced cell death and reduces immunopathology in XLP-1. Sci Transl Med 8:321ra327
Sakane F, Yamada K, Kanoh H, Yokoyama C, Tanabe T (1990) Porcine diacylglycerol kinase sequence has zinc finger and E-F hand motifs. Nature 344:345–348
Sanchez Chinchilla D, Pinto S, Hoppe B, Adragna M, Lopez L, Justa Roldan ML, Pena A, Lopez Trascasa M, Sanchez-Corral P, Rodriguez de Cordoba S (2014) Complement mutations in diacylglycerol kinase-epsilon-associated atypical hemolytic uremic syndrome. Clin J Am Soc Nephrol 9:1611–1619
Sanjuan MA, Jones DR, Izquierdo M, Merida I (2001) Role of diacylglycerol kinase alpha in the attenuation of receptor signaling. J Cell Biol 153:207–220
Sanjuan MA, Pradet-Balade B, Jones DR, Martinez AC, Stone JC, Garcia-Sanz JA, Merida I (2003) T cell activation in vivo targets diacylglycerol kinase alpha to the membrane: a novel mechanism for Ras attenuation. J Immunol 170:2877–2883
Shin JJ, Loewen CJ (2011) Putting the pH into phosphatidic acid signaling. BMC Biol 9:85
Shirai Y, Saito N (2014) Diacylglycerol kinase as a possible therapeutic target for neuronal diseases. J Biomed Sci 21:28
Shirai Y, Kouzuki T, Kakefuda K, Moriguchi S, Oyagi A, Horie K, Morita SY, Shimazawa M, Fukunaga K, Takeda J et al (2010) Essential role of neuron-enriched diacylglycerol kinase (DGK), DGKbeta in neurite spine formation, contributing to cognitive function. PLoS One 5: e11602
Simons M, Gault WJ, Gotthardt D, Rohatgi R, Klein TJ, Shao Y, Lee HJ, Wu AL, Fang Y, Satlin LM et al (2009) Electrochemical cues regulate assembly of the Frizzled/Dishevelled complex at the plasma membrane during planar epithelial polarization. Nat Cell Biol 11:286–294
Singh BK, Kambayashi T (2016) The immunomodulatory functions of diacylglycerol kinase zeta. Front Cell Dev Biol 4:96
Solimini NL, Luo J, Elledge SJ (2007) Non-oncogene addiction and the stress phenotype of cancer cells. Cell 130:986–988
Soto-Nieves N, Puga I, Abe BT, Bandyopadhyay S, Baine I, Rao A, Macian F (2009) Transcriptional complexes formed by NFAT dimers regulate the induction of T cell tolerance. J Exp Med 206:867–876
Stace CL, Ktistakis NT (2006) Phosphatidic acid- and phosphatidylserine-binding proteins. Biochim Biophys Acta 1761:913–926
Szendroedi J, Yoshimura T, Phielix E, Koliaki C, Marcucci M, Zhang D, Jelenik T, Muller J, Herder C, Nowotny P et al (2014) Role of diacylglycerol activation of PKCtheta in lipid-induced muscle insulin resistance in humans. Proc Natl Acad Sci U S A 111:9597–9602
Tabet R, Moutin E, Becker JA, Heintz D, Fouillen L, Flatter E, Krezel W, Alunni V, Koebel P, Dembele D et al (2016) Fragile X mental retardation protein (FMRP) controls diacylglycerol kinase activity in neurons. Proc Natl Acad Sci U S A 113:E3619–E3628
Takeishi K, Taketomi A, Shirabe K, Toshima T, Motomura T, Ikegami T, Yoshizumi T, Sakane F, Maehara Y (2012) Diacylglycerol kinase alpha enhances hepatocellular carcinoma progression by activation of Ras-Raf-MEK-ERK pathway. J Hepatol 57:77–83
Tam WL, Weinberg RA (2013) The epigenetics of epithelial-mesenchymal plasticity in cancer. Nat Med 19:1438–1449
Torres-Ayuso P, Daza-Martin M, Martin-Perez J, Avila-Flores A, Merida I (2014) Diacylglycerol kinase alpha promotes 3D cancer cell growth and limits drug sensitivity through functional interaction with Src. Oncotarget 5:9710–9726
Torres-Ayuso P, Tello-Lafoz M, Merida I, Avila-Flores A (2015) Diacylglycerol kinase-zeta regulates mTORC1 and lipogenic metabolism in cancer cells through SREBP-1. Oncogene 4: e164
Valdor R, Macian F (2013) Induction and stability of the anergic phenotype in T cells. Semin Immunol 25:313–320
Valinciute G, Weigel C, Veldwijk MR, Oakes CC, Herskind C, Wenz F, Plass C, Schmezer P, Popanda O (2017) BET-bromodomain inhibitors modulate epigenetic patterns at the

diacylglycerol kinase alpha enhancer associated with radiation-induced fibrosis. Radiother Oncol 125:168–174

van der Zanden LF, van Rooij IA, Feitz WF, Knight J, Donders AR, Renkema KY, Bongers EM, Vermeulen SH, Kiemeney LA, Veltman JA et al (2011) Common variants in DGKK are strongly associated with risk of hypospadias. Nat Genet 43:48–50

Veillette A, Perez-Quintero LA, Latour S (2013) X-linked lymphoproliferative syndromes and related autosomal recessive disorders. Curr Opin Allergy Clin Immunol 13:614–622

Verrier E, Wang L, Wadham C, Albanese N, Hahn C, Gamble JR, Chatterjee VK, Vadas MA, Xia P (2004) PPARgamma agonists ameliorate endothelial cell activation via inhibition of diacylglycerol-protein kinase C signaling pathway: role of diacylglycerol kinase. Circ Res 94:1515–1522

Weber H, Kittel-Schneider S, Gessner A, Domschke K, Neuner M, Jacob CP, Buttenschon HN, Boreatti-Hummer A, Volkert J, Herterich S et al (2011) Cross-disorder analysis of bipolar risk genes: further evidence of DGKH as a risk gene for bipolar disorder, but also unipolar depression and adult ADHD. Neuropsychopharmacology 36:2076–2085

Weigel C, Veldwijk MR, Oakes CC, Seibold P, Slynko A, Liesenfeld DB, Rabionet M, Hanke SA, Wenz F, Sperk E et al (2016) Epigenetic regulation of diacylglycerol kinase alpha promotes radiation-induced fibrosis. Nat Commun 7:10893

Wheeler ML, Dong MB, Brink R, Zhong XP, DeFranco AL (2013) Diacylglycerol kinase zeta limits B cell antigen receptor-dependent activation of ERK signaling to inhibit early antibody responses. Sci Signal 6:ra91

Woodham EF, Machesky LM (2014) Polarised cell migration: intrinsic and extrinsic drivers. Curr Opin Cell Biol 30:25–32

Yanagisawa K, Yasuda S, Kai M, Imai S, Yamada K, Yamashita T, Jimbow K, Kanoh H, Sakane F (2007) Diacylglycerol kinase alpha suppresses tumor necrosis factor-alpha-induced apoptosis of human melanoma cells through NF-kappaB activation. Biochim Biophys Acta 1771:462–474

Yang J, Seo J, Nair R, Han S, Jang S, Kim K, Han K, Paik SK, Choi J, Lee S et al (2011) DGKiota regulates presynaptic release during mGluR-dependent LTD. EMBO J 30:165–180

Yang E, Singh BK, Paustian AM, Kambayashi T (2016) Diacylglycerol kinase zeta is a target to enhance NK cell function. J Immunol 197:934–941

You JS, Lincoln HC, Kim CR, Frey JW, Goodman CA, Zhong XP, Hornberger TA (2014) The role of diacylglycerol kinase zeta and phosphatidic acid in the mechanical activation of mammalian target of rapamycin (mTOR) signaling and skeletal muscle hypertrophy. J Biol Chem 289:1551–1563

Young BP, Shin JJ, Orij R, Chao JT, Li SC, Guan XL, Khong A, Jan E, Wenk MR, Prinz WA et al (2010) Phosphatidic acid is a pH biosensor that links membrane biogenesis to metabolism. Science 329:1085–1088

Zamani A, Decker C, Cremasco V, Hughes L, Novack DV, Faccio R (2015) Diacylglycerol kinase zeta (DGKzeta) is a critical regulator of bone homeostasis via modulation of c-Fos levels in osteoclasts. J Bone Miner Res 30:1852–1863

Zeng Z, Wang T, Li T, Li Y, Chen P, Zhao Q, Liu J, Li J, Feng G, He L, Shi Y (2011) Common SNPs and haplotypes in DGKH are associated with bipolar disorder and schizophrenia in the Chinese Han population. Mol Psychiatry 16:473–475

Zha Y, Marks R, Ho AW, Peterson AC, Janardhan S, Brown I, Praveen K, Stang S, Stone JC, Gajewski TF (2006) T cell anergy is reversed by active Ras and is regulated by diacylglycerol kinase-alpha. Nat Immunol 7:1166–1173

Zheng Y, Zha Y, Driessens G, Locke F, Gajewski TF (2012) Transcriptional regulator early growth response gene 2 (Egr2) is required for T cell anergy in vitro and in vivo. J Exp Med 209:2157–2163

Zheng Y, Zha Y, Spaapen RM, Mathew R, Barr K, Bendelac A, Gajewski TF (2013) Egr2-dependent gene expression profiling and ChIP-Seq reveal novel biologic targets in T cell anergy. Mol Immunol 55:283–291

Functions of Nuclear Polyphosphoinositides

Manuel Olazabal-Morán, Ana González-García, and Ana C. Carrera

Contents

Abstract

Despite interest in phosphoinositide (PtdIns) kinases, such as PtdIns 3 kinases (PI3K), as targets for controlling plasma membrane PtdIns levels in disease, the PtdIns have another less well-known site of action in the cell nucleus.

Recent studies show that PtdIns use a variety of strategies to alter DNA responses. Here, we provide an overview of these newly identified forms of gene expression control, which should be considered when studying the therapeutic use of PtdIns-directed compounds. As PI3K is one of the most important clinical targets in recent years, we will focus on two polyphosphoinositides, the PI3K substrate PtdIns(4,5)di-phosphate (PI4,5P_2) and its product PtdIns(3,4,5)tri-phosphate (PI3,4,5P_3).

M. Olazabal-Morán · A. González-García · A. C. Carrera (✉)
Department of Immunology and Oncology, Centro Nacional de Biotecnología/CSIC, Madrid, Spain
e-mail: acarrera@cnb.csic.es

J. Gomez-Cambronero, M. A. Frohman (eds.), *Lipid Signaling in Human Diseases*, Handbook of Experimental Pharmacology 259, https://doi.org/10.1007/164_2019_219

Keywords
Chromatin remodeling · Gene expression · Lipid transport proteins · Nuclear lipids · Nuclear phosphoinositide · Phosphoinositide transport proteins · $PI3,4,5P_3$ · PI3K · $PI4,5P_2$

1 Phosphoinositide 3-Kinase Enzymes: An Overview

The PtdIns are a subset of phospholipids with inositol, a hydrophilic cyclic polyalcohol, in the third carbon of diacylglycerol. The inositol polar head can be phosphorylated at positions 3, 4, and 5, giving rise to seven possible PtdIns with diverse cellular functions. The distinct organelles of the cell each have a unique lipid composition that includes a specific set of PtdIns.

PtdIns are components of the plasma membrane (PM) lipid bilayer. The classical pathways regulated by these lipids act at the PM or in the cytosol. At the PM, phosphorylated PtdIns trigger recruitment of signaling proteins with PtdIns-binding domains, thereby initiating the signaling cascades needed to induce cell responses. Protein domains that recognize PtdIns include the pleckstrin homology (*PH*), PX (phagocytic oxidase; phox), PHD (plant homeodomain), and FERM (four-point-one, ezrin, radixin, moesin) domains. Arrays of lysines and arginines also mediate PtdIns binding (Shah et al. 2013). Although some PtdIns-initiated signaling cascades affect transcription factor (TF) function in the nucleus, these regulatory cascades were initially reported in the cytosol; for example, the PI3K effector AKT (also termed PKB) phosphorylates the FOXO TF and triggers its cytosolic retention (Fig. 1) and, therefore, its functional inactivation (Alvarez et al. 2001).

PI3K enzymes transfer phosphate to the 3 OH-position of the inositol ring of membrane PtdIns. Depending on their structure and substrate preference, they are classified as class I, II, or III. Class I PI3Ks are heterodimeric enzymes composed of a p110 catalytic and either a p85-like regulatory subunit (p85α, p55α, p50α, p85β, p55γ) (class I_A) or a distinct, unrelated p101 or p87 regulatory partner (class I_B). The *PIK3CA*, *PIK3CB*, *PIK3CC*, and *PIK3CD* genes encode four very similar p110 catalytic subunits (PI3Kα, PI3Kβ, PI3Kγ, and PI3Kδ). The class I PI3K catalytic subunits use $PI4,5P_2$ as their preferred substrate in vivo. Class I PI3Ks are activated by growth factor receptors (tyrosine kinase and G protein-coupled receptors) and regulate cell survival, division, migration, and metabolism (reviewed in García et al. 2006; Vanhaesebroeck et al. 2010).

Class II PI3Ks produce phosphatidylinositol 3-phosphate (PI3P) in vivo, the same product generated by class III PI3K. The distinct proteins that bind to class II or class III PI3K and the distinct subcellular localization of these molecules confer specificity on these two classes (Vanhaesebroeck et al. 2010). The class II PI3K catalytic subunits (PI3K-C2α, PI3K-C2β, and PI3K-C2γ) are large enzymes ($>$170 kDa) composed of an extended N-terminal region and a C-terminal region with a PX and a C2 (similar to PKC-C2) domain; they lack associated regulatory subunits. The mechanism of PI3K-C2 activation is poorly known; these enzymes control processes

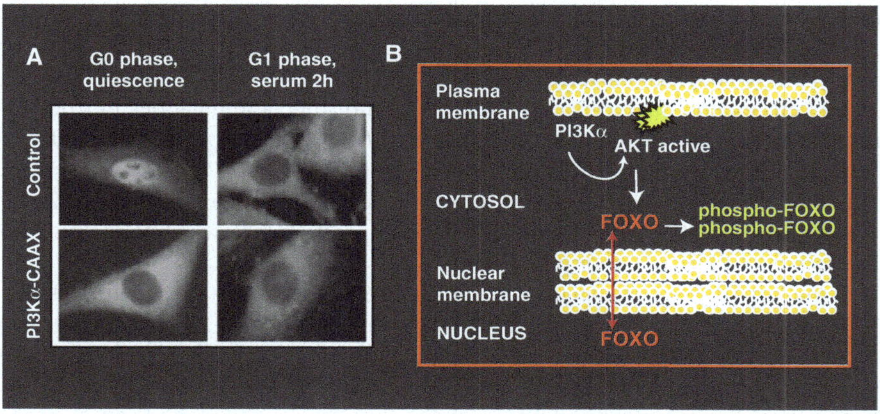

Fig. 1 FOXO transcription factors are inactivated by PI3K/AKT. (**a**) Representative immunofluorescence staining of the FOXO transcription factor (TF) FKHRL1 in NIH3T3 cells, control or expressing the constitutive active form of PI3Kα (PI3Kα-CAAX). NIH3T3 cells are arrested in G0 and are untreated or treated with serum for 2 h (G1). In control cells, FKHRL1 is located in the nucleus in G0 and accumulates in the cytosol after serum addition. Constitutive activation of PI3K triggers FKHRL1 cytosolic retention, even in the absence of stimulus (adapted from Alvarez et al. 2001). (**b**) Scheme showing the steps for PI3K/AKT control of FOXO TF localization. In quiescence, FOXO TF concentrates in the nucleus; following PI3K activation by serum or by PI3K-α-CAAX expression, AKT is activated and phosphorylates FOXO TF, which is retained in the cytosol by association to 14-3-3 proteins

such as endocytosis, exocytosis, and autophagy (Di Paolo and De Camilli 2006; Falasca and Maffucci 2012; Devereaux et al. 2013).

The class III PI3K, Vps34, was first identified in yeast. Vps34 only modifies PtdIns and is probably responsible for producing most of the cellular PI3P in the endosomal compartment. Vps34 forms a heterodimer with the vesicular protein-sorting protein Vps15p. Glucose, amino acids, G protein-coupled receptors, and several large multimolecular complexes activate the Vps34/Vps15p dimer, which is conserved across eukaryotes. Vps34 participates in the regulation of vesicle traffic/protein sorting and in induction of autophagy (Lindmo and Stenmark 2006; Funderburk et al. 2010; Devereaux et al. 2013; Carpentier et al. 2013).

The products of class I (p110), class II (PI3K-C2), and class III PI3K (Vps34) are found in the nucleus. A number of kinases and phosphatases regulate formation of other PtdIns, some of which also have nuclear functions (see below). In addition, phosphorylated inositols, generated by phospholipase (PLC)-mediated cleavage of PtdIns, have been shown to regulate nuclear processes and are reviewed elsewhere (Monserrate and York 2010).

2 Phosphoinositide Enzymes in Human Disease

Class I PI3K enzymes enhance glycolysis, cell survival, division, and migration; cancer cells exploit these capacities through gain-of-function mutations in *PIK3CA* and *PIK3R1* or loss-of-function mutations in *PTEN,* the phosphatase that reduces PI3,4,$5P_3$ levels. The combined frequency of *PIK3CA*, *PIK3R1*, and *PTEN* mutations in cancer cells is slightly less than that of the tumor suppressor *TP53* (Kandoth et al. 2013; Martincorena and Campbell 2015), which indicates the importance of PI3K in tumor progression.

In the last 10 years, tremendous effort has been directed to implementing class I PI3K inhibitors for clinical use; the advances and limitations of these treatments were recently reviewed by Fruman et al. (2017). In brief, PI3K-directed compounds are active as inhibitors in vivo and have been useful for treating some cancer types. Nonetheless, the complexity of PI3K feedback pathways and acquisition of resistance necessitate a continued search for optimal therapeutic combinations for most tumor types.

PI3K inhibitors have also been useful in the treatment of several recently defined *overgrowth syndromes* caused by activation of the class I PI3K pathway. These include the CLOVES syndrome (congenital lipomatous overgrowth, vascular malformation, and epidermal nevi and skeletal anomalies), which is caused by activating *PIK3CA*, *TORC1*, or *S6K* mutations; APDS (activated PI3Kδ syndrome), caused by *PIK3CD* gain of function; and APDS2, caused by *PIK3R1* mutations (Fruman et al. 2017).

In addition to diseases that arise from PI3,4,$5P_3$ homeostasis defects, some *human neuropathies and myopathies* are linked to germ-line mutations in the PI3P phosphatase myotubularin or in the PI3P 5-kinase FAB1 (reviewed in Nicot and Laporte 2008). Vps34 has been implicated in *schizophrenia*, whereas Vps34, PI3K-C2α, and PI3K-C2β are linked to cell survival and growth in some *cancer* types (reviewed in Di Paolo and De Camilli 2006) (Table 1).

The enzymes that control PtdIns turnover are potential targets for several human diseases. Knowledge of PtdIns function in the nucleus could help to predict the in vivo action of inhibitory compounds that target PtdIns substrates or products.

3 PI4,5P2 and PI3,4,5P3 in the Nucleus

Given the amphipathic nature of phospholipids, their localization to sites other than a lipid bilayer is puzzling. PtdIns in solution generally form micelles, with their hydrophobic regions interacting with each other and the hydrophilic polar heads facing the aqueous phase. In addition to PtdIns, nuclear membranes and nucleoplasm contain other hydrophobic or amphipathic lipids such as fatty acids, sterols, and sphingosines, which indicates that these lipids find mechanisms for solubilization (Hamann and Blind 2018).

The presence of PI4,$5P_2$ in the nucleus has long been known (reviewed in Martelli et al. 2004; Cocco et al. 1988). Immunofluorescence (IF) experiments

Table 1 Selected human diseases related to phosphoinositide-modifying enzymes

Disease	Gene	Enzyme	Function	PtdIns substrate	PtdIns product
Lowe syndrome	*OCRL1* (Attree et al. 1992)	5-Phosphatase	Phosphatase	PI 4,5P2	PI 4P
Schizophrenia and bipolar disorders	*PIK3C3* (Stopkova et al. 2004)	VPS34	Kinase	PI PI 4P	PI 3P PI3,4P2
Myotubular myopathy	*MTM1* (Laporte et al. 1996)	Myotubularin 1	Phosphatase	PI 3P PI 3,5P2	PI PI 5P
Charcot-Marie-tooth type 4B1 neuropathy	*MTMR2* (Bolino et al. 2000)	Myotubularin-related protein 2	Phosphatase	PI 3P PI 3,5P2	PI PI 5P
Cancer (combined gene alterations ≈30%)	*PIK3CA* (rev. in Liu et al. 2009)	Class I PI3K p110α	Kinase	PI 4,5P2	PI 3,4,5P3
	PIK3R1 (rev. in Liu et al. 2009)	Class I PI3K p85α	Regulatory	PI 4,5P2	PI3,4,5P3
	PTEN (rev. in Liu et al. 2009)	PI3,4,5P3 phosphatase	Phosphatase	PI 3,4,5P3	PI4,5P2
CLOVES syndrome[a]	*PIK3CA* (Kurek et al. 2012)	Class I PI3K p110α	Kinase	PI 4,5P2	PI 3,4,5P3
APDS[b]	*PIK3CD* (Angulo et al. 2013)	Class I PI3K p110δ	Kinase	PI 4,5P2	PI3,4,5P3
APDS2[c]	*PIK3R1* (Dornan et al. 2017)	Class I PI3K p85α	Regulatory	PI 4,5P2	PI3,4,5P3

[a]Congenital lipomatous overgrowth-vascular malformation-epidermal nevi-spinal anomaly syndrome
[b]Activated PI3K-delta syndrome
[c]Activated PI3K-delta syndrome 2

showed that this lipid localizes not only to the nuclear membrane but also to the internal region at locations compatible with chromatin and interchromatin domains. $PI4,5P_2$ concentrates in nuclear speckles, structures that are found in chromatin and are enriched in mRNA-splicing and export factors as well as PtdIns enzymes, and in which mRNA modification takes place (Boronenkov et al. 1998; Smith et al. 1999). Many of the enzymes that participate in the classic PtdIns cycle, including kinases necessary for synthesis of $PI4,5P_2$, PtdIns-PLC, and DAG (diacylglycerol) kinase, are also found in the nucleus; the $PI4,5P_2$ effector PLCβ1 controls DNA replication, differentiation, and resumption of meiosis (Martelli et al. 2004).

$PI3,4,5P_3$ localization to the nucleus was more difficult to show than that of $PI4,5P_2$. Whereas IF staining of $PI4,5P_2$ gives a prominent signal in the nuclear membrane and the nuclear matrix, IF using anti-$PI3,4,5P_3$ antibodies yields only a modest specific signal, with a punctate pattern at the nuclear membrane and a few dots in the chromatin. This signal is less extended than that of $PI4,5P_2$ (Fig. 2) (Kumar et al. 2010; Redondo-Muñoz et al. 2015). The nuclear $PI3,4,5P_3$ signal was tested using specific inhibitors; in the case of DNA damage, specificity was suggested by the precise localization of PI3Kβ and a $PI3,4,5P_3$-specific PH domain confined to the site of DNA damage (Fig. 2) (Kumar et al. 2010; Redondo-Muñoz et al. 2015).

Nuclear extracts obtained after nuclear membrane digestion have PI3K activity (Kim 1998). High performance liquid chromatography detection of fatty acid specimens of $PI4,5P_2$ and $PI3,4,5P_3$ from purified nuclear extracts showed high levels of $PI4,5P_2$, at least 10^3 times those of its $PI3,4,5P_3$ counterpart, similar to levels in the PM. Nuclear $PI3,4,5P_3$ is increased following growth factor receptor stimulation [our unpublished observations]. Assays using nuclear extracts nonetheless do not distinguish external nuclear membrane (or closely attached endoplasmic reticulum; ER) from a true intranuclear location. Localization of the of PI3K class I_A regulatory subunit p85 (Zini et al. 1996; Lu et al. 1998; Neri et al. 1999) gives a pattern similar to that of anti-$PI3,4,5P_3$ (Kumar et al. 2010), which supports the presence of a small amount of $PI3,4,5P_3$ in the nucleus.

PIKE (PI3K enhancer) is a brain-specific nuclear GTPase that concentrates around the nuclear envelope. An elegant set of experiments in neuronal cells showed that after *NGF* (neuronal growth factor) treatment, *PIKE* associates with and activates nuclear PI3K (p85/p110 complexes), thereby affecting cyclin D1 expression in response to NGF (Ye et al. 2000). *PIKE* activation of nuclear PI3K might act in a manner similar to Ras in cytosolic PI3K. *NGF* treatment also promotes 4.1N translocation to the nucleus with later kinetics than PI3K activation; PIKE binding to 4.1N reduces nuclear PI3K activation in neurons, showing that PIKE upregulates nuclear PI3K transiently (Ye et al. 2000).

Additional evidence for $PI3,4,5P_3$ in the nuclear matrix was obtained by on-section labeling with the purified PH domain of GRP1 ($PI3,4,5P_3$-specific), followed by quantitative electron microscopy. This analysis showed intense labeling of the PM, which was more discreet at nuclear membranes, and an even lower $PI3,4,5P_3$ signal in the nuclear matrix (Lindsay et al. 2006). *IPMK* (inositol polyphosphate multikinase) is a nuclear enzyme able to phosphorylate soluble inositols as well as $PI4,5P_2$ (to produce $PI3,4,5P_3$); IPMK is insensitive to PI3K inhibitors (Resnick et al. 2005). As both pools of nuclear $PI3,4,5P_3$ detected with GRP1-PH were sensitive to PI3K inhibitors, the authors concluded that nuclear $PI3,4,5P_3$ is not produced by IPMK (Lindsay et al. 2006). Only $PI3,4,5P_3$ membrane pools were regulated by PTEN (Lindsay et al. 2006), which indicates that it acts optimally only at membrane surfaces or that inner nuclear $PI3,4,5P_3$ might be masked to PTEN action.

Whereas a large amount of $PI4,5P_2$ is found at the nuclear envelope and nuclear matrix, only a small amount of $PI3,4,5P_3$ is detected in the nucleus, similar to the

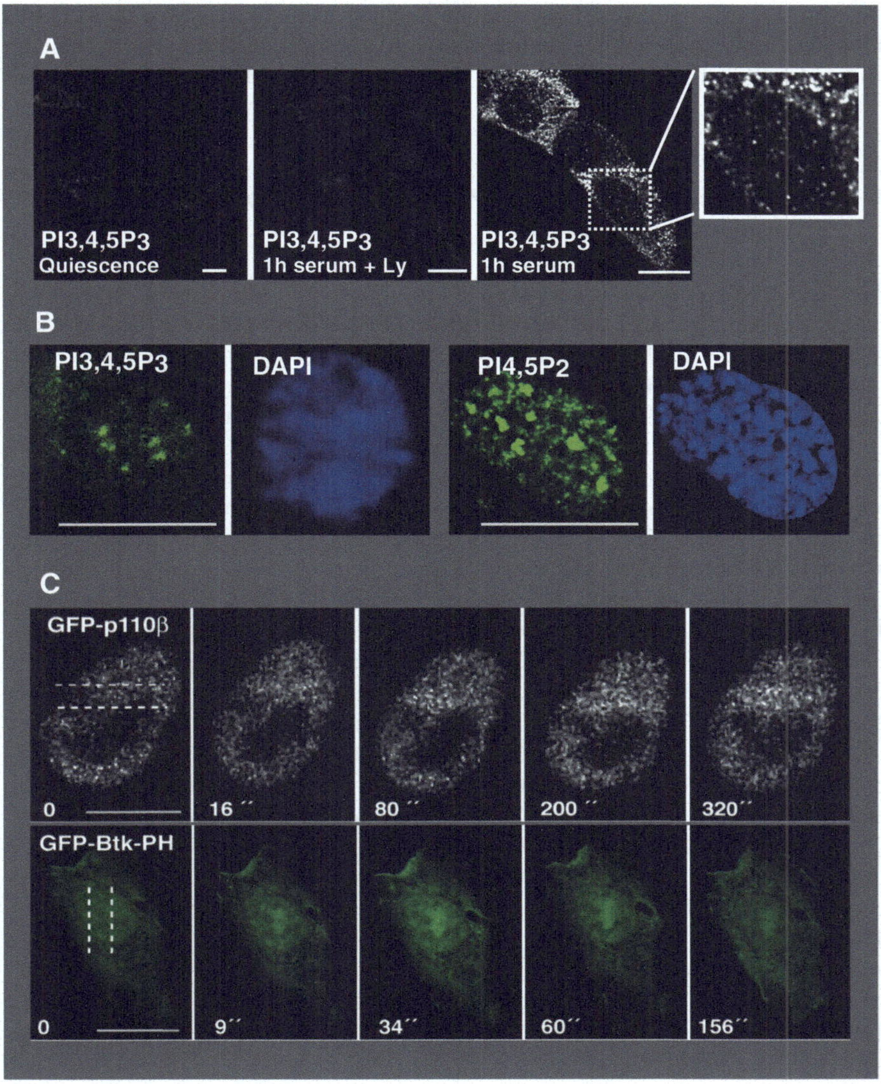

Fig. 2 PI3,4,5P$_3$ signal in the nucleus. (**a**) NIH3T3 cells were incubated without serum (16 h) and then serum-activated for 1 h or were pretreated with the pan-PI3K inhibitor Ly294002 (Ly; 10 μM) prior to serum activation. Cells were stained with anti-PI3,4,5P$_3$ antibody; representative sections. Bars, 12 μm (adapted from Redondo-Muñoz et al. 2015). (**b**) NIH3T3 cells were irradiated (5 Gy); 30 cells were examined with anti-PI3,4,5P$_3$ or anti-PI4,5P$_2$ antibodies and DAPI. Bars, 15 μm. (**c**) Real-time GFP (green fluorescent protein)-PI3Kβ or GFP-Btk-PH translocation to the DNA damage region. NIH3T3 cells expressing GFP-PI3Kβ (top row) were micro-irradiated with a UV laser; dotted lines indicate laser paths. Bottom, GFP-Btk-PH-transfected U2OS cells (24 h) were micro-irradiated and examined as above. Bars, 15 μm. (**a–c**) Immunofluorescence, GFP and DNA (DAPI) signals were examined by confocal microscopy (Kumar et al. 2010)

$PI4,5P_2$/$PI3,4,5P_3$ ratios in plasma membrane. It remains unclear how these PtdIns solubilize in the inner nucleus, but recent observations of phosphoinositide-binding protein function might help understand how these lipids localize to the nucleoplasm.

4 Phospholipid-Binding Proteins Solubilize Lipids in Aqueous Phases

The distinct cell organelles each have a unique lipid composition (including different PtdIns species). In many cases, these lipids cannot be transported from one organelle to another in vesicles. Lipid transport proteins (LTPs) have come to be considered as players in lipid homeostasis and signal transduction. A number of recent reports describe the role of LTP in promoting lipid exchange between different organelles.

Lipids tend to be hydrophobic or amphipathic, and LTPs can accommodate a lipid molecule within a hydrophobic pocket and bear it from one membrane to another through the aqueous phase. As an example of exchange between the *ER* and the *PM,* several LTPs were found to transport lipids at close membrane contact sites (MCS) between these subcellular compartments. LTP are grouped in families according to their structure; these include the SEC14 (*Saccharomyces cerevisiae* 14)-like, StAR-related lipid transfer domain (START), glycolipid-transfer proteins (GLTP), sterol carrier protein 2 (SCP2), oxysterol-binding proteins (OSBP), oxysterol-related proteins (ORP), extended synaptotagmins, and tubular lipid-binding proteins (TULIP) (Balla 2005; D'Angelo et al. 2008; Alva and Lupas 2016).

A subfamily of the LTPs are those that transfer PtdIns (PITPs). The PITPs bind preferentially to PtdIns in its hydrophobic pocket and show structural conservation that permits their classification as mainly SEC14- or START-like proteins (Nile et al. 2010). Several studies highlight the contribution of PITPs to cell physiology. For instance, Lees et al. (2017) reported a new function for TMEM24, an ER protein that concentrates at ER-PM contact sites where it contacts the two lipid bilayers. TMEM24 belongs to the family of TULIP LTPs, which have a lipid-binding domain with preferential affinity for PtdIns. TMEM24 transports PtdIns from its synthesis site in the ER to the PM, where it is transformed into $PI4,5P_2$ and $PI3,4,5P_3$. TMEM24 capacity to replenish PtdIns at the PM is essential for control of insulin secretion (Lees et al. 2017).

TIPE proteins (tumor necrosis factor-alpha-induced protein 8) are lipid-binding proteins; they have a lipid-binding pocket reminiscent of the LTP lipid-binding domain. This TH (TIPE2 homology) domain accommodates $PI4,5P_2$ and $PI3,4,5P_3$. TIPE3 expression is increased in various tumor types and its over-expression promotes tumorigenesis. TIPE3 localizes in the cytosol and promotes transfer of $PI4,5P_2$ to the PM, and it enhances PI3K activation after PDGF (platelet-derived growth factor) addition by facilitating $PI4,5P_2$ phosphorylation by class I PI3K (Fayngerts et al. 2014). For this activity, TIPE3 requires its lipid-binding pocket and an acidic N-terminal region (Fayngerts et al. 2014). TIPE3 therefore acts as a soluble $PI4,5P_2$ carrier that is able to transfer poly-PtdIns to the PM (Fig. 3).

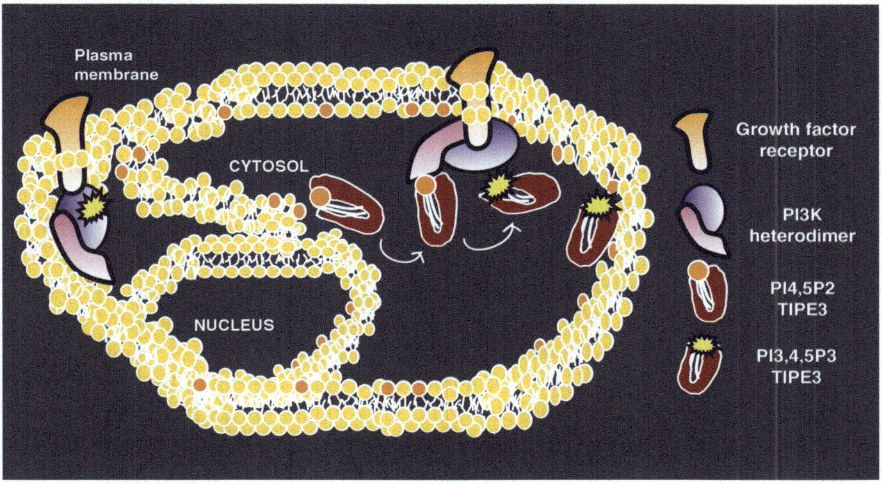

Fig. 3 TIPE3 acts as a soluble $PI4,5P_2$ and $PI3,4,5P_3$ carrier and is able to transfer poly-PtdIns to the plasma membrane. Scheme showing the role of TIPE3 protein, which is able to bind $PI4,5P_2$ and $PI3,4,5P_3$. TIPE3 binding to $PI4,5P_2$ facilitates class I_A PI3K action and increases $PI3,4,5P_3$ levels at PM (Fayngerts et al. 2014). One of the nuclear membranes is omitted for clarity

Although TIPE3 acts primarily at the PM, the homologous *TIPE2* molecule localizes in the nucleus and can act in a similar manner there (Goldsmith and Chen 2017).

These findings show that hydrophobic and amphipathic lipids can be found not only in lipid bilayers but also in complex with lipid transport proteins that solubilize them in aqueous phases.

5 Phosphoinositide-Binding Proteins Control Gene Expression

Several nuclear proteins have been found to interact with $PI4,5P_2$. Among these are RNA polymerase I (Pol I) (Yildirim et al. 2013), the polyadenylate polymerase Star-PAP (Mellman et al. 2008), and nuclear receptors such as steroidogenic factor 1 (SF-1 or NR5A1) or liver receptor homolog 1 (LRH-1 or NR5A2), which bind $PI4,5P_2$ and other PtdIns (Krylova et al. 2005; Blind et al. 2014).

Pol I transcription is essential for ribosome biogenesis and thus for cell cycle progression, cell growth, and protein synthesis in eukaryotes. Initiation of transcription by Pol I requires formation of a complex between the TATA-binding protein (TBP) and three TBP-associated factors specific for Pol I; this complex is termed SL1 (selective factor 1). Ribosomal RNA (rRNA) transcription is driven by Pol I after binding to the *UBF* (upstream binding factor) and the SL1 complex at the rDNA enhancer region (Hempel et al. 1996). $PI4,5P_2$ binds to UBF in complex with Pol I and enhances rRNA transcription. $PI4,5P_2$ also binds directly to fibrillarin (Fib), a pre-rRNA processing factor, and co-localizes with nascent transcripts in the nucleolus. $PI4,5P_2$ binding to UBF and Fib governs their respective binding to DNA and RNA and thereby regulates RNA Pol I transcription (Yildirim et al. 2013).

mRNA maturation involves its modification following transcription. One of these modifications is the addition of a chain of adenosines at its 3′ end; polyadenylation enhances mRNA stability. mRNA adenylation is induced by polyadenylate polymerases (PAP). Mellman et al. (2008) reported that noncanonical *Star-PAP* (speckle targeted PIPKIalpha regulated-poly(A) polymerase), which modifies a specific set of mRNAs, is regulated by $PI4,5P_2$ in the nucleus. PIPKIα, a PI4P 5-kinase that triggers PI4P conversion to $PI4,5P_2$, interacts and co-localizes with *Star-PAP* at nuclear speckles; the activity of Star-PAP is regulated by $PI4,5P_2$ binding (Mellman et al. 2008). Thus, $PI4,5P_2$ by regulating Star-PAP controls mRNA polyadenylation and stabilization.

The steroidogenic factor 1 (SF-1) is a nuclear receptor important for the control of adrenal and reproductive organ development. *SF-1* mutations are the basis of several human monogenic disorders. SF-1 binds $PI4,5P_2$; mutations that affect SF-1 lipid-binding pocket result in reduced transcriptional activity (Sablin et al. 2009), showing that $PI4,5P_2$ binding regulates SF-1 transcriptional activity. Like the TIPE proteins, SF-1 envelops the phospholipid, leaving the head group exposed. In the case of SF-1, IPMK, but not class I PI3K, converts the *SF-1*-bound $PI4,5P_2$ into $PI3,4,5P_3$. Silencing of IPMK, or overexpression of PTEN, reduces *SF-1* transcriptional activity (Blind et al. 2012). This indicates that $PI3,4,5P_3$ binding to *SF-1* enhances its activity. As IPMK is expressed predominantly in fetal organs (brain, heart, liver), this mechanism might be critical during embryonic development.

With respect to nuclear proteins that bind $PI3,4,5P_3$ directly, several proteomic analyses using solid-bound, micelle-bound PtdIns, or activity probes have identified a number of DNA regulatory proteins that bind to and might be regulated by $PI3,4,5P_3$ (Zhu et al. 2001; Bidlingmaier and Liu 2007; Catimel et al. 2009; Gallego et al. 2010; Rowland et al. 2011; Jungmichel et al. 2014). Only a few of these candidates have been examined in detail; functional studies are needed for each of these to demonstrate that $PI3,4,5P_3$ binding controls their activities.

ALY (ally of AML-1 and LEF-1) is a $PI3,4,5P_3$-binding nuclear protein that localizes to nuclear speckles and is implicated in mRNA export. $PI3,4,5P_3$ binding is necessary for correct *ALY* localization at nuclear speckles. Both Akt-mediated phosphorylation of ALY and its binding to $PI3,4,5P_3$ reduce mRNA export (Okada et al. 2008), which shows that ALY binding to $PI3,4,5P_3$ modulates mRNA export. The role of $PI3,4,5P_3$ in enhancing mRNA export is supported by additional studies (Quaresma et al. 2013; Redondo-Muñoz et al. 2015).

Nucleophosmin/*NPM/B23* is a major nucleolar phosphoprotein with an essential role in ribosome biogenesis. NPM is a multifunctional protein found in nucleoli. It moves between the nucleus and cytoplasm and has additional functions outside of nucleoli (reviewed in Grisendi et al. 2006). In nucleoli, NPM endoribonuclease activity processes the 32S rRNA precursor to the 28S mature rRNA, and as a chaperone, it can prevent rRNA and ribosomal protein aggregation; in addition, NPM transports ribosomal subunits to the cytoplasm (Grisendi et al. 2006). By associating directly with Arf in nucleoli, NPM also regulates the p53 pathway

(Grisendi et al. 2006). NPM recruits the ubiquitin-specific protease USP36 to nucleoli, where it regulates the levels of several nucleolar proteins (Endo et al. 2009). In addition to ribosome biogenesis control, NPM acts as an anti-apoptotic molecule in several cellular settings; in PC12 neuronal cells, it mediates the NFG anti-apoptotic effect by inhibiting DNA fragmentation by caspase-activated DNase. NPM binds to PI3,4,5P_3, and prevention of this binding eliminates the anti-apoptotic effect of NFG in the nucleus (Ahn et al. 2005).

These observations show that RNA polymerase I and Star-PAP, among other enzymes, are regulated by PI4,5P_2 binding, whereas the actions of the mRNA export protein ALY, the nuclear receptor *SF-1*, and nucleophosmin are controlled by binding to PI3,4,5P_3. In several cases, these PtdIns-binding proteins have a structural pocket that accommodates the hydrophobic head of PtdIns and thus resemble the structure of LTPs. This mechanism probably enables poly-PtdIns transport through the nucleus. Binding of these PtdIns within these pockets facilitates their solubility in the inner nucleus.

The larger amount of PI4,5P_2 in the nucleoplasm compared to that of PI3,4,5P_3 supports the idea that the former could bind to a larger number of effectors or to a more common protein partner than PI3,4,5P_3. It remains to be determined whether PI4,5P_2 functions in the nuclear matrix in regions distinct from nuclear speckles.

6 PI5P Action in Gene Expression Control

In addition to PI3,4,5P_3 and PI4,5P_2, other PtdIns have been shown to control gene expression. This is the case for PI5P. The *ING* (inhibitor of growth) are nuclear adaptor proteins with tumor suppressor functions; they have a highly conserved PHD motif that binds to PI5P. ING2 functions as a core component of the chromatin remodeling complex Sin3a-HDAC1, which explains many ING2 actions such as p53 regulation or histone acetylation in response to cell stress. UV irradiation blocks PI5P conversion to PI4,5P_2 via p38 kinase-mediated attenuation of 4-kinase (PIP4K2B) activity; this leads to an increase in PI5P levels. The increase in nuclear PI5P enhances ING2 association with chromatin (Jones et al. 2006).

The basal transcription complex component *TAF3* (TBP-associated factor 3) also responds to PI5P binding. Analysis of TAF3 mutants that do not bind PI5P show that they are able to promote expression of only a fraction of the TAF3 target genes during myocyte differentiation (Stijf-Bultsma et al. 2015), suggesting that PI5P binding to TAF3 regulates the specificity of TAF3-regulated promoters.

UHRF1 (ubiquitin-like with PHD and RING finger domains 1) is an E3 ubiquitin ligase that binds to specific DNA sequences and recruits a histone deacetylase at these sites; *UHRF1* is upregulated in various tumors. *UHRF1* is important for G1 > S transition, as it controls topoisomerase IIa and retinoblastoma protein expression. Nuclear PI5P also regulates access of the trimethylated lysine residue of histone 3 (H3K9me3) to UHRF1 (Gelato et al. 2014).

These findings indicate that specific PtdIns are able to modulate gene expression; this is the case for PI5P, which regulates association of various gene expression regulators with chromatin.

7 Phosphoinositide Actions in Chromatin Remodeling

DNA wraps around histone octamers (formed by two sets of H2A, H2B, H3, and H4 histones) to form the basic unit of the chromatin, the nucleosome. Nucleosome arrays are further packaged into more compact DNA structures. Histone 1 occupies the space between nucleosomes and contributes to chromatin compaction. The different proteins that bind or act on DNA must gain access to the nucleic acid through at least two mechanisms, modification of histones or alteration of chromatin structure through ATP-consuming DNA remodeling complexes. In this section, we discuss the role of PtdIns in chromatin remodeling.

The first hint as to how phospholipids alter chromatin structure came from electron microscopy studies showing that phospholipid addition alters nuclear ultrastructure (Maraldi et al. 1984). In the case of PtdIns, PI4P and $PI4,5P_2$ were reported to be among the phospholipids that can be obtained from purified nuclei and whose levels change following growth factor addition or stress induction (reviewed in Shah et al. 2013). Several mechanisms have recently been described that highlight PtdIns action in chromatin structure.

One of the first findings to suggest potential PtdIns action on chromatin was that $PI4,5P_2$ binds to histones H1 and H3 in vitro. As histone H1 reduces transcription, the authors tested the effect of adding $PI4,5P_2$ in a transcription assay; $PI4,5P_2$ binding to histone H1 (like histone H1 phosphorylation) released its transcriptional inhibition in vitro (Yu et al. 1998). PTEN also binds histone H1, thereby helping to maintain a closed chromatin conformation, although this does not require its $PI3,4,5P_3$ phosphatase activity (Chen et al. 2014).

Several chromatin remodeling complexes in yeast, *Drosophila*, and mammals contain actin and actin-related proteins; the role of actin in these complexes is not known. The mammalian *SWI/SNF*-like *BAF* chromatin remodeling complex component *BRG1* (Brahma-related gene 1) binds to $PI4,5P_2$ in micelles; $PI4,5P_2$ in turn enhances actin recruitment to BAF complexes in vitro (Rando et al. 2002). These results identify the BAF complex as a possible mediator of matrix localization for $PI4,5P_2$; the physiological formation of these complexes in cells remains to be determined.

IPMK is an enzyme that phosphorylates multiple sites on the inositol phosphate ring and generates $PI3,4,5P_3$ from $PI4,5P_2$ in the nucleus (Resnick et al. 2005). IPMK acts as a transcriptional coactivator by binding the histone acetyltransferase CBP (CREB-binding protein); it regulates histone modification, transcriptional regulation of nuclear receptors, and mRNA export (Hamann and Blind 2018). For these functions, IPMK might use the inositol phosphates or $PI4,5P_2$ conversion to $PI3,4,5P_3$. $PI4,5P_2$ action in open chromatin compartments is supported by localization of *PLCβ1* (which has a $PI4,5P_2$-specific PH domain) at DNA replication sites and its capacity to trigger DNA synthesis (Poli et al. 2016). These observations support PLCβ1 action (and potentially that of its product $PI4,5P_2$) in DNA replication.

p85α (class I_A PI3K regulatory subunit) associates with *BRD7* (bromodomain-containing protein 7), a PBAF (polybromo-associated BAF)-specific SWI/SNF subunit with many cell functions that include regulation of p53-mediated p21 transcription and gene activation (or repression) in embryonic stem cells. Whereas *BRD7/p85α* complex formation triggers p85α nuclear entry and reduces cytosolic PI3K activity, in cells that lack p85α and/or p85β, BRD7 is still able to induce p21 expression (Chiu et al. 2014). p85 is thus dispensable for BRD7 regulatory function in p53 transcriptional activity.

PI3Kβ is a class I_A PI3K isoform that generates $PI3,4,5P_3$ in response to growth factor receptor stimulation (tyrosine kinase as well as G protein-coupled receptors). In contrast to PI3Kα, which is mainly cytosolic, PI3Kβ has an NLS (nuclear localization signal) and can localize to the nucleus in complex with p85β (Kumar et al. 2011). PI3Kβ depletion markedly reduces DNA synthesis in S phase and DNA homologous recombination after double-strand DNA breakage (Marqués et al. 2009; Kumar et al. 2010). Assembly of a functional DNA damage response therefore requires expression of a nuclear PI3Kβ (a cytosolic PI3Kβ mutant does not rescue survival in *PIK3CB*-depleted cells) (Kumar et al. 2011). Inhibition (rather than depletion) of PI3Kβ also reduces DNA synthesis and repair, which suggests that both PI3Kβ kinase activity and scaffold function facilitate these events (Fig. 4). PI3Kβ also regulates chromosome segregation and nuclear envelope formation in an activity- and scaffold-dependent manner (Silió et al. 2012; Redondo-Muñoz et al. 2015). These studies show that the PI3Kβ scaffold functions controls DNA events through PI3Kβ-specific binding to protein partners such as PCNA and NBS1 (Redondo-Muñoz et al. 2014). How PI3Kβ-activity contributes to these events remains to be elucidated. Both PI3Kβ-associated proteins and kinase activity thus control DNA synthesis and repair.

In prostate cancer cells, PI3Kβ inhibition and depletion reduce androgen receptor-triggered histone H3 Lys4 dimethylation (H3K4me2), a modification associated with transcriptional activation (Pang et al. 2017). The capacity of PI3Kβ kinase activity to regulate H3K4me2 levels provides a mechanism for $PI3,4,5P_3$ action in chromatin remodeling in prostate cancer cells.

H3K4me2/H3K4me3 also increases in breast tumors driven by an activated *PIK3CA* (PI3Kα) allele (Spangle et al. 2016). The authors reported that AKT phosphorylates the H3K4-demethylase *KDM5A* and induces its cytoplasmic localization, thereby increasing H3K4me2/H3K4me3 nuclear levels (Spangle et al. 2016). Both PI3Kα and PI3Kβ thus increase the H3K4me2 associated with transcriptional activation.

The anionic head group of $PI4,5P_2$ and $PI3,4,5P_3$ bound to DNA regulatory enzymes could help displace the histones (cationic), which would provide enzyme access to the DNA. Poly-PtdIns interaction with histones has been shown to occur in vitro (Lete et al. 2014). Using turbidimetric studies, these authors showed that different isolated histone preparations including H1, H2AH2B, H3H4, and histone

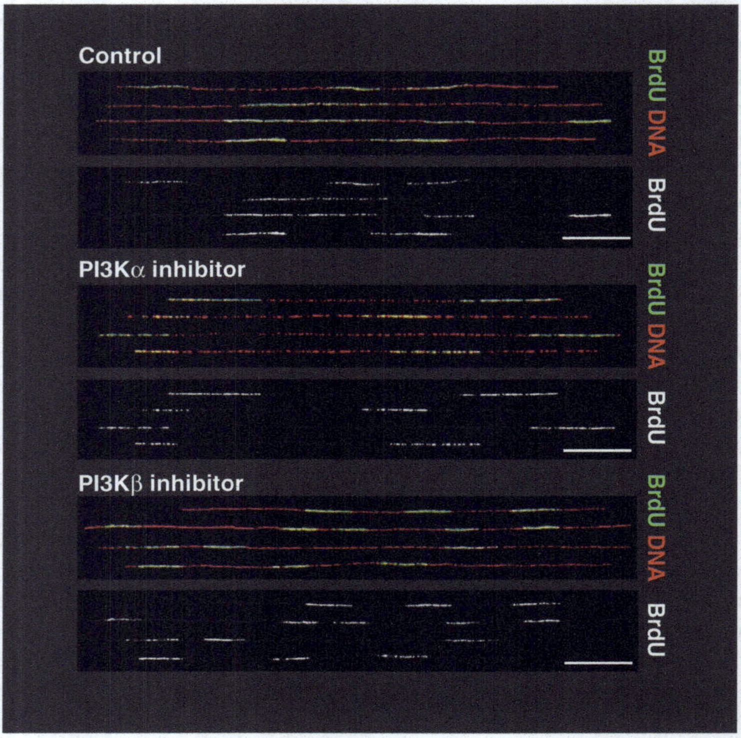

Fig. 4 Inhibition of class I_A PI3Kβ reduces DNA synthesis. G0-synchronized NIH3T3 cells treated with PI3Kα (PIK75) or PI3Kβ (TGX221) inhibitors were pulse-labeled (20 min) with BrdU and collected. DNA replication was tested by single-molecule analysis using genomic DNA fiber extraction; fibers were stretched by DNA combing, and newly replicated DNA was detected by immunofluorescence with an anti-BrdU antibody (green); DNA fibers were counterstained with anti-DNA antibody (red). Representative fibers are shown. Bar, 50 Kb (from Marqués et al. 2009)

octamers led to dose-dependent aggregation of phosphatidylcholine vesicles containing the negatively charged phospholipids PIP or PI. Aggregation was observed even when vesicles contained as little as 5% PIP (a larger proportion of PI was needed for aggregation). DNA addition disassembled the histone-PIP vesicle aggregates (Lete et al. 2014). These results suggest that a complex interplay of histones, DNA, and PtdIns could take place in the nucleoplasm. The authors propose that this might occur at nuclear envelope invaginations, although whether these interactions occur in vivo is still not known.

These reports support the concept that $PI4,5P_2$ and $PI3,4,5P_3$ modulate chromatin structure. In the case of $PI4,5P_2$, these changes take place through its direct binding to histones or to chromatin remodeling complexes, or when it is produced by PLCβ1 (which triggers DNA replication). In the case of $PI3,4,5P_3$, the data support an effect on DNA structure including alteration of H3K4me2 levels by PI3Kα and PI3Kβ activities, as well as a contribution by PI3Kβ nuclear activity in DNA replication and repair.

8 Concluding Remarks

Taken together, these observations show that a number of interactions between nuclear proteins and poly-PtdIns take place in the nucleoplasm. Considering the amphipathic nature of PtdIns, these lipids should not reside spontaneously (by themselves) in the nucleoplasm. They can nonetheless localize to the inner nucleus in microvesicles, associated to lipid-binding proteins, or by penetrating the nucleus in nuclear membrane invaginations that reach the chromatin (Fig. 5). In the latter case, PtdIns in membrane invaginations could associate with chromatin at close contact sites. The observation that $PI4,5P_2$ binds to histones H1 and H3, and that histone combinations can induce aggregation of PI- or PIP-containing lipid vesicles (which are disassembled by DNA), suggests that by sequestering histones from DNA, PtdIns could facilitate accessibility of PtdIns-bound DNA regulators to DNA. The large amount of $PI4,5P_2$ detected in the nucleoplasm by IF supports that this lipid might solubilize bound to an abundant nuclear protein (actin, histone, etc.).

Although future studies could rule out some of these possibilities, these lipids clearly appear to regulate gene expression. This is shown by $PI4,5P_2$ capacity to modulate RNA pol I-mediated transcription, to bind Star-PAP and thus control mRNA polyadenylation/stabilization, and to increase the transcriptional activity of nuclear receptors *SF-1* or LRH-1. In the case of $PI3,4,5P_3$, this regulation is suggested by its control of mRNA export and nucleoplasmin action on rRNA synthesis.

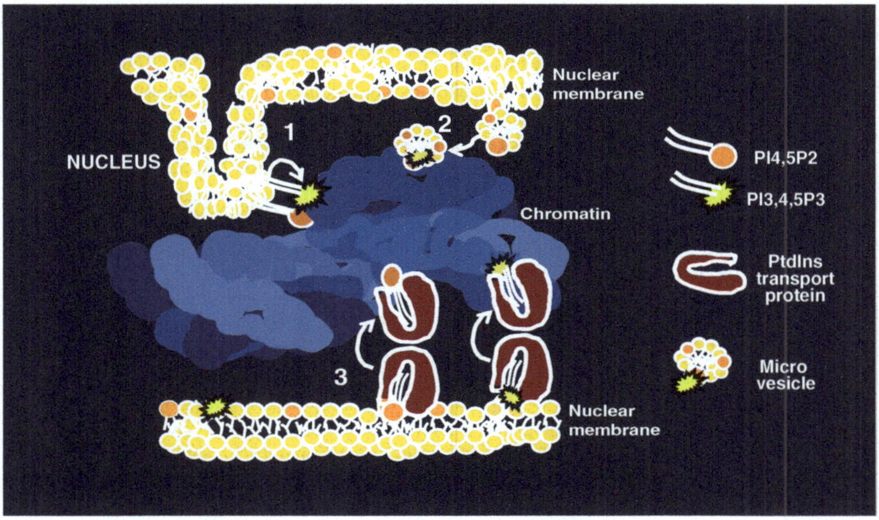

Fig. 5 Models for PtdIns localization in the nucleoplasm. Due to their amphipathic nature, PtdIns do not reside spontaneously in the nucleoplasm. They can localize in the inner nucleus through several mechanisms: (1) inclusion in nuclear membrane invaginations that reach the chromatin in the nucleoplasm; (2) entry into deep nuclear sites via microvesicles; or (3) association to PtdIns transfer proteins

$PI4,5P_2$'s ability to bind histone 1 and enhance transcription, or to bind the SWI/SNF-like BAF remodeling complex to induce actin recruitment, supports a role for $PI4,5P_2$ in the control of chromatin conformation. $PI3,4,5P_3$ also regulates chromatin conformation, as indicated by the increase in DNA transcriptional activity via histone modifications (such as H3K4me2/H3K4me3) mediated by PI3Kα and PI3Kβ kinase activities; in addition, PI3Kβ activity enhances processes that need an open DNA chromatin conformation (such as replication and double-strand DNA break repair).

PI5P also regulates gene expression, as it controls tumor suppressor ING2 association to chromatin, it modulates promoter occupancy by basal transcription complex, and it induces binding of inactive chromatin regions (with the H3K9me3 mark) to UHRF1-histone deacetylases. Whereas PI5P action in chromatin organization is well characterized, the functions of nuclear of $PI3,4,5P_3$ and $PI4,5P_2$ require further research. The studies described here show that these lipids assist in the control of chromatin structure and of gene expression, which should be considered in the context of therapies that modify PtdIns levels.

References

Ahn JY, Liu X, Cheng D et al (2005) Nucleophosmin/B23, a nuclear PI (3,4,5)P3 receptor, mediates the antiapoptotic actions of NGF by inhibiting CAD. Mol Cell 18:435–445

Alva V, Lupas AN (2016) The TULIP superfamily of eukaryotic lipid-binding proteins as a mediator of lipid sensing and transport. Biochem Biophys Acta 1861:913–923

Alvarez B, Martínez-A C, Burgering B et al (2001) Forkhead transcription factors contribute to the execution of the mitotic program in mammals. Nature 413:744–747

Angulo I, Vadas O, Garçon F et al (2013) Phosphoinositide 3-kinase δ gene mutation predisposes to respiratory infection and airway damage. Science 342:866–871

Attree O, Olivos IM, Okabe I et al (1992) The Lowe's oculocerebrorenal syndrome gene encodes a protein highly homologous to inositol polyphosphate-5-phosphatase. Nature 358:239–242

Balla T (2005) Inositol-lipid binding motifs: signal integrators through protein-lipid and protein-protein interactions. J Cell Sci 118:2093–2104

Bidlingmaier S, Liu B (2007) Interrogating yeast surface-displayed human proteome to identify small molecule-binding proteins. Mol Cell Proteomics 11:2012–2020

Blind RD, Suzawa M, Ingraham HA (2012) Direct modification and activation of a nuclear receptor-PIP2 complex by the inositol lipid kinase IPMK. Sci Signal 5:ra44

Blind RD, Sablin EP, Kuchenbecker KM et al (2014) The signaling phospholipid PIP3 creates a new interaction surface on the nuclear receptor SF-1. Proc Natl Acad Sci U S A 111:15054–15059

Bolino A, Muglia M, Conforti FL et al (2000) Charcot-Marie-Tooth type 4B is caused by mutations in the gene encoding myotubularin-related protein-2. Nat Genet 25:17–19

Boronenkov IV, Loijens JC, Umeda M et al (1998) Phosphoinositide signaling pathways in nuclei are associated with nuclear speckles containing pre-mRNA processing factors. Mol Biol Cell 9:3547–3560

Carpentier S, N'Kuli F, Grieco G et al (2013) Class III phosphoinositide 3-kinase/VPS34 and dynamin are critical for apical endocytic recycling. Traffic 14:933–948

Catimel B, Yin MX, Schieber C et al (2009) PI(3,4,5)P3 interactome. J Proteome Res 8:3712–3726

Chen ZH, Zhu M, Yang J et al (2014) PTEN interacts with histone H1 and controls chromatin condensation. Cell Rep 8:2003–2014

Chiu YH, Lee JY, Cantley LC (2014) BRD7, a tumor suppressor, interacts with p85α and regulates PI3K activity. Mol Cell 54:193–202
Cocco L, Martelli AM, Gilmour RS et al (1988) Rapid changes in phospholipid metabolism in the nuclei of Swiss 3T3 cells induced by treatment of the cells with insulin-like growth factor I. Biochem Biophys Res Commun 154:1266–1272
D'Angelo G, Vicinanza M, De Matteis MA (2008) Lipid-transfer proteins in biosynthetic pathways. Curr Opin Cell Biol 20:360–370
Devereaux K, Dall'Armi C, Alcazar-Roman A et al (2013) Regulation of mammalian autophagy by class II and III PI 3-kinases through PI3P synthesis. PLoS One 8:e76405
Di Paolo G, De Camilli P (2006) Phosphoinositides in cell regulation and membrane dynamics. Nature 443:651–657
Dornan GL, Siempelkamp BD, Jenkins ML et al (2017) Conformational disruption of PI3Kδ regulation by immunodeficiency mutations in PIK3CD and PIK3R1. Proc Natl Acad Sci U S A 118:1982–1987
Endo A, Kitamura N, Komada M (2009) Nucleophosmin/B23 regulates ubiquitin dynamics in nucleoli by recruiting deubiquitylating enzyme USP36. J Biol Chem 284:27918–27923
Falasca M, Maffucci T (2012) Regulation and cellular functions of class II phosphoinositide 3-kinases. Biochem J 443:587–601
Fayngerts SA, Wu J, Oxley CL et al (2014) TIPE3 is the transfer protein of lipid second messengers that promote cancer. Cancer Cell 26:465–478
Fruman DA, Chiu H, Hopkins BD et al (2017) The PI3K pathway in human disease. Cell 170:605–635
Funderburk SF, Wang QJ, Yue Z (2010) The Beclin 1-VPS34 complex--at the crossroads of autophagy and beyond. Trends Cell Biol 20:355–362
Gallego O, Betts MJ, Gvozdenovic-Jeremic J et al (2010) A systematic screen for protein-lipid interactions in *Saccharomyces cerevisiae*. Mol Syst Biol 6:430
García Z, Kumar A, Marqués M et al (2006) PI3K controls early and late events in mammalian cell division. EMBO J 25:655–661
Gelato KA, Tauber M, Ong MS et al (2014) Accessibility of different histone H3-binding domains of UHRF1 is allosterically regulated by phosphatidylinositol 5-phosphate. Mol Cell 54:905–919
Goldsmith JR, Chen YH (2017) Regulation of inflammation and tumorigenesis by the TIPE family of phospholipid transfer proteins. Cell Mol Immunol 14:482–487
Grisendi S, Mecucci C, Falini B et al (2006) Nucleophosmin and cancer. Nat Rev Cancer 6:493–505
Hamann BL, Blind RD (2018) Nuclear phosphoinositide regulation of chromatin. J Cell Physiol 233:107–123
Hempel WM, Cavanaugh AH, Hannan RD et al (1996) The species-specific RNA polymerase I transcription factor SL-1 binds to upstream binding factor. Mol Cell Biol 16:557–563
Jones DR, Bultsma Y, Keune WJ et al (2006) Nuclear PtdIns5P as a transducer of stress signaling: an in vivo role for PIP4Kbeta. Mol Cell 23:685–695
Jungmichel S, Sylvestersen KB, Choudhary C et al (2014) Specificity and commonality of the phosphoinositide-binding proteome analyzed by quantitative mass spectrometry. Cell Rep 6:578–591
Kandoth C, McLellan MD, Vandin F et al (2013) Mutational landscape and significance across 12 major cancer types. Nature 502:333–339
Kim SJ (1998) Insulin rapidly induces nuclear translocation of PI3-kinase in HepG2 cells. Biochem Mol Biol Int 46:187–196
Krylova IN, Sablin EP, Moore J et al (2005) Structural analyses reveal phosphatidyl inositols as ligands for the NR5 orphan receptors SF-1 and LRH-1. Cell 120:343–355
Kumar A, Fernadez-Capetillo O, Carrera AC (2010) Nuclear phosphoinositide 3-kinase beta controls double-strand break DNA repair. Proc Natl Acad Sci U S A 107:7491–7496

Kumar A, Redondo-Muñoz J, Perez-García V et al (2011) Nuclear but not cytosolic phosphoinositide 3-kinase beta plays an essential function in cell survival. Mol Cell Biol 31:2122–2133
Kurek KC, Luks VL, Ayturk UM et al (2012) Somatic mosaic activating mutations in PIK3CA cause CLOVES syndrome. Am J Hum Genet 90:1108–1115
Laporte J, Hu LJ, Kretz C et al (1996) A gene mutated in X-linked myotubular myopathy defines a new putative tyrosine phosphatase family conserved in yeast. Nat Genet 13:175–182
Lees JA, Messa M, Sun EW et al (2017) Lipid transport by TMEM24 at ER-plasma membrane contacts regulates pulsatile insulin secretion. Science 355(6326):eaah6171
Lete MG, Sot J, Ahyayauch H et al (2014) Histones and DNA compete for binding polyphosphoinositides in bilayers. Biophys J 106:1092–1100
Lindmo K, Stenmark H (2006) Regulation of membrane traffic by phosphoinositide 3-kinases. J Cell Sci 119:605–614
Lindsay Y, McCoull D, Davidson L et al (2006) Localization of agonist-sensitive PtdIns(3,4,5)P3 reveals a nuclear pool that is insensitive to PTEN expression. J Cell Sci 119:5160–5168
Liu P, Cheng H, Roberts TM et al (2009) Targeting the phosphoinositide 3-kinase pathway in cancer. Nat Rev Drug Discov 8:627–644
Lu PJ, Hsu AL, Wang DS et al (1998) Phosphoinositide 3-kinase in rat liver nuclei. Biochemistry 37:5738–5745
Maraldi NM, Capitani S, Caramelli E et al (1984) Conformational changes of nuclear chromatin related to phospholipid induced modifications of the template availability. Adv Enzym Regul 22:447–464
Marqués M, Kumar A, Poveda AM et al (2009) Specific function of phosphoinositide 3-kinase beta in the control of DNA replication. Proc Natl Acad Sci U S A 106:7525–7530
Martelli AM, Manzoli L, Cocco L (2004) Nuclear inositides: facts and perspectives. Pharmacol Ther 101:47–64
Martincorena I, Campbell PJ (2015) Somatic mutation in cancer and normal cells. Science 349:1483–1489
Mellman DL, Gonzales ML, Song C et al (2008) A PtdIns4,5P2-regulated nuclear poly (A) polymerase controls expression of select mRNAs. Nature 451:1013–1017
Monserrate JP, York JD (2010) Inositol phosphate synthesis and the nuclear processes they affect. Curr Opin Cell Biol 22:365–373
Neri LM, Martelli AM, Borgatti P et al (1999) Increase in nuclear phosphatidylinositol 3-kinase activity and phosphatidylinositol (3,4,5) trisphosphate synthesis precede PKC-f translocation to the nucleus of NGF-treated PC12 cells. FASEB J 13:2299–2310
Nicot AS, Laporte J (2008) Endosomal phosphoinositides and human diseases. Traffic 9:1240–1249
Nile AH, Bankaitis VA, Grabon A (2010) Mammalian diseases of phosphatidylinositol transfer proteins and their homologs. Clin Lipidol 5:867–897
Okada M, Jang SW, Ye K (2008) Akt phosphorylation and nuclear phosphoinositide association mediate mRNA export and cell proliferation activities by ALY. Proc Natl Acad Sci U S A 105:8649–8654
Pang J, Yang YW, Huang Y et al (2017) p110β inhibition reduces histone H3K4 Di-methylation in prostate cancer. Prostate 77:299–308
Poli A, Billi AM, Mongiorgi S et al (2016) Nuclear phosphatidylinositol signaling: focus on phosphatidylinositol phosphate kinases and phospholipases C. J Cell Physiol 231:1645–1655
Quaresma AJ, Sievert R, Nickerson JA (2013) Regulation of mRNA export by the PI3 kinase/AKT signal transduction pathway. Mol Biol Cell 24:1208–1221
Rando OJ, Zhao K, Janmey P et al (2002) Phosphatidylinositol-dependent actin filament binding by the SWI/SNF-like BAF chromatin remodeling complex. Proc Natl Acad Sci U S A 99:2824–2829
Redondo-Muñoz J, Pérez-García V, Carrera AC (2014) Phosphoinositide 3-kinase beta: when a kinase is more than a kinase. Trends Cell Mol Biol 8:83–92

Redondo-Muñoz J, Pérez-García V, Rodríguez MJ et al (2015) Phosphoinositide 3-kinase beta protects nuclear envelope integrity by controlling RCC1 localization and ran activity. Mol Cell Biol 35:249–263

Resnick AC, Snowman AM, Kang B et al (2005) Inositol polyphosphate multikinase is a nuclear PI3-kinase with transcriptional regulatory activity. Proc Natl Acad Sci U S A 102:12783–12788

Rowland MM, Bostic HE, Gong D et al (2011) Phosphatidylinositol 3,4,5-trisphosphate activity probes for the labeling and proteomic characterization of protein binding partners. Biochemistry 50:11143–11161

Sablin EP, Blind RD, Krylova IN et al (2009) Structure of SF-1 bound by different phospholipids: evidence for regulatory ligands. Mol Endocrinol 23:25–34

Shah ZH, Jones DR, Sommer L et al (2013) Nuclear phosphoinositides and their impact on nuclear functions. FEBS J 280:6295–6310

Silió V, Redondo-Muñoz J, Carrera AC (2012) Phosphoinositide 3-kinase beta regulates chromosome segregation in mitosis. Mol Biol Cell 23:4526–4542

Smith KP, Moen PT, Wydner KL et al (1999) Processing of endogenous pre-mRNAs in association with SC-35 domains is gene specific. J Cell Biol 144:617–629

Spangle JM, Dreijerink KM, Groner AC et al (2016) PI3K/AKT signaling regulates H3K4 methylation in breast cancer. Cell Rep 15:2692–2704

Stijf-Bultsma Y, Sommer L, Tauber M et al (2015) The basal transcription complex component TAF3 transduces changes in nuclear phosphoinositides into transcriptional output. Mol Cell 58:453–467

Stopkova P, Saito T, Papolos DF et al (2004) Identification of PIK3C3 promoter variant associated with bipolar disorder and schizophrenia. Biol Psychiatry 55:981–988

Vanhaesebroeck B, Guillermet-Guibert J, Graupera M et al (2010) The emerging mechanisms of isoform-specific PI3K signalling. Nat Rev Mol Cell Biol 11:329–341

Ye K, Hurt KJ, Wu FY et al (2000) Pike. A nuclear gtpase that enhances PI3kinase activity and is regulated by protein 4.1N. Cell 103:919–930

Yildirim S, Castano E, Sobol M et al (2013) Involvement of phosphatidylinositol 4,5-bisphosphate in RNA polymerase I transcription. J Cell Sci 126:2730–2739

Yu H, Fukami K, Watanabe Y et al (1998) Phosphatidylinositol 4,5-bisphosphate reverses the inhibition of RNA transcription caused by histone H1. Eur J Biochem 251:281–287

Zhu H, Bilgin M, Bangham R et al (2001) Global analysis of protein activities using proteome chips. Science 293:2101–2105

Zini N, Ognibene A, Bavelloni A et al (1996) Cytoplasmic and nuclear localization sites of phosphatidylinositol 3-kinase in human osteosarcoma sensitive and multidrug-resistant Saos-2 cells. Histochem Cell Biol 106:457–464

Part IV

Bioactive Lipids in Health and Disease

Platelet-Activating Factor as an Effector for Environmental Stressors

Jeffrey B. Travers

Contents

Abstract

Environmental stressors exert a profound effect on humans. Many environmental stressors have in common the ability to induce reactive oxygen species. The goal of this chapter is to present evidence that the potent lipid mediator platelet-activating factor (PAF) is involved in the effects of many stressors ranging from cigarette smoke to ultraviolet B radiation. These environmental stressors can generate PAF enzymatically as well as PAF-like lipids produced by free radical-mediated attack of glycerophosphocholines. Inasmuch as PAF exerts both

J. B. Travers (✉)
Department of Pharmacology and Toxicology, Wright State University, Dayton, OH, USA

Dayton Veterans Administration Medical Center, Dayton, OH, USA
e-mail: jeffrey.travers@wright.edu

J. Gomez-Cambronero, M. A. Frohman (eds.), *Lipid Signaling in Human Diseases*, Handbook of Experimental Pharmacology 259, https://doi.org/10.1007/164_2019_218

acute inflammation and delayed immunosuppressive effects, involvement of the PAF system can provide an explanation for many consequences of environmental stressor exposures.

Keywords
Immunosuppression · Microvesicle particles · Platelet-activating factor · Reactive oxygen species · Skin · Ultraviolet radiation

1 Introduction

Environmental influences upon the human host are profound. For example, ultraviolet radiation from sunlight not only is needed for plant photosynthesis, but ultraviolet B radiation (UVB) is necessary for human vitamin D synthesis (Wacker and Holick 2013; Leitenberger et al. 2007). Yet, many environmental agents exert pro-carcinogenic effects. In particular, UVB is responsible for the majority of skin cancers, including malignant melanoma (Leitenberger et al. 2007; Ullrich 2005). Polycyclic aromatic hydrocarbons (e.g., benzo[a]pyrene) found in coal tar and in the atmosphere from combustion of petrochemicals and wood have also been demonstrated to be both a mutagen and highly carcinogenic (Ramesh et al. 2004; Haritash and Kaushik 2009). It should be noted that the polycyclic aromatic hydrocarbons were among the first agents associated with cancer from the increased incidence of scrotal carcinomas among British chimney sweepers in the 1700s. Other pro-carcinogenic environmental agents from sunlight to cigarette smoke have also been shown to induce immunosuppression (Walterscheid et al. 2002; Wolf et al. 2006; Zhang et al. 2008; Sahu et al. 2013; Ferracini et al. 2015). The exact mechanisms through which environmental stressors generate both beneficial and injurious outcomes remain under active investigation.

Though environmental agents are a heterogeneous group, many agents with harmful effects have in common the ability to generate and/or bind to reactive oxygen species (ROS). As will be detailed in this review, the class of glycerophosphocholine-based lipid mediators collectively known as platelet-activating factor (PAF) can serve effectors between many pro-oxidative stressors and the human host. In particular, PAF agonists have the ability to be produced rapidly in response to numerous stimuli that have in common ROS and/or cell membrane disruption. PAF agonists generate both an early pro-inflammatory and a delayed immunosuppressive response, which provides many opportunities for them to serve as effectors for environmental agents, especially pro-oxidative stressors.

2 PAF Generation

PAF is the term coined by Jacques Benveniste and colleagues in the early 1970s to the substance released by activated leukocytes that induced platelet aggregation (Benveniste et al. 1972). The structure of this activity was elucidated in 1979 and found to be a glycerophosphocholine with a short-chained fatty acid at the *sn-2* position (Demopoulos et al. 1979). With respect to structure-activity relationships, maximal PAF activity is observed when a long-chained saturated fatty acid (hexadecyl or octadecyl) is at the *sn-1* position and a short-chained saturated fatty acid (usually acetate) is at the *sn-2* position. Glycerophosphocholines with *sn-1* acyl groups have approximately 1–10% of the biological activity of the alkyl-containing species (Demopoulos et al. 1979; Braquet et al. 1987). Regarding *sn-2* species, a 3-carbon ester appears to be as potent as a 2-carbon one, with decreased activity for 4- or 5-carbon *sn-2* species.

2.1 Enzymatic Synthesis

PAF is synthesized enzymatically via two distinct pathways (Braquet et al. 1987; Nakanishi et al. 2006; Shimizu 2009; Morimoto et al. 2010). The remodeling pathway (see Fig. 1), which is associated with cellular stimulation from a variety of sources, consists of PLA_2 (often cytosolic PLA_2) followed by an acetyl-CoA-dependent acetyltransferase (LPCAT) that acetylates a lyso-PAF intermediate to form PAF. Two LPCATs have been implicated in PAF biosynthesis, with LPCAT1 more constitutively active and LPCAT2 more associated with inflammatory cells (Shimizu 2009; Morimoto et al. 2010). Cellular stimuli that activate PAF biosynthesis via the remodeling pathway usually do so through induction of intracellular calcium mobilization. The ability of PAF to be generated rapidly in response

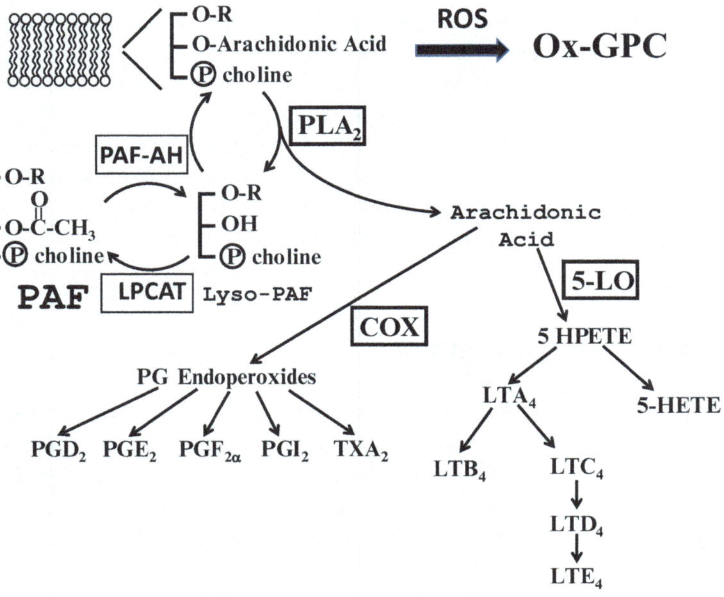

Fig. 1 Biosynthesis of PAF and eicosanoids via the remodeling pathway

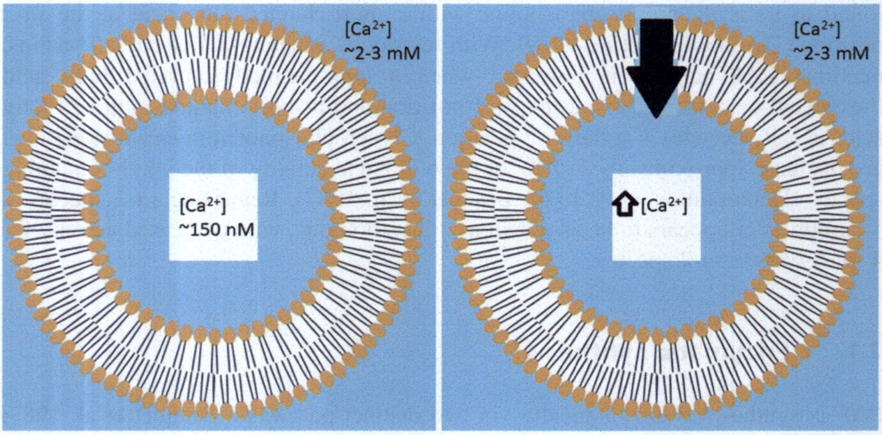

Fig. 2 Model for how acute damage elevates intracellular calcium levels. Resting intracellular Ca^{2+} levels are at least 10,000× lower than extracellular levels. Disruption of the cellular membrane results in an increase in intracellular Ca^{2+} that then activates numerous enzymes including phospholipases that can stimulate eicosanoids and PAF

to intracellular calcium provides an important mechanism through which a cell can respond rapidly to disruption of the cellular membrane, which creates a >10,000-fold gradient from extracellular calcium at millimolar levels to intracellular calcium which is 100–250 nanomolar. As shown in Fig. 2, damage to cellular membranes can serve as a rapid mechanism to increase levels of PAF agonists. Many cellular receptors, including G-protein-coupled receptors such as the PAF receptor, can also stimulate PAF biosynthesis (Travers et al. 1996).

PAF can also be synthesized through a de novo pathway that consists of three enzymes: 1-alkyl-2-lyso-sn-glycero-3-phosphate (alkyllyso-GP):acetyl-CoA acetyltransferase, 1-alkyl-2-acetyl-sn-glycero-3-phosphate phosphohydrolase, and 1-alkyl-2-acetyl-sn-glycerol (alkylacetyl-G):CDP-choline cholinephosphotransferase. This de novo pathway appears to be constitutively active, although it can be further stimulated by phorbol esters (Shimizu 2009; Snyder et al. 1996).

2.2 Nonenzymatic Synthesis

PAF agonists can also be generated nonenzymatically via direct attack of free radicals on the *sn-2* long-chained unsaturated fatty acids in glycerophosphocholines (Marathe et al. 2001; Konger et al. 2008). Oxidation of esterified fatty acyl residues introduces oxy functions, rearranges bonds, and results in the fragmentation of carbon–carbon bonds by β-scission that generates a myriad of phospholipid reaction products including ones that exert PAFR agonistic activity. In this regard, cellular and potentially nuclear membranes serve as the source of oxidized phospholipids and are thus the sources of reactive oxygen species (ROS)-mediated PAFR agonist formation. In contrast to the tightly regulated enzymatic PAF production, generation of oxidized glycerophosphocholines (Ox-GPC) is relatively unregulated. The likely factors in Ox-GPC generation include the nature and amount of ROS, the host antioxidant defenses, and the amounts of sn-2 unsaturated fatty acids (associated with diet). Only a handful of these Ox-GPC PAFR agonists have been structurally characterized (Marathe et al. 2001; Konger et al. 2008). Stimuli that have been demonstrated to generate Ox-GPC include cigarette smoke (Sahu et al. 2013), chemotherapeutic agents (Sahu et al. 2014), chronic ethanol exposure (Yang et al. 2010), radiation therapy (Sahu et al. 2016), and ultraviolet B radiation (Marathe et al. 2005).

2.3 PAF Metabolism

Though glycerophosphocholines can be metabolized via multiple phospholipases (e.g., PLA_1, PLA_2, PLC, PLD), PAF and Ox-GPC are inactivated predominantly via removal of the *sn-2* group by specialized PLA_2 enzymes known as PAF-acetylhydrolases (PAF-AH). The major types relevant for PAF metabolism are the serum form, PAF-AH type I, and cell-associated PAF-AH type II. Genetic deficiencies in PAF-AH type I (also known as lipoprotein-associated PLA_2) have been associated with pathologies including atherosclerotic disease (Rosenson and Stafforini 2012; Zalewski and Macphee 2005; Min et al. 2001; Yamada and Yokota 1997). Consistent with PAF elevation in various disorders, PAF-AH type I levels have been demonstrated to be decreased following sepsis or acute allergic reactions in humans (Franck Trimoreau et al. 2000; Vadas et al. 2008).

3 PAF Receptor

The PAF receptor (PAFR) is a member of the G protein-coupled receptor family (Shimizu 2009; Honda et al. 1991). The PAFR is widely expressed, including in cells of the immune system (e.g., neutrophils, eosinophils, mast cells, macrophages, B cells) as well as in other cell types (e.g., keratinocytes, fibroblasts, platelets). Creation of PAFR knockout mice confirmed that a single receptor mediates all PAF effects (Ishii et al. 1998). Two different PAFR mRNA transcripts with open identical reading frames are generated via the use of separate promoters. Expression of transcript I is regulated by estrogen and transcript II by the PKC-NFkB pathway. Consistent with the ability of the PAFR to activate a myriad of responses, this receptor is coupled to G proteins Gi, Gq, and G12/13. In addition, the PAFR has been demonstrated to transactivate the epidermal growth factor (EGF) receptor through its ability to release heparin-binding EGF (Marques et al. 2002). Activation of the PAFR results in intracellular calcium mobilization, activation of mitogen-activated protein kinases, NF-kB pathway activation, and inhibition of cyclic AMP formation. In addition to PAFR effects alone, activation of the PAFR synergizes with other stimuli ranging from ultraviolet radiation to retinoids (Wolverton et al. 2010). It has been hypothesized that PAFR on the cellular membrane that appears to be coupled to Gq and PAFR on the nuclear membrane receptor that appears to be coupled to Gi/o activate distinct signaling pathways (Bazan et al. 1994; Marrache et al. 2002). A mutant PAFR has been reported wherein the alanine residue at position 224 is substituted by aspartic acid (A224D) in the putative third intracellular loop. This mutation is observed at a 7.8% allele frequency in Japanese populations (Fukunaga et al. 2001). The functional consequences of this structural alteration as inferred from cellular in vitro studies have been suggested to involve impaired coupling to G-proteins. Thus, this receptor mutation may serve as a basis for interindividual variation in PAFR-related processes, including physiological responses, disease predisposition or phenotypes, and drug responsiveness.

4 Acute PAF Effects

Inasmuch as the PAFR is expressed in endothelial, inflammatory, and innate immunity cells, it is not surprising that activation of the PAFR is linked to acute inflammation. Engagement of PAFR induces multiple biochemical pathways. These include phosphatidylinositol turnover, increase in intracellular calcium, activation of kinases and anti-apoptotic pathways, and transcription of several genes coding for pro- and anti-inflammatory cytokines as well as for cyclooxygenase-2 (COX-2) and inducible nitric oxide synthase (iNOS) (Travers et al. 1996; Honda et al. 1991; Marques et al. 2002; Zimmerman et al. 2002). PAFR activation also induces eicosanoids and PAF production, indicating a positive feed-forward loop. The cellular response to PAFR activation seems to depend on the type of G protein linked to the receptor. The cellular membrane PAFR is coupled to Gq and the nuclear membrane receptor to Gi/o, allowing a single receptor type to trigger distinct signaling pathways (Bazan et al. 1994; Marrache et al. 2002). It has been suggested that activation of the cell membrane receptor linked to Gq generates early pro-inflammatory responses and synthesis of PAF that in turn activate nuclear PAFR linked to Gi/o to induce transcription of genes for COX-2, iNOS, and cytokines (Zimmerman et al. 2002). Moreover, the cell response to PAFR also depends on the type of ligand and on the interaction with other receptors. This response may be adverse or beneficial; indeed, during infections, production of PAF has been shown to mediate resistance to various pathogens including *Leishmania amazonensis* (Lonardoni et al. 2000), *Trypanosoma cruzi* (Aliberti et al. 1999), and gram-negative bacterial *Klebsiella pneumoniae* (Soares et al. 2002). Pharmacologic inhibitors of the PAFR have been reported to increase local and systemic infection in these model systems. Of note, PAFR KO mice infected with *T. cruzi* exhibit higher blood parasitemia, parasite load in the lymph nodes and spleen, and mortality (Talvani et al. 2003). The emerging view is that endogenous PAF appears vital for controlling certain infections in part via facilitation of optimal macrophage activation. It should be noted that concomitant activation of PAFR and other receptor types such as Toll-like receptors (TLRs) results in augmented pro-inflammatory effects. Thus, the PAFR can act in cooperation with other macrophage receptors to induce either suppression or activation, affecting both innate and adaptive immunity (Lefebvre et al. 2010).

Injection of low doses of PAF into the skin triggers urticarial eruption in both rodents and humans (Archer et al. 1984; Hellewell and Williams 1989; Travers et al. 1998a). PAF injection also induces itching and pain in these models. Of interest, PAF has been reported to be measurable in the blood of patients with active cold urticaria (Grandel et al. 1985). Systemic PAF exerts acute effects on the cardiopulmonary system and has been shown to mimic sepsis. Of interest, PAFR KO mice are protected against LPS-induced lethality (Ishii et al. 1998). PAF can be found in association with multiple acute inflammatory states ranging from sepsis to the blistering disease bullous pemphigoid (Travers et al. 1998b; Mallet and Cunningham 1985). Hence, PAF in theory could contribute to all of the classic acute inflammatory features of calor (heat), rubor (redness), tumor (swelling), and dolor (pain).

5 Chronic PAF Effects

In contrast to the overall "pro-inflammatory" effects ascribed to acute PAF, chronic effects of PAF appear to be more "anti-inflammatory." For example, PAF has been demonstrated to inhibit delayed-type hypersensitivity reactions to *Candida* antigens and the chemical dinitrofluorobenzene (Walterscheid et al. 2002; Zhang et al. 2008). This process has been studied in some detail and appears to be due to PAF interacting with the mast cell PAFR, resulting in upregulation of regulatory T cells (Treg) in a COX-2-dependent manner (Chacon-Salinas et al. 2014). As will be detailed elsewhere in this review, this PAF→Mast cell→Treg process appears to be responsible for the systemic immunosuppressive effects of multiple environmental stressors ranging from cigarette smoke (Sahu et al. 2013) to ultraviolet B radiation (Walterscheid et al. 2002; Zhang et al. 2008).

In addition to the immune effects of chronic PAF exposure, several studies have implicated PAF in chronic ethanol toxicity. In particular, chronic ethanol administration in rats and mice results in increased levels of oxidized glycerophosphocholines and PAF in plasma (Yang et al. 2010; Liu et al. 2013). Moreover, PAFR-deficient mice are protected from chronic ethanol-mediated kidney damage (Latchoumycandane et al. 2015). In these chronic ethanol models, nonenzymatic oxidized glycerophosphocholine PAF agonists appear to play important roles. Finally, PAF has been identified in multiple chronic conditions involving numerous organ types including experimental cerebral malaria (Lacerda-Queiroz et al. 2012) and necrotizing enterocolitis (Lefebvre et al. 2010). Thus, the PAF system has been implicated in both pro- and anti-inflammatory chronic pathologies.

6 PAF System and Environmental Stressors

Given that PAF and Ox-GPC PAFR agonists are generated in response to multiple environmental stressors, this class of lipid mediators could play important roles in the effects of these agents. This review will focus on recent findings providing evidence that links the PAF system with the pro-oxidative stressors UVB, photodynamic therapy, and cigarette smoke. The potential implications of PAF in how the host interacts with these stressors will be outlined, with an eye toward translational modulation.

6.1 Ultraviolet B Radiation

Ultraviolet B radiation (290–320 nm; UVB) is a pro-oxidative stressor that has profound effects upon human skin (Wacker and Holick 2013; Leitenberger et al. 2007). These "burning rays" of sunlight are critical for vitamin D metabolism yet also induce sunburns as well as both melanoma and non-melanoma skin cancer (Ullrich 2005). Given that UVB generates anti-inflammatory effects in skin, phototherapy is used clinically to treat a myriad of skin diseases including psoriasis (Leitenberger et al. 2007). UVB stimulates the production of PAF and Ox-GPC with PAFR agonistic activity (Marathe et al. 2005). PAFR signaling is involved in two separate aspects of photobiology. First, PAFR activation appears important in the early acute responses of UVB. In a murine model of photosensitivity due to deficiency of the DNA repair enzyme xeroderma pigmentosum type A (XPA), UVB treatment results in increased levels of PAF and Ox-GPC formation (Yao et al. 2012). Moreover, the exaggerated pro-inflammatory response to UVB in XPA-deficient mice is blocked by PAFR antagonists (Yao et al. 2012). It should be noted that PAFR-deficient mice exhibit decreased acute inflammation as well as decreased production of cytokines such as tumor necrosis factor in response to UVB (Yao et al. 2012; Travers et al. 2008). Second, the systemic immunosuppression induced by UVB has been demonstrated to involve PAFR signaling via Ox-GPCs (Walterscheid et al. 2002; Zhang et al. 2008). Of interest, UVB can induce both local immunosuppression (where the UVB-treated site is anergic) and systemic immunosuppression (i.e., at a non-treated UVB site). Local immunosuppression appears to involve decreasing dendritic cell function, whereas systemic immunosuppression involves mast cells and Tregs (see Fig. 3). It has been demonstrated that UVB-induced systemic immunosuppression is defective in PAFR-deficient mice (Zhang et al. 2008). However, local immunosuppression is normal in PAFR KO mice (Sahu et al. 2012a). Finally, systemic PAFR antagonists inhibit tumor formation in a murine model of UVB photocarcinogenesis (Sreevidya et al. 2008).

Other agents such as organic solvents found in jet fuel have also been demonstrated to act upon the skin to induce systemic immunosuppression via PAF/Ox-GPC PAFR agonists (Ramos et al. 2004). Thus, PAFR signaling appears to play an important role in inflammatory processes in the skin, and this system can be activated by a wide range of pro-oxidative stressors.

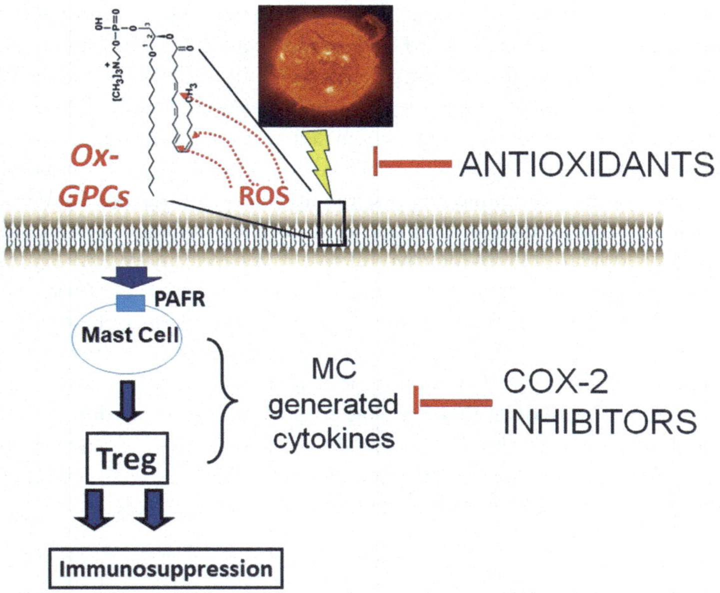

Fig. 3 Model for how environmental stressors can induce immunosuppression via PAFR-mediated generation of regulatory T cells

6.2 Photodynamic Therapy

Photodynamic therapy (PDT) combines the phototoxic effects of porphyrin and a compatible light source. Photodynamic therapy using topical 5-aminolevulinic acid is a commonly used procedure in dermatology to treat patients with extensive areas of actinic damage (precancerous actinic keratosis) and also has efficacy against superficial basal cell carcinomas (BCC) (Lee and Baron 2011; Gold 2011). Regular PDT treatments have also been championed as a strategy for management of high-risk populations, including immunosuppressed (e.g., organ transplant recipients) due to their tremendous burden of actinic neoplasia (Basset-Seguin et al. 2013). However, relatively little is known regarding PDT, in particular the long-term effects of this treatment modality that thousands of patients are being exposed to annually.

Acute responses to PDT include a potent phototoxic reaction. Studies have demonstrated that PDT is immunosuppressive in both mice (Ferracini et al. 2015; Hayami et al. 2007) and humans (Matthews and Damian 2010; Frost et al. 2011). Consistent with PDT being immunosuppressive, there are reports of skin cancers and herpes simplex recurrences developing following PDT (Gogia et al. 2013; Varma et al. 2000; Fiechter et al. 2012; Wolf et al. 1997; Nobbe et al. 2011). However, under certain conditions, PDT can be immune enhancing (St Denis et al. 2011; Krosl et al. 1996; Kabingu et al. 2009). In particular, Dr. Sandra Gollnick's group has reported that PDT of skin BCC generated a cytotoxic immune response with enhanced gamma-interferon production against the BCC-associated protein Hedgehog-interacting protein 1 (Hip1) (Kabingu et al. 2009). Inasmuch as PDT is a commonly used procedure, investigations as to its effects on the human skin immune system and their consequences and potential manipulation to allow enhanced therapeutic effects are highly warranted. Our group has discovered that PDT of keratinocytes is a potent inducer of PAFR agonists and that standard doses of PDT result in systemic immunosuppression in wild-type but not PAFR-deficient mice (Ferracini et al. 2015). Additionally, studies in humans suggest that high-fluence rates of topical PDT (which would likely generate more PAF agonists) are more immunosuppressive than lower rates (Frost et al. 2011). Moreover, PDT appears less effective in patients who are already immunosuppressed (Dragieva et al. 2004). Of interest, a few reports using preclinical models have shown that COX-2 inhibitors augment PDT antitumor responses (Ferrario and Gomer 2010; Makowski et al. 2003). Given that PAF-induced immunosuppression is blocked by COX-2 inhibitors (Walterscheid et al. 2002; Wolf et al. 2006; Zhang et al. 2008; Sahu et al. 2013), it is indeed possible that the PAF agonists produced as a by-product of PDT could be exerting immunomodulatory effects.

6.3 Cigarette Smoke

Affecting approximately one in six humans, tobacco smoke is one of the most significant environmental exposures (Hatsukami et al. 2008; Stampfli and Anderson 2009). The many adverse effects of cigarette smoke (CS) on immune responses have far-reaching consequences, such as increased infections, vaccine failures, and tumor generation (Stampfli and Anderson 2009; Finklea et al. 1971; Esber et al. 1973; Suclu-Foca et al. 1974; Winter et al. 1994). Cigarette smoke generates isoprostanes in humans that can be blocked by vitamin C (Pryor and Stone 1993; Morrow et al. 1995; Lehr et al. 1997; Obwegeser et al. 1999; Imaizumi et al. 1991; Dietrich et al. 2002; Geng et al. 1996; Dillon et al. 2002; Revathikumar et al. 2016). As isoprostanes are prostaglandin-like compounds formed by the free radical-catalyzed peroxidation of arachidonic acid nonenzymatically, this fits with the notion that CS can generate enough ROS to induce lipid oxidation (and thus Ox-GPC formation). Indeed, PAFR agonistic activity has been identified in both hamsters and humans following CS exposure (Morrow et al. 1995; Lehr et al. 1997; Obwegeser et al. 1999; Imaizumi et al. 1991). Vitamin C supplementation blocked this PAFR agonistic activity in hamsters, suggesting Ox-GPC PAFR agonist involvement. Our group has reported that CS generates PAFR agonistic activity in mice, which can be blocked by placement of the mice on an experimental diet of vitamin C-enriched (10 g/kg) chow and 5 mM N-acetylcysteine (NAC) in water for 10 days prior to CS exposure (Sahu et al. 2013). CS exposure also inhibits CHS conversion to DNFB in PAFR-positive but not PAFR KO mice (Sahu et al. 2013). Of importance, CS-induced immunosuppression was blocked by antioxidants and COX-2 inhibitors, as well as by depleting Tregs (Sahu et al. 2013).

Though nicotine has been implicated in some aspects of CS-mediated immunosuppression (Dillon et al. 2002; Revathikumar et al. 2016; Reale et al. 2015; Nouri-

Shirazi et al. 2015), nicotine itself has been reported to not exert systemic immunosuppressive effects in humans. It should be noted that our preclinical studies revealed that CS derived from low-nicotine cigarettes resulted in levels of PAF agonists that were similar to those seen for normal cigarettes (Sahu et al. 2013).

The proposed mechanism by which CS generates PAFR agonists via ROS suggests that many other potential environmental exposures (e.g., *air pollutants*) could also exert similar effects. Further studies are warranted to determine how lung tumors associated with CS use evade immune-mediated clearance and how host and environmental factors influence this process.

7 PAF System and Cancer Therapy

The immune system plays an important role in cancer development and progression [reviewed in (Marin-Acevedo et al. 2018; Passarelli et al. 2017)]. Indeed, therapeutics designed to enhance immunity such as CTLA4 and PD-1 inhibitors are now being used to treat cancers, especially melanoma. We have demonstrated that systemic exposure of PAF augments experimental tumor growth in mice (Sahu et al. 2012b, 2014). Similar to systemic immunosuppressive effects of PAFR activation, PAF-augmented tumor growth is blocked by COX-2 inhibitors and is dependent upon Tregs. Thus, systemic PAFR activation inhibits tumor immunity.

Chemotherapeutic agents are known to act as pro-oxidative stressors. We have demonstrated that chemotherapeutic agents including etoposide, dacarbazine, cisplatin, and melphalan all generate PAF and Ox-GPC PAFR agonists (Sahu et al. 2014). Consistent with the ability of these chemotherapeutic agents to induce ROS, this PAF agonist generation is partially inhibited by antioxidants. Of importance, chemotherapeutic agent-induced PAF is increased in tumor cells expressing a PAFR (Sahu et al. 2014). Using a novel model system of subcutaneous placement of two B16F10 syngeneic melanoma tumors, intratumoral injection of etoposide or melphalan into one tumor resulted in the enhanced growth of the second tumor, a process not seen in PAFR KO mice (Sahu et al. 2014). These findings fit with the notion that PAF agonists produced by the chemotherapy-treated tumor inhibit tumoral immunity. Of translational importance, high levels of PAF are measured in human subjects undergoing regional chemotherapy with melphalan (Sahu et al. 2014).

Radiation therapy is also commonly used to treat tumors (Citrin 2017). Localized radiation therapy has been demonstrated to exert immunosuppressive effects (Wara 1977; Wara et al. 1975). Moreover, radiation can induce Tregs (Schaue et al. 2012). Recently, radiation therapy was demonstrated to induce PAF agonists both in cell lines in experimental tumors and in human patients undergoing localized radiation to tumors (Sahu et al. 2016). Similar to the two-tumor model used to study intratumoral chemotherapy (Sahu et al. 2014), localized radiation of one tumor resulted in increased growth of the second tumor in a PAFR-dependent manner (Sahu et al. 2016). Again, COX-2 inhibitors blocked this PAFR-dependent inhibition of antitumor immunity.

8 PAF and Microvesicle Particles

Microvesicle particles (MVP) are defined as submicron vesicles generated from cellular membranes via exocytosis. They are irregularly shaped and range from ~100 to 1,000 nm in size. MVP generation occurs in response to various stimuli, many involving intracellular calcium mobilization (Xiao et al. 2015; Camussi et al. 2010). Once released into the circulation (blood and urine), MVP can then exert functional effects on various cell types. MVP have different functions that depend on the cell of origin and stimuli. Moreover, MVP are thought to be able to target other cell types through surface membrane interactions that then allow fusion of the MVP to the target cell membrane and subsequent delivery of the intravesicular contents. The pathways by which MVP are released from cells are cellular- and stimulus-dependent (Norling and Dalli 2013). For example, in endothelial cells, MVP release in response to agents like TNF-α is due to P38 MAPK signaling, whereas in THP-1 monocytes, both Erk 1/2 (p42/44) and P38 MAPK pathways are involved (Norling and Dalli 2013; Vion et al. 2013; Li et al. 2010; Herring et al. 2013). Ceramides appear to play an important role in MVP generation and release. In particular, blocking the enzyme acid sphingomyelinase via either pharmacologic tools or genetic strategies inhibits MVP generation (Serban et al. 2016).

The functions of various MVP in physiological and pathological processes depend on the contents they bear (proteins, lipids, and nucleic acids) (Camussi et al. 2010). One advantage of this arrangement is that metabolically unstable compounds inside MVP can be protected from enzymatic degradation in the extracellular milieu. Studies have reported that circulating MVP are increased in inflammatory skin diseases such as psoriasis in which many cytokines are also elevated (Tamagawa-Mineoka et al. 2010; Liu et al. 2016; Takeshita et al. 2014). In translational studies, elevated levels of MVP have been documented in vascular diseases and correlated with the severity of disease.

Recent studies by our group have demonstrated that activation of the keratinocyte PAFR induces MVP release (Bihl et al. 2016; Fahy et al. 2017). Of interest, UVB radiation also induces MVP in a PAFR-dependent manner (see Fig. 4). These studies indicate that MVP could serve as effectors linking environmental stressors that act upon the skin, with the PAF system playing an intermediary role. If this is the case, then, novel therapeutic strategies aimed at MVP could be useful in conditions such as photosensitivity.

9 Future Directions

Environmental stressors play important roles in human biology and pathology. Accumulating evidence links PAF with multiple stressors, which have in common the ability to generate cell damage and ROS. Given that PAF agonists are produced in response to multiple therapeutic agents, it is possible that this could be exploited. For example, chemotherapy-generated PAF agonists could be exerting adverse effects on cancer patients by blocking antitumor immunity. If this is the case, then

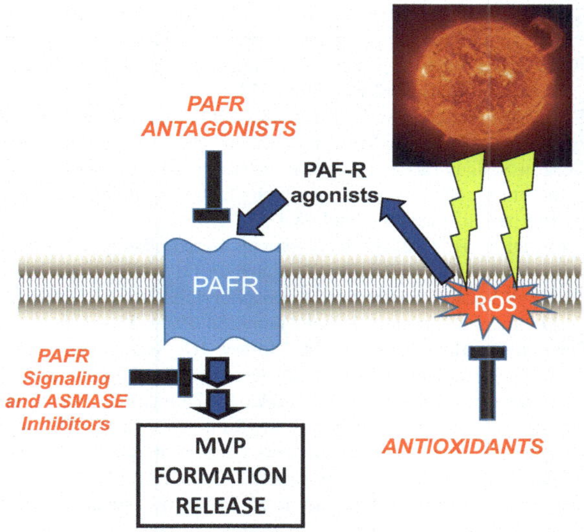

Fig. 4 Model for how UVB and potentially other environmental stressors can generate microvesicle particles via PAFR signaling in a process dependent upon the enzyme acid sphingomyelinase

strategies such as antioxidants to block PAF agonist generation or COX-2 inhibitors to block the downstream pathways that induce Tregs could be valuable adjuncts for chemotherapy. Another potential strategy to modulate effects of PAF agonists could be to further study MVP as potential carriers of metabolically labile PAF agonists. Thus, future directions in this arena will be to first define the PAF system as it relates to human-based interactions with environmental agents to assess whether this could be exploited pharmacologically.

Acknowledgments The PI wishes to acknowledge the support by grants from the National Institutes of Health grant R01 HL062996, R21 AR070010, and Veteran's Administration Merit Award 5I01BX000853.

References

Aliberti JC, Machado FS, Gazzinelli RT, Teixeira MM, Silva JS (1999) Platelet-activating factor induces nitric oxide synthesis in Trypanosoma cruzi-infected macrophages and mediates resistance to parasite infection in mice. Infect Immun 67(6):2810–2814

Archer CB, Page CP, Morley JP, MacDonald DM (1984) Inflammatory characteristics of platelet-activating factor (Pafacether) in human skin. Br J Dermatol 110:45–49

Basset-Seguin N et al (2013) Photodynamic therapy for actinic keratosis in organ transplant patients. J Eur Acad Dermatol Venereol 27(1):57–66

Bazan NG, Fletcher BS, Herschman HR, Mukherjee PK (1994) Platelet-activating factor and retinoic acid synergistically activate the inducible prostaglandin synthase gene. Proc Natl Acad Sci U S A 91(12):5252–5256

Benveniste J, Henson PM, Cochrane CG (1972) Leukocyte-dependent histamine release from rabbit platelets. The role of IgE, basophils, and a platelet-activating factor. J Exp Med 136 (6):1356–1377

Bihl JC, Rapp CM, Chen Y, Travers JB (2016) UVB generates microvesicle particle release in part due to platelet-activating factor signaling. Photochem Photobiol 92(3):503–506

Braquet P, Touqui L, Shen TY, Vargaftig BB (1987) Perspectives in platelet-activating factor research. Pharmacol Rev 39:97–145

Camussi G, Deregibus MC, Bruno S, Cantaluppi V, Biancone L (2010) Exosomes/microvesicles as a mechanism of cell-to-cell communication. Kidney Int 78(9):838–848

Chacon-Salinas R, Chen L, Chavez-Blanco AD, Limon-Flores AY, Ma Y, Ullrich SE (2014) An essential role for platelet-activating factor in activating mast cell migration following ultraviolet irradiation. J Leukoc Biol 95:139–148

Citrin DE (2017) Recent developments in radiotherapy. N Engl J Med 377(11):1065–1075

Demopoulos CA, Pinckard RN, Hanahan DJ (1979) Platelet-activating factor. Evidence for 1-O-alkyl-2-acetyl-sn-glyceryl-3-phosphorylcholine as the active component (a new class of lipid chemical mediators). J Biol Chem 254(19):9355–9358

Dietrich M, Block G, Hudes M, Morrow JD, Norkus EP, Traber MG, Cross CE, Packer L (2002) Antioxidant supplementation decreases lipid peroxidation biomarker F(2)-isoprostanes in plasma of smokers. Cancer Epidemiol Biomarkers Prev 11(1):7–13

Dillon SA, Lowe GM, Billington D, Rahman K (2002) Dietary supplementation with aged garlic extract reduces plasma and urine concentrations of 8-iso-prostaglandin F(2 alpha) in smoking and nonsmoking men and women. J Nutr 132(2):168–171

Dragieva G, Hafner J, Dummer R et al (2004) Topical photodynamic therapy in the treatment of actinic keratosis and Bowen's disease in transplant recipients. Transplantation 77:115–121

Esber HJ, Menninger FF Jr, Bogden AE, Mason MM (1973) Immunological deficiency associated with cigarette smoke inhalation by mice. Primary and secondary hemagglutinin response. Arch Environ Health 27(2):99–104

Fahy K, Langni L, Rapp CM, Borchers C, Bihl JC, Chen Y, Simman R, Travers JB (2017) UVB-generated microvesicle particles: a novel pathway by which a skin-specific stimulus could exert systemic effects. Photochem Photobiol 93(4):937–942

Ferracini M, Sahu RP, Harrison KA, Waeiss RA, Murphy RC, Jancar S, Konger RL, Travers JB (2015) Topical photodynamic therapy induces systemic immunosuppression via generation of platelet-activating factor agonists. J Investig Dermatol 135:321–323

Ferrario A, Gomer CJ (2010) Targeting the tumor microenvironment using photodynamic therapy combined with inhibitors of cyclooxygenase-2 or vascular endothelial growth factor. Methods Mol Biol 635:121–132

Fiechter ZS, Skaria A, Nievergelt H et al (2012) Facial basal cell carcinomas recurring after photodynamic therapy: a retrospective analysis of histological subtypes. Dermatology 224:346–351

Finklea JF, Hasselblad V, Riggan WB, Nelson WB, Hammer DI, Newall VA (1971) Cigarette smoking and hemagglutination inhibition response to influenza after natural disease and immunization. Am Rev Respir Dis 104:368–372

Franck Trimoreau CA, Bruno F, Desachy A, Besse F, Vignon P, Denizot Y (2000) Platelet-activating factor acetylhydrolase and haemophagocytosis in the sepsis syndrome. Mediators Inflamm 9:197–200

Frost GA, Halliday GM, Damian DL (2011) Photodynamic therapy-induced immunosuppression in humans is prevented by reducing the rate of light delivery. J Investig Dermatol 131(4):962–968

Fukunaga K, Ishii S, Asano K, Yokomizo T, Shiomi T, Shimizu T, Yamaguchi K (2001) Single nucleotide polymorphism of human platelet-activating factor receptor impairs G-protein activation. J Biol Chem 276(46):43025–43030

Geng Y, Savage SM, Razani-Boroujerdi S, Sopori ML (1996) Effects of nicotine on the immune response. II. Chronic nicotine treatment induces T cell anergy. J Immunol 156(7):2384–2390

Gogia R, Grekin RC, Shinkai K (2013) Eruptive self-resolving keratoacanthomas developing after treatment with photodynamic therapy and microdermabrasion. Dermatol Surg 39 (11):1717–1720

Gold MH (2011) Photodynamic therapy. Curr Probl Dermatol 42:181–192

Grandel KE, Farr RS, Wanderer AA, Eisenstadt TC, Wasserman SI (1985) Association of platelet-activating factor with primary acquired cold urticaria. N Engl J Med 313(7):405–409
Haritash AK, Kaushik CP (2009) Biodegradation aspects of polycyclic aromatic hydrocarbons (PAHs): a review. J Hazard Mater 169(1–3):1–15
Hatsukami DK, Stead LF, Gupta PC (2008) Tobacco addiction. Lancet 371(9629):2027–2038
Hayami J, Okamoto H, Sugihara A et al (2007) Immunosuppressive effects of photodynamic therapy by topical aminolevulinic acid. J Dermatol 34:320–327
Hellewell PG, Williams TJ (1989) Antagonism of PAF-induced oedema formation in rabbit skin: a comparison of different antagonists. Br J Pharmacol 97(1):171–180
Herring JM, McMichael MA, Smith SA (2013) Microparticles in health and disease. J Vet Intern Med 27:1020–1033
Honda Z, Nakamura M, Miki I, Minami M, Watanabe T, Seyama Y, Okado H, Toh H, Ito K, Miyamoto T (1991) Cloning by functional expression of platelet-activating factor receptor from guinea-pig lung. Nature 349(6307):342–346
Imaizumi T, Satoh K, Yoshida H, Kawamura Y, Hiramoto M, Takamatsu S (1991) Effect of cigarette smoking on the levels of platelet-activating factor-like lipid(s) in plasma lipoproteins. Atherosclerosis 87(1):47–55
Ishii S, Kuwaki T, Nagase T, Maki K, Tashiro F, Sunaga S, Cao WH, Kume K, Fukuchi Y, Ikuta K, Miyazaki J, Kumada M, Shimizu T (1998) Impaired anaphylactic responses with intact sensitivity to endotoxin in mice lacking a platelet-activating factor receptor. J Exp Med 187:1779–1788
Kabingu E, Oseroff AR, Wilding GE, Gollnick SO (2009) Enhanced systemic immune reactivity to a basal cell carcinoma associated antigen following photodynamic therapy. Clin Cancer Res 15:4460–4466
Konger RL, Marathe GK, Yao Y, Zhang Q, Travers JB (2008) Oxidized glycerophosphocholines as biologically active mediators for ultraviolet radiation-mediated effects. Prostaglandins Other Lipid Mediat 87(1–4):1–8
Krosl G, Korbelik M, Krosl J, Dougherty GJ (1996) Potentiation of photodynamic therapy-elicited antitumor response by localized treatment with granulocyte-macrophage colony-stimulating factor. Cancer Res 56(14):3281–3286
Lacerda-Queiroz N, Rodrigues DH, Vilela MC, Rachid MA, Soriani FM, Sousa LP, Campos RD, Quesniaux VF, Teixeira MM, Teixeira AL (2012) Platelet-activating factor receptor is essential for the development of experimental cerebral malaria. Am J Pathol 180(1):246–255
Latchoumycandane C, Nagy LE, McIntyre TM (2015) Myeloperoxidase formation of PAF receptor ligands induces PAF receptor-dependent kidney injury during ethanol consumption. Free Radic Biol Med 86:179–190
Lee Y, Baron ED (2011) Photodynamic therapy: current evidence and applications in dermatology. Semin Cutan Med Surg 30(4):199–209
Lefebvre JS, Marleau S, Milot V, Lévesque T, Picard S, Flamand N, Borgeat P (2010) Toll-like receptor ligands induce polymorphonuclear leukocyte migration: key roles for leukotriene B4 and platelet-activating factor. FASEB J 24(2):637–647
Lehr HA, Weyrich AS, Saetzler RK, Jurek A, Arfors KE, Zimmerman GA, Prescott SM, McIntyre TM (1997) Vitamin C blocks inflammatory platelet-activating factor mimetics created by cigarette smoking. J Clin Investig 99(10):2358–2364
Leitenberger J, Jacobe HT, Cruz PD Jr (2007) Photoimmunology – illuminating the immune system through photobiology. Semin Immunopathol 29:65–70
Li M, Yu D, Williams KJ, Liu ML (2010) Tobacco smoke induces the generation of procoagulant microvesicles from human monocytes/macrophages. Arterioscler Thromb Vasc Biol 30 (9):1818–1824
Liu J, Li W, Chen R, McIntyre TM (2013) Circulating biologically active oxidized phospholipids show on-going and increased oxidative stress in older male mice. Redox Biol 1:110–114
Liu M-L, Williams KJ, Werth VP (2016) Chapter four-microvesicles in autoimmune diseases. Adv Clin Chem 77:125–175

Lonardoni MV, Russo M, Jancar S (2000) Essential role of platelet-activating factor in control of Leishmania (Leishmania) amazonensis infection. Infect Immun 68(11):6355–6361

Makowski M et al (2003) Inhibition of cyclooxygenase-2 indirectly potentiates antitumor effects of photodynamic therapy in mice. Clin Cancer Res 9(14):5417–5422

Mallet AI, Cunningham FM (1985) Structural identification of platelet-activating factor in psoriatic scale. Biochem Biophys Res Commun 126:192–196

Marathe GK, Prescott SM, Zimmerman GA, McIntyre TM (2001) Oxidized LDL contains inflammatory PAF-like phospholipids. Trends Cardiovasc Med 11:139–142

Marathe GK, Johnson C, Billings SD, Southall MD, Pei Y, Spandau D, Murphy RC, Zimmerman GA, McIntyre TM, Travers JB (2005) Ultraviolet B radiation generates platelet-activating factor-like phospholipids underlying cutaneous damage. J Biol Chem 280:35448–35457

Marin-Acevedo JA, Soyano AE, Dholaria B, Knutson KL, Lou Y (2018) Cancer immunotherapy beyond immune checkpoint inhibitors. J Hematol Oncol 11(1):8. https://doi.org/10.1186/s13045-017-0552-6

Marques SA, Dy L, Southall MD, Yi Q, Smietana E, Kapur R, Marques M, Travers JB, Spandau D (2002) The platelet-activating factor receptor activates the ERK MAP kinase and induces proliferation of epidermal cells through an EGF receptor-dependent pathway. J Pharmacol Exp Ther 300:1026–1035

Marrache AM, Gobeil F, Bernier SG, Stankova J, Rola-Pleszczynski M, Choufani S, Bkaily G, Bourdeau A, Sirois MG, Vazquez-Tello A et al (2002) Proinflammatory gene induction by platelet-activating factor mediated via its cognate nuclear receptor. J Immunol 169(11):6474–6481

Matthews YJ, Damian DL (2010) Topical photodynamic therapy is immunosuppressive in humans. Br J Dermatol 162(3):637–641

Min JH, Wilder C, Aoki J, Arai H, Inoue K, Paul L, Gelb MH (2001) Platelet-activating factor acetylhydrolases: broad substrate specificity and lipoprotein binding does not modulate the catalytic properties of the plasma enzyme. Biochemistry 40(15):4539–4549

Morimoto R, Shindou H, Oda Y, Shimizu T (2010) Phosphorylation of lysophosphatidylcholine acyltransferase 2 at Ser^{34} enhances platelet-activating factor production in endotoxin-stimulated macrophages. J Biol Chem 285:29857–29862

Morrow JD, Frei B, Longmire AW, Gaziano JM, Lynch SM, Shyr Y, Strauss WE, Oates JA, Roberts LJ 2nd. (1995) Increase in circulating products of lipid peroxidation (F2-isoprostanes) in smokers. Smoking as a cause of oxidative damage. N Engl J Med 332(18):1198–1203

Nakanishi H, Shindou H, Hishikawa D, Harayama T, Ogasawara R, Suwabe A, Taguchi R, Shimizu T (2006) Cloning and characterization of mouse lung-type acyl-CoA:lysophosphatidylcholine acyltransferase 1 (LPCAT1). Expression in alveolar type II cells and possible involvement in surfactant production. J Biol Chem 281(29):20140–20147

Nobbe S, Trueb RM, French LE, Hofbauer GFL (2011) Herpes simplex virus reactivation as a complication of photodynamic therapy. Photodermatol Photoimmunol Photomed 27:51–52

Norling LV, Dalli J (2013) Microparticles are novel effectors of immunity. Curr Opin Pharmacol 13:570–575

Nouri-Shirazi M, Kahlden C, Nishino P, Guinet E (2015) Nicotine exposure alters the mRNA expression of Notch ligands in dendritic cells and their response to Th1-/Th2-promoting stimuli. Scand J Immunol 81(2):110–120

Obwegeser R, Oguogho A, Ulm M, Berghammer P, Sinzinger H (1999) Maternal cigarette smoking increases F2-isoprostanes and reduces prostacyclin and nitric oxide in umbilical vessels. Prostaglandins Other Lipid Mediat 57(4):269–279

Passarelli A, Mannavola F, Stucci LS, Tucci M, Silvestris F (2017) Immune system and melanoma biology: a balance between immunosurveillance and immune escape. Oncotarget 8(62):106132–106142

Pryor WA, Stone K (1993) Oxidants in cigarette smoke. Ann N Y Acad Sci 686:12–28

Ramesh A, Walker SA, Hood DB, Guillén MD, Schneider K, Weyand EH (2004) Bioavailability and risk assessment of orally ingested polycyclic aromatic hydrocarbons. Int J Toxicol 23 (5):301–333

Ramos G, Kazimi N, Nghiem DX, Walterscheid JP, Ullrich SE (2004) Platelet activating factor receptor binding plays a critical role in jet fuel-induced immune suppression. Toxicol Appl Pharmacol 195(3):331–338

Reale M, Di Bari M, Di Nicola M, D'Angelo C, De Angelis F, Velluto L, Tata AM (2015) Nicotinic receptor activation negatively modulates pro-inflammatory cytokine production in multiple sclerosis patients. Int Immunopharmacol 29(1):152–157

Revathikumar P, Bergqvist F, Gopalakrishnan S, Korotkova M, Jakobsson PJ, Lampa J, Le Maître E (2016) Immunomodulatory effects of nicotine on interleukin 1β activated human astrocytes and the role of cyclooxygenase 2 in the underlying mechanism. J Neuroinflammation 13(1):256

Rosenson RS, Stafforini DM (2012) Modulation of oxidative stress, inflammation, and atherosclerosis by lipoprotein-associated phospholipase A2. J Lipid Res 53(9):1767–1782

Sahu RP, Yao Y, Konger RL, Travers JB (2012a) Platelet-activating factor does not mediate UVB-induced local immune suppression. Photochem Photobiol 88:490–493

Sahu RP, Turner MJ, DaSilva SC, Rashid BM, Ocana JA, Perkins SM, Konger KL, Touloukian CE, Kaplan MH, Travers JB (2012b) The environmental stressor ultraviolet radiation inhibits murine anti-tumor immunity through its ability to generate platelet-activating factor agonists. Carcinogenesis 33(7):1360–1367

Sahu RP et al (2013) Cigarette smoke exposure inhibits contact hypersensitivity via the generation of platelet-activating factor agonists. J Immunol 190(5):2447–2454

Sahu RP, Ocana JA, Harrison KA, Ferracini M, Touloukian CE, Al-Hassani M, Sun L, Loesch M, Murphy RC, Althouse SK, Perkins SM, Speicher PJ, Tyler DS, Konger RL, Travers JB (2014) Chemotherapeutic agents subvert tumor immunity by generating agonists of platelet-activating factor. Cancer Res 74(23):7069–7078

Sahu RP, Harrison KA, Weyerbacher J, Murphy RC, Konger RL, Garrett JE, Chin-Sinex HJ, Johnston ME II, Dynlacht JR, Mendonca M, McMullen K, Li G, Spandau DF, Travers JB (2016) Radiation therapy generates immunosuppressive platelet-activating factor agonists. Oncotarget 7:20788–20800

Schaue D, Ratikan JA, Iwamoto KS, McBride WH (2012) Maximizing tumor immunity with fractionated radiation. Int J Radiat Oncol Biol Phys 83:1306–1310

Serban KA, Rezania S, Petrusca DN, Poirier C, Cao D, Justice MJ, Patel M, Tsvetkova I, Kamocki K, Mikosz A, Schweitzer KS, Jacobson S, Cardoso A, Carlesso N, Hubbard WC, Kechris K, Dragnea B, Berdyshev EV, McClintock J, Petrache I (2016) Structural and functional characterization of endothelial microparticles released by cigarette smoke. Sci Rep 6:31596

Shimizu T (2009) Lipid mediators in health and disease: enzymes and receptors as therapeutic targets for the regulation of immunity and inflammation. Annu Rev Pharmacol Toxicol 49:123–150

Snyder F, Fitzgerald V, Blank ML (1996) Biosynthesis of platelet-activating factor and enzyme inhibitors. Adv Exp Med Biol 416:5–10

Soares AC, Pinho VS, Souza DG, Shimizu T, Ishii S, Nicoli JR, Teixeira MM (2002) Role of the platelet-activating factor (PAF) receptor during pulmonary infection with gram negative bacteria. Br J Pharmacol 137(5):621–628

Sreevidya CS, Khaskhely NM, Fukunaga A, Khaskina P, Ullrich SE (2008) Inhibition of photocarcinogenesis by platelet-activating factor or serotonin receptor antagonists. Cancer Res 68(10):3978–3984

St Denis TG, Aziz K, Waheed AA et al (2011) Combination approaches to potentiate immune response after photodynamic therapy for cancer. Photochem Photobiol Sci 10(5):792–801

Stampfli MR, Anderson GP (2009) How cigarette smoke skews immune responses to promote infection, lung disease and cancer. Nat Rev Immunol 9(5):377–384

SucIu-Foca N, Molinaro A, Buda J, Reemtsma K (1974) Cellular immune responsiveness in cigarette smokers. Lancet 1:1062–1064

Takeshita J, Mohler ER, Krishnamoorthy P, Moore J, Rogers WT, Zhang L, Gelfand JM, Mehta NN (2014) Endothelial cell-, platelet-, and monocyte/macrophage-derived microparticles are elevated in psoriasis beyond cardiometabolic risk factors. J Am Heart Assoc 3(1):e000507

Talvani A, Santana G, Barcelos LS, Ishii S, Shimizu T, Romanha AJ, Silva JS, Soares MB, Teixeira MM (2003) Experimental Trypanosoma cruzi infection in platelet-activating factor receptor-deficient mice. Microbes Infect 5:789–796

Tamagawa-Mineoka R, Katoh N, Kishimoto S (2010) Platelet activation in patients with psoriasis: increased plasma levels of platelet-derived microparticles and soluble P-selectin. J Am Acad Dermatol 62:621–626

Travers JB, Harrison KA, Johnson CA, Clay KL, Morelli JG, Murphy RC (1996) Platelet-activating factor biosynthesis induced by various stimuli in human HaCaT keratinocytes. J Invest Dermatol 107:88–94

Travers JB, Pei Y, Morin M, Hood A (1998a) Antiinflammatory effects of the platelet- activating factor receptor antagonist A85783. Arch Dermatol Res 290:569–573

Travers JB, Murphy RC, Johnson CA, Pei Y, Morin SM, Barber LA, Clay K, Hood AF, Morelli JG, Williams DA (1998b) Identification and pharmacological characterization of PAF and 1-acyl species found in human inflammatory blistering diseases. Prostaglandins 56:305–324

Travers JB, Edenberg HJ, Zhang Q, Al-Hassani M, Yi Q, Baskaran S, Konger RL (2008) Augmentation of UVB radiation-mediated early gene expression by the epidermal platelet-activating factor receptor. J Invest Dermatol 128(2):455–460

Ullrich SE (2005) Mechanisms underlying UV-induced immune suppression. Mutat Res 571:185–205

Vadas P, Gold M, Perelman B, Liss GM, Lack G, Blyth T, Simons FER, Simons KJ, Cass D, Yeung J (2008) Platelet-activating factor, PAF acetylhydrolase, and severe anaphylaxis. N Engl J Med 358:28–35

Varma S, Holt PJ, Anstey AV (2000) Erythroplasia of queyrat treated by topical aminolaevulinic acid photodynamic therapy: a cautionary tale. Br J Dermatol 142:825–826

Vion A-C, Ramkhelawon B, Loyer X et al (2013) Shear stress regulates endothelial microparticle release. Circ Res 112:1323–1333

Wacker M, Holick MF (2013) Sunlight and vitamin D. Dermato-Endocrinol 5(1):51–108

Walterscheid JP, Ullrich SE, Nghiem DX (2002) Platelet-activating factor, a molecular sensor for cellular damage, activates systemic immune suppression. J Exp Med 195:171–179

Wara WM (1977) Immunosuppression associated with radiation therapy. Int J Radiat Oncol Biol Phys 2:593–596

Wara WM, Phillips TL, Wara DW, Ammann AJ, Smith V (1975) Immunosuppression following radiation therapy for carcinoma of the nasopharynx. Am J Roentgenol Radium Ther Nucl Med 123:482–485

Winter AP, Follett EA, McIntyre J, Stewart J, Symington IS (1994) Influence of smoking on immunological responses to hepatitis B vaccine. Vaccine 12(9):771–772

Wolf P, Fink-Puches R, Reimann-Weber A et al (1997) Development of malignant melanoma after repeated topical photodynamic therapy with 5-aminolevulinic acid at the exposed site. Dermatology 194:53–54

Wolf P et al (2006) Platelet-activating factor is crucial in psoralen and ultraviolet A-induced immune suppression, inflammation, and apoptosis. Am J Pathol 169(3):795–805

Wolverton JE, Al-Hassani M, Yao Y, Travers JB (2010) Epidermal platelet-activating factor activation and ultraviolet B radiation result in synergistic tumor necrosis factor alpha production. Photochem Photobiol 86:231–235

Xiao X, Ma X, Liu L, Wang J, Bi K, Liu Y, Fan R, Zhao B, Chen Y, Bihl JC (2015) Cellular membrane microparticles: potential targets of combinational therapy for vascular disease. Curr Vasc Pharmacol 13(4):449–458

Yamada Y, Yokota M (1997) Loss of activity of plasma platelet-activating factor acetylhydrolase due to a novel Gln281-->Arg mutation. Biochem Biophys Res Commun 236(3):772–775

Yang L et al (2010) Chronic alcohol exposure increases circulating bioactive oxidized phospholipids. J Biol Chem 285(29):22211–22220

Yao Y, Harrison KA, Al-Hassani M, Murphy RC, Rezania S, Konger RL, Travers JB (2012) Platelet-activating factor agonists mediate xeroderma pigmentosum A photosensitivity. J Biol Chem 287:9311–9321

Zalewski A, Macphee C (2005) Role of lipoprotein-associated phospholipase A2 in atherosclerosis: biology, epidemiology, and possible therapeutic target. Arterioscler Thromb Vasc Biol 25 (5):923–931

Zhang Q, Yao Y, Konger RL, Sinn AL, Cai S, Pollok KE, Travers JB (2008) UVB radiation-mediated inhibition of contact hypersensitivity reactions is dependent on the platelet-activating factor system. J Invest Dermatol 128:1780–1787

Zimmerman GA, McIntyre TM, Prescott SM, Stafforini DM (2002) The platelet-activating factor signaling system and its regulators in syndromes of inflammation and thrombosis. Crit Care Med 30(5 Suppl):S294–S301

Phospholipase D and Choline Metabolism

Fredrick O. Onono and Andrew J. Morris

Contents

Abstract

Phospholipases D (PLDs) catalyze hydrolysis of the diester bond of phospholipids to generate phosphatidic acid and the free lipid headgroup. In mammals, PLD enzymes comprise the intracellular enzymes PLD1 and PLD2 and possibly the proteins encoded by related genes, as well as a class of cell surface and secreted enzymes with structural homology to ectonucleotide phosphatases/ phosphodiesterases as typified by autotaxin (ENPP2) that have lysoPLD activities. Genetic and pharmacological loss-of-function approaches implicate these enzymes in intra- and intercellular signaling mediated by the lipid products phosphatidic acid, lysophosphatidic acid, and their metabolites, while the possibility that the water-soluble product of their reactions is biologically relevant has received far less attention. PLD1 and PLD2 are highly selective for phosphatidylcholine (PC), whereas autotaxin has broader substrate specificity for

F. O. Onono · A. J. Morris (✉)
Division of Cardiovascular Medicine, The Gill Heart and Vascular Institute, University of Kentucky College of Medicine, Lexington, KY, USA

Lexington Veterans Affairs Medical Center, Lexington, KY, USA
e-mail: fred.onono@uky.edu; a.j.morris@uky.edu

J. Gomez-Cambronero, M. A. Frohman (eds.), *Lipid Signaling in Human Diseases*, Handbook of Experimental Pharmacology 259, https://doi.org/10.1007/164_2019_320

lysophospholipids but by virtue of the high abundance of lysophosphatidylcholine (LPC) in extracellular fluids predominantly hydrolyses this substrate. In all cases, the water-soluble product of these PLD activities is choline. Although choline can be formed de novo by methylation of phosphatidylethanolamine, this activity is absent in most tissues, so mammals are effectively auxotrophic for choline. Dietary consumption of choline in both free and esterified forms is substantial. Choline is necessary for synthesis of the neurotransmitter acetylcholine and of the choline-containing phospholipids PC and sphingomyelin (SM) and also plays a recently appreciated important role as a methyl donor in the pathways of "one-carbon (1C)" metabolism. This review discusses emerging evidence that some of the biological functions of these intra- and extracellular PLD enzymes involve generation of choline with a particular focus on the possibility that these choline and PLD dependent processes are dysregulated in cancer.

Keywords
Choline · One carbon metabolism · Phospholipase D

1 Overview of Choline Metabolism

Figure 1 summarizes the pathways of choline metabolism that are discussed in detail in the following sections. Choline is a ubiquitous metabolite present in tissues, plasma, and other biological fluids. Humans can synthesize small amounts of choline by sequential methylation of phosphatidylethanolamine (PE) to form phosphatidylcholine (PC) in the liver (Gibellini and Smith 2010). Hence, choline is considered an essential nutrient that must be obtained from the diet to supplement this smaller endogenously/de novo synthesized pool (Zeisel and da Costa 2009). Choline is therefore derived from three major sources: (1) dietary choline, as free base or as a constituent of phospholipids present within many foods; (2) endogenous synthesis, principally in the liver; and (3) liberation from choline-containing phospholipids, which are major constituents of all cell membranes. The most abundant sources of esterified choline, phosphatidylcholine and sphingomyelin, are essential for both the structural integrity of cellular membranes and for lipid-dependent signaling pathways, both of which are required for cancer cell growth (Institute of Medicine USA Standing Committee on the Scientific Evaluation of Dietary Reference Intakes and its Panel on Folate, Other B Vitamins, and Choline 1998). Free choline is released from esterified choline containing lipid sources by hydrolysis catalyzed by phospholipase D enzymes. Dietary choline is absorbed by enterocytes in the lumen of the small intestine which is mediated by choline transporter proteins (Institute of Medicine USA Standing Committee on the Scientific Evaluation of Dietary Reference Intakes and its Panel on Folate, Other B Vitamins, and Choline 1998). Free choline enters the portal circulation of the liver, whereas PC enters the circulation via lymph as a phospholipid constituent of triglyceride-rich chylomicrons. Choline can be phosphorylated to phosphocholine or oxidized to form betaine by the gut microbiota, or in some cell types such as hepatocytes, to feed into the choline biosynthetic pathway and one-carbon metabolism (Zeisel 2009). It is also

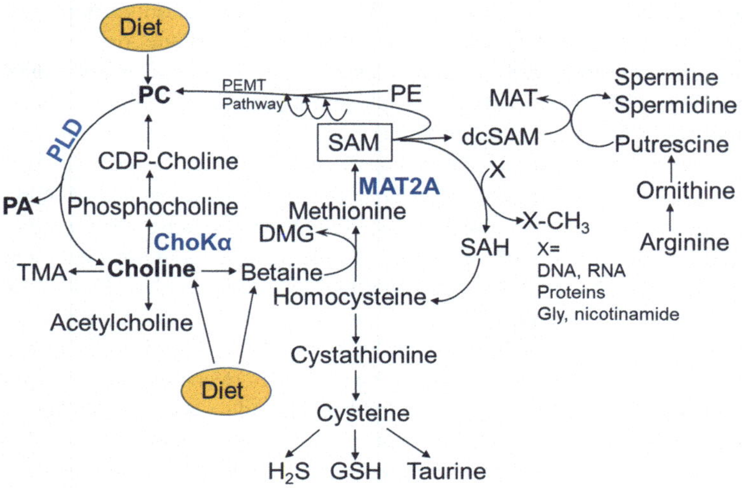

Fig. 1 Role of diet and phospholipase D in choline metabolism and choline-mediated 1C metabolism. Phospholipase D (PLD) catalyzes release of choline from either diet-derived or endogenously synthesized phosphatidylcholine (PC). Choline is a substrate for the synthesis of acetylcholine, trimethylamine (TMA), and phosphatidylcholine (PC) via cytidine diphosphate choline (CDP-choline). Formation of phosphocholine catalyzed by choline kinase α (ChoKα) is the initial step of de novo PC synthesis. Choline can also be oxidized to betaine. The oxidation of choline to betaine links PLD activity to 1C metabolism through de novo synthesis of methionine from homocysteine. The by-product of this reaction, dimethylglycine (DMG), is also a potential methyl donor. The methionine product is utilized for synthesis of S-adenosylmethionine (SAM) catalyzed by methionine adenosyltransferase 2A (MAT2A). SAM is the universal methyl donor for a wide range of substrates including phosphatidylethanolamine (PE), DNA, RNA, and proteins including histones and for generating S-adenosyl-L-homocysteine (SAH). SAH is hydrolyzed to homocysteine which couples 1C metabolism to the transsulfuration pathway involving sequential synthesis of cystathionine and cysteine and ultimately forming glutathione, taurine, and hydrogen sulfide (H_2S). SAM can also be decarboxylated to decarboxylated S-adenosylmethionine (dc-SAM) which supports synthesis of the polyamines, spermine, and spermidine. The by-product, 5-methylthioadenosine (MTA) is salvaged back to methionine for SAM generation. The highlighted enzymes PLD, ChoKα, and MAT2A are attractive therapeutic targets for treatment of cancer

a precursor to the neurotransmitter acetylcholine. Although choline plays essential roles, it is also implicated, either directly or indirectly via its metabolites, in chronic noncommunicable diseases including cardiovascular diseases, and cancers.

2 Dietary Sources of Choline

Dietary choline can be obtained from a wide variety of foods and supplements. Because de novo synthesis of choline alone is not sufficient to meet human requirements, choline was officially recognized as an essential nutrient by the

Institute of Medicine in 1998 (Institute of Medicine USA Standing Committee on the Scientific Evaluation of Dietary Reference Intakes and its Panel on Folate, Other B Vitamins, and Choline 1998). It is available in foods as both water-soluble (free choline, phosphocholine, and glycerophosphocholine) and lipid-soluble forms (phosphatidylcholine and sphingomyelin) (Zeisel 2012a). The main dietary sources of choline in the USA are animal products such as meat – especially beef liver, poultry, eggs, fish, and dairy products (McGuire 2016). Other sources rich in choline include cruciferous vegetables such as cauliflower and broccoli, nuts, seeds, certain beans, and whole grains. Additives and supplements containing choline are also readily available. The most common choline-containing food additive, lecithin, is usually derived from sunflower seeds, eggs, or soybeans. Lecithin is used as an emulsifying agent in routinely consumed processed foods such as salad dressings, gravies, and margarine. It can also be purchased as an over-the-counter supplement. Other forms of supplements high in choline include choline chloride, cytidine diphosphate-choline (CDP-choline), and glycero phosphocholine (alpha-GPC). The choline oxidation product, betaine, is also available as a supplement.

The Food and Nutrition Board of the Institute of Medicine recommends daily intake of choline of 425 and 550 mg for adult females and males, respectively (Institute of Medicine USA Standing Committee on the Scientific Evaluation of Dietary Reference Intakes and its Panel on Folate, Other B Vitamins, and Choline 1998). The tolerable upper intake level for adults is estimated at 3.5 g/day. Dietary choline intake is calculated based on estimates of the free choline and phosphatidylcholine content of foods. There are no reliable estimates of the frequency of use or amount of these dietary supplements consumed by individuals in the USA and Canada. However, there are reports suggesting that the average dietary intake of choline in adults could be higher and is underreported (Fischer et al. 2005). According to the USA Dietary Guidelines Advisory Committee (DGAC) 2015–2020 report, eggs provide the most abundant source of choline for individuals whose intake is at or above the recommended levels. Egg yolks provide 680 mg of choline per 100 g (Zeisel and da Costa 2009).

Choline insufficiency in the diet can lead to liver damage, muscle damage, and nonalcoholic fatty liver disease (NAFLD or hepatosteatosis) (Sherriff et al. 2016). Furthermore, choline deficiency is one of the few single-nutrient deficiencies that causes increased spontaneous carcinogenesis (Zeisel 2012b). In rats and mice, diets low in choline and other methyl-group donors such as folate, methionine, serine, vitamin B12, and betaine result in spontaneous hepatocarcinomas or sensitize rodents to hepatic carcinogens such as aflatoxin B1 (Schrager et al. 1990). Oral administration of lecithin (containing esterified choline) or free choline for a prolonged period of time has been shown to increase plasma choline levels (Buchman et al. 1992, 1995). High dietary intake of choline causes adverse effects such as hypotension, fishy body odor, vomiting, excessive sweating and salivation, and liver toxicity (Davis et al. 1975; Growdon et al. 1977; Lawrence et al. 1980; Wood and Allison 1982). High choline consumption also increases the production of trimethylamine oxide (TMAO), a choline metabolite that has been linked to a higher risk of cardiovascular disease, in a dose-dependent manner in adults (Wang et al.

2011). The association between dietary intake of choline and cancers is less clear. Overall, the recognition of dietary association with cancer incidence has only began to be appreciated. For example, the USA DGAC concluded in 2010 that there was not sufficient evidence to acknowledge the effects of dietary patterns and cancer risk (Van Horn 2010). It was not until very recently in 2015 that DGAC officially recognized diet as a risk factor for colon and postmenopausal breast cancer risk (McGuire 2016). However, there is no clear consensus on the effects of high choline consumption on cancer.

3 Choline and Phospholipid Synthesis

Choline is an important dietary nutrient that supports the synthesis of the most abundant glycerophospholipid PC via the cytidine diphosphate (CDP)-choline pathway. Up to 95% of the total choline pool in most tissues is used in the synthesis of PC (Zeisel and Blusztajn 1994; Zeisel et al. 2003). First described in 1956, Kennedy and Weiss elucidated a pathway for the de novo biosynthesis of PC and PE using rat liver as source of enzyme activities (Kennedy and Weiss 1956). Hence, there are two branches of the Kennedy pathway: CDP-choline pathway and the analogous pathway for PE called the CDP-ethanolamine pathway (Sundler and Akesson 1975). The CDP-choline pathway consists of three enzymatic steps. Initially, choline kinase catalyzes the ATP-dependent phosphorylation of choline to form phosphocholine. In the second step, CDP-choline is formed from phosphocholine and Cytidine triphosphate (CTP) catalyzed by CTP/phosphocholine cytidylyltransferase. The final step of PC synthesis involves CDP-choline and a lipid anchor such as diacylglycerol (DAG) or alkyl-acylglycerol (AAG) (Sundler and Akesson 1975). The Kennedy pathway enzymes are found ubiquitously in eukaryotes (Lykidis 2007). PC synthesis is required for lipoprotein secretion from the liver (Li and Vance 2008). It is also a major source of the second messengers DAG, phosphatidic acid, lysophosphatidic acid, and arachidonic acid, which can be further metabolized to other signaling molecules (Li and Vance 2008).

4 Choline and One-Carbon Metabolism

One-carbon (1C) metabolism comprises a complex network of biochemical reactions that facilitates the transfer of 1C moieties in the form of methenyl, formyl, and methyl groups to support the synthesis of molecules that are required for cellular processes (Shane and Stokstad 1985; Stipanuk 2004; Stover 2004). The carbon unit cycle is essential for multiple physiological processes including cellular biosynthesis (purines and thymidine), amino acid homeostasis (glycine, serine, and methionine), methylation (PC biosynthesis, epigenetic maintenance), and regulation of redox status (Ducker and Rabinowitz 2017). Three pathways are involved: the folate cycle, methionine remethylation, and transsulfuration pathways. The most important metabolites through which cells refuel one-carbon metabolism are folic acid, serine, glycine, and choline. Essentially, two major one-carbon donors are involved in the biosynthetic reactions: tetrahydrofolate (THF) derived from folate and S-adenosylmethionine (SAM) derived from methionine (Mentch and Locasale 2016).

In mammalian cells, choline contributes to regeneration of methionine from homocysteine via its oxidation product, betaine, catalyzed by the enzyme betaine-homocysteine methyltransferase (BHMT) (Pajares and Perez-Sala 2006). After donating a methyl group to homocysteine, the by-product of this reaction, dimethylglycine, can also yield additional 1C units through its utilization for synthesis of THF (Ueland 2011). Expression of BHMT is restricted to the liver and kidney. Methionine synthase is expressed globally, thus enabling homocysteine remethylation to occur throughout the body. Methionine is the substrate for S-adenosylmethionine (SAM) synthetase which produces SAM. The reactive methyl carrier, SAM, is the second most common enzymatic cofactor after ATP (Su et al. 2016). SAM plays a major role in DNA methylation-dependent epigenetic mechanisms of gene regulation; biosynthetic processes including phosphatidylcholine, creatine, and polyamine synthesis; and sulfur metabolism. It is believed that phosphatidylcholine synthesis from phosphoethanolamine using SAM is likely the largest 1C sink in adult mammals (Stead et al. 2006). During the PC synthesis from PE, SAM donates three methyl groups via phosphatidylethanolamine methyltransferase (PEMT), an enzyme expressed principally in the liver. The impact of the intake of the 1C donor choline on these processes is less studied, and the associations between choline consumption and disease are not clear.

5 Role of Phospholipase D in Choline Metabolism

Phospholipase D (PLD) and phospholipase C (PLC) are the major enzymes responsible for the release of choline and phosphocholine, respectively, from the most abundant phospholipid PC. Choline can also be released from the lyso-derivative of PC, lysoPC (LPC), by autotaxin, an enzyme that has lysophospholipase D activity. Although no mammalian PC-specific PLC isoforms have been sequenced or cloned, PLD is well characterized and is highly expressed in breast cancers as well as in colorectal, renal, gastric, ovarian, prostate, and non-small cell lung cancers (McDermott et al. 2004; Morris 2007). Mammalian PLD constitutes an enzyme superfamily with six members, PLD1–6. Each PLD isoform has unique patterns of subcellular localization and roles in cellular processes. PLD1 and PLD2 are the most widely studied PLD isoforms and are expressed in most tissues at varying basal levels. Human PLD1 and PLD2 share 50% amino acid identity and display a similar protein structure (Pettitt et al. 2001). The PLD1 (120 kDa) isoform is mainly found in the inner membranes of mammalian cells including lysosomes, secretory endosomes, the Golgi complex, and endosomes (Nanjundan and Possmayer 2003). It is readily transported to the plasma membrane subsequent to extracellular stimulation (Choi et al. 2002). PLD2 (106 kDa), on the other hand, most commonly localizes to the plasma membrane (Zhao et al. 2007). Whereas PLD1 exhibits low intrinsic activity, i.e., does not transduce extracellular signaling in its basal state, PLD2 has relatively high basal catalytic activity. However, the available evidence shows that PLD2 displays the same enzymatic activity as PLD1, catalyzing the hydrolysis of PC to produce free choline and phosphatidic acid (PA). A single nucleotide polymorphism associated with increased risk of non-small cell lung cancer has been observed in the PLD1 gene, while polymorphisms in the PLD2 gene are associated with risk of colorectal cancer (Ahn et al. 2012; Yamada et al. 2003). Overexpression of PLD1 or PLD2 in murine fibroblasts or in breast cancer xenograft models alters cell growth and leads to primary tumor initiation and metastasis (Henkels et al. 2013; Min et al. 2001). The signaling lipid PA has pleiotropic effects (Cruchaga et al. 2014). It can facilitate membrane vesicle trafficking, endocytosis/exocytosis, and also function as a lipid anchor to recruit PA-binding proteins to localize to sites of signal transduction. PA is also known to activate proteins such as phosphatidylinositol 4-phosphate 5-Kinase (PI4P5K) and mTOR to regulate cellular processes such as cell hypertrophy, survival, and differentiation (Cho and Han 2017). Furthermore, PA can be dephosphorylated by Lipin to produce diacylglycerol (DAG) or hydrolyzed by phospholipase A (PLA) to produce LysoPA (LPA) (Baba et al. 2014). Because of its significance to disease, PLD has been studied both in vitro using cultured cells and animal models. Mice with genetic ablation of PLD1 are viable and fertile with no reported abnormalities (Zhang and Frohman 2014). When studied in a model of spontaneous intestinal cancer, PLD1-deficient mice showed significantly reduced intestinal tumorigenesis and increased survival (Dall'Armi et al. 2010). In contrast, deficiency of the related isoform PLD2 does not significantly reduce tumorigenesis. Similarly, in a syngeneic melanoma cancer model, loss of PLD1 by genetic knockout or use of the PLD1/2 small molecule inhibitor, 5-fluoro-2-indolyl des-chlorohalopemide (FIPI) (Su et al. 2009), decreased tumor size and weight and decreased metastasis (Chen et al. 2012). These reports suggest that PLD1 could be a promising target for breast cancer therapy. Furthermore, an interdependency has been reported between the PLD1 isoform and choline kinase α enzymes in terms of protein expression (Gadiya et al. 2014). PLD1 silencing increases CHKA expression and vice versa. Interestingly, novel findings from recent microbiota studies show that several gut microorganisms also express and possibly secrete PLD enzymes that hydrolyze PC as the preferred substrate to produce free choline for downstream metabolism (Chittim et al. 2019). Although Chittim et al. (2019) demonstrated in their work that the released choline is utilized in the production of trimethylamine (TMA) by other gut microorganisms, these findings support the idea that gut microbiota PLD-released choline could also be substrate for choline kinase and subsequent systemic metabolic pathways.

6 Dysregulated Choline Metabolism in Cancer Cells

Cancer is a dynamic disease with phenotypic and functional heterogeneity arising from genetic changes, environmental differences, and reversible changes in cellular properties (Meacham and Morrison 2013). Common pathways are rare in cancer. However, dysregulated choline metabolism, a fairly new metabolic hallmark of cancer, is a common feature in nearly all cancers (Cheng et al. 2016; Glunde et al. 2011). Elevated levels of choline, phosphocholine, and glycerophosphocholine have been consistently observed in cancer cells and tumor tissues (Glunde et al. 2015).

Comparative studies in cancer cells and rapidly proliferating non-cancerous epithelial cells have identified malignant transformation rather than just cell proliferation as the cause of abnormal choline metabolism in cancer (Aboagye and Bhujwalla 1999; Daly et al. 1987). Enzymes involved in choline metabolism are proving to be an attractive and effective strategy for cancer treatment. For example, choline kinase α (CHKA), the first enzyme in the CDP-pathway, is expressed in a large diversity of human tumors including breast, lung, colorectal, bladder, prostate, ovary, endometrial, and T-cell lymphoma (Ramirez de Molina et al. 2002a, b). Overexpression of CHKA has oncogenic potential and synergizes with other known oncogenes to drive cancer progression. As a result, several groups have made attempts to design small molecules as new inhibitors of its enzymatic activity and characterize their activity as anticancer drugs under in vitro and in vivo conditions (Al-Saffar et al. 2006; Lacal 2001). Among these, TCD-717, a second generation of CHKA inhibitors, has completed a first-in-human, phase I clinical trial (http://clinicaltrials.gov/ct2/show/NCT01215864) (Lacal and Campos 2015). An interdependency has been reported between the PLD1 isoform and choline kinase α enzymes in terms of protein expression that suggests compensatory effects between these two main choline-regulating enzymes (Gadiya et al. 2014). Numerous studies with cells, animal models, and humans have established the value of magnetic resonance spectroscopy (MRS) measurements for total choline-containing compounds (tCho) for detection of cancers and determining response to therapy (Daly et al. 1987). In addition, dietary manipulations that may impact on choline metabolism, especially methionine restriction, have been shown to attenuate tumor development, suggesting a viable approach to cancer management through nutritional intervention (Hanley et al. 2016; Kadaveru et al. 2012; Lamming et al. 2015). Choline metabolites have also been implicated in oncogenesis and tumor progression through roles in phospholipid synthesis and 1C metabolism (Glunde et al. 2011).

7 Pharmacological Targeting of Phospholipase D and One Carbon Metabolism

Because of their roles in generating phosphatidic acid (PA), which regulates many cellular processes and is also a precursor to many bioactive lipid signaling molecules, PLD1 and PLD2 have emerged as drug targets for various diseases such as cancer, cardiovascular diseases, infectious diseases, and neurodegenerative conditions (Parkinson's and Alzheimer's disease). Initially, primary alcohols (e.g., *n*-butanol) were the most commonly used molecules to inhibit PLD-catalyzed production of PA by promoting the formation of phosphatidyl alcohols which are presumed to be biologically inactive (Brown et al. 2017; Selvy et al. 2011). This approach generally results in only incomplete attenuation of PLD- dependent PA production. High-throughput screening approaches enabled discovery of small molecules that could be used to target the two PLD isoenzymes. The first compounds described were halopemide and its derivatives notably 5-fluoro-2-indolyl des-chlorohalopemide (FIPI) (Monovich et al. 2007; Su et al. 2009). Halopemide and its derivatives were initially reported to be PLD2 inhibitors but were later found to also inhibit PLD1 with even greater potency (Scott et al. 2009; Su et al. 2009). Using halopemide as a base, isoenzyme-selective PLD inhibitors with improved ancillary pharmacology and drug metabolism and pharmacokinetics profiles were later developed. A series of highly selective PLD1 inhibitors such as VU0359595 have been reported (Lewis et al. 2009). VU0359595 is approximately 1,700 times more selective for PLD1 compared to PLD2. On the other hand, the first highly selective PLD2 inhibitor identified by the same group, VU0364739, has 75-fold selectivity for PLD2 versus PLD1 (Lavieri et al. 2010). In attempts to further develop even more selective PLD2 inhibitors, ML298 and ML395 were synthesized using triazaspirone as the core of the molecules (O'Reilly et al. 2013). The halopemide-derived and triazaspirone-based series were potent inhibitors of mammalian PLD enzymes but were inactive against both the bacterial *Pseudomonas aeruginosa* PLD (PldA) and the endocannabinoid generating NAPE-PLD (Scott et al. 2015). This prompted the development of PLD inhibitors based on selective estrogen receptor modulators (SERMs) which had previously displayed off-target inhibition of PLD enzymes (Eisen and Brown 2002). One of the best characterized SERMs, desketoraloxifene, has comparable inhibitory activity against mammalian PLD1 and PLD2, and bacterial PldA (Scott et al. 2015).

As mentioned elsewhere in this review and shown in Fig. 1, the free headgroup (choline) generated by PLD enzymes can be used for de novo synthesis of phosphatidylcholine or enter 1C metabolism via its oxidized product, betaine. Therefore inhibitors of PC biosynthetic pathway or 1C metabolism might be complementary or synergistic with PLD inhibitors. Two of the enzymes targeted with potential anticancer agents are choline kinase α (ChoKα) and methyl adenosyltransferase (MAT2A). ChoKα catalyzes the phosphorylation of choline which is the first step in the choline pathway for synthesis of PC. As with PLD inhibitors, the first inhibitors of ChoKα included alcohols such as propanol and butanol (Mehendale et al. 1966). Other earlier inhibitors of ChoKα to be synthesized were methyl-substituted derivatives of choline. Hemicholinium-3 (HC-3), structural homologs of choline, was later developed and demonstrated potent antitumor effects (Daly et al. 1987; Hamza et al. 1983). This was followed by a series of bis-quinolinium compounds which are less toxic derivatives of HC-3. The first generation of these compounds was MN58b (Hernandez-Alcoceba et al. 1999). With further improvement for tolerability, RSM-932A, a more potent bis-quinolinium with a better therapeutic window and improved safety profile, was developed (Lacal and Campos 2015). RSM-932A (also called TCD-717) became the first ChoKα inhibitor to be tested in humans when it entered phase I clinical trials (Lacal and Campos 2015). MAT2A catalyzes the biosynthesis of the universal methyl donor S-adenosylmethionine (SAM) from methionine and ATP. SAM is required for many methyl transfer reactions and polyamine biosynthesis. Inhibitors of MAT2A have been developed that bind to either an allosteric site or to the catalytic subunit of MAT2A. A family of fluorinated N,N-dialkylaminostilbene (FIDAS) agents and their analogs have been developed that directly target the catalytic subunit of MAT2A (Zhang et al. 2013). On the other hand, Pfizer developed a MAT2A inhibitor, PF-9366, that binds and allosterically regulates the activity of MAT2A (Quinlan et al. 2017). The MAT2A inhibitor AG-270 developed by Agios

Pharmaceuticals as a first-in-class MAT2A inhibitor is being tested in patients with advanced solid tumors or lymphoma characterized by the homozygous deletion of the MTAP gene which plays a critical role in methionine salvage and consequently when absent renders cells highly dependent on MT2A-dependent methionine synthesis (Marjon et al. 2016). Collectively, continued development of the classes of inhibitors discussed above is expected to result in compounds with improved specificity, potency, and tolerability. These compounds will continue to be valuable tools for analyzing the role of PLD, ChoKα, and MAT2A enzymes in normal physiology and disease. These tools can be used to complement genetic knockout approaches in studies targeting distinct PLD isoenzymes and other pathways that utilize products of PLD activity. In addition, these small molecules can be utilized in cases where genetic ablation would be difficult to achieve or in settings where deletion of the aforementioned enzymes would have effects distinct from those of short-term inhibition. Although presently not used clinically, it is likely that small molecule inhibitors of PLD isoenzymes will be tested for efficacy in diseases, especially those where currently available therapeutics are limited. PLD inhibitors could be used in combination with novel ChoKα and MAT2A inhibitors or with standard chemotherapy to target pathways of 1C metabolism that are known to be critical for development and progression of some cancers.

8 Concluding Comments

Although substantial advances have been made in understanding the molecular mechanisms that drive aberrant choline metabolism in cancer, the role of diet-derived choline in this process is unclear. A number of epidemiologic studies examining the relationship between dietary choline intake and cancer have yielded conflicting findings. Therefore, investigating the idea that high consumption of dietary lipids, rich in esterified choline, promotes the abnormal choline metabolism leading to cancer progression and metastasis would be worthwhile. This could be done using mouse models of cancer and rodent diets formulated with exogenous phosphatidylcholine as the major source of dietary choline. PLD-deficient animal models have been generated and characterized. Development of small molecule inhibitors targeting PLD is ongoing. With the interest and rapid increase in gut microbiome research over the last several years, the discovery of widespread PLD activity among gut bacteria with a likely role in generation of free choline from dietary esterified sources provides additional opportunities for therapeutic intervention. Together, these tools present an excellent opportunity to unravel the missing link between PLD and diet in contributing to choline and one-carbon metabolism. It would be possible, for example, to test the hypothesis that PLD expression and higher consumption of dietary PC support the abnormal choline metabolism in cancer.

Acknowledgments Research in the author's laboratories is supported by grants from the NIH and the Department of Veterans Affairs. FOO is the recipient of an NIH/NCI Mentored Research Scientist Development Award K01CA197073.

References

Aboagye EO, Bhujwalla ZM (1999) Malignant transformation alters membrane choline phospholipid metabolism of human mammary epithelial cells. Cancer Res 59:80–84

Ahn MJ et al (2012) A single nucleotide polymorphism in the phospholipase D1 gene is associated with risk of non-small cell lung cancer. Int J Biomed Sci 8:121–128

Al-Saffar NM et al (2006) Noninvasive magnetic resonance spectroscopic pharmacodynamic markers of the choline kinase inhibitor MN58b in human carcinoma models. Cancer Res 66:427–434. https://doi.org/10.1158/0008-5472.Can-05-1338

Baba T et al (2014) Phosphatidic acid (PA)-preferring phospholipase A1 regulates mitochondrial dynamics. J Biol Chem 289:11497–11511. https://doi.org/10.1074/jbc.M113.531921

Brown HA, Thomas PG, Lindsley CW (2017) Targeting phospholipase D in cancer, infection and neurodegenerative disorders. Nat Rev Drug Discov 16:351–367. https://doi.org/10.1038/nrd.2016.252

Buchman AL et al (1992) Lecithin increases plasma free choline and decreases hepatic steatosis in long-term total parenteral nutrition patients. Gastroenterology 102:1363–1370

Buchman AL et al (1995) Choline deficiency: a cause of hepatic steatosis during parenteral nutrition that can be reversed with intravenous choline supplementation. Hepatology 22:1399–1403

Chen Q et al (2012) Key roles for the lipid signaling enzyme phospholipase D1 in the tumor microenvironment during tumor angiogenesis and metastasis. Sci Signal 5:ra79. https://doi.org/10.1126/scisignal.2003257

Cheng M, Bhujwalla ZM, Glunde K (2016) Targeting phospholipid metabolism in cancer. Front Oncol 6:266. https://doi.org/10.3389/fonc.2016.00266

Chittim CL, Martinez Del Campo A, Balskus EP (2019) Gut bacterial phospholipase Ds support disease-associated metabolism by generating choline. Nat Microbiol 4:155–163. https://doi.org/10.1038/s41564-018-0294-4

Cho JH, Han JS (2017) Phospholipase D and its essential role in cancer. Mol Cell 40:805–813. https://doi.org/10.14348/molcells.2017.0241

Choi WS, Chahdi A, Kim YM, Fraundorfer PF, Beaven MA (2002) Regulation of phospholipase D and secretion in mast cells by protein kinase A and other protein kinases. Ann N Y Acad Sci 968:198–212. https://doi.org/10.1111/j.1749-6632.2002.tb04336.x

Cruchaga C et al (2014) Rare coding variants in the phospholipase D3 gene confer risk for Alzheimer's disease. Nature 505:550–554. https://doi.org/10.1038/nature12825

Dall'Armi C et al (2010) The phospholipase D1 pathway modulates macroautophagy. Nat Commun 1:142. https://doi.org/10.1038/ncomms1144

Daly PF, Lyon RC, Faustino PJ, Cohen JS (1987) Phospholipid metabolism in cancer cells monitored by 31P NMR spectroscopy. J Biol Chem 262:14875–14878

Davis KL, Berger PA, Hollister LE (1975) Letter: choline for tardive dyskinesia. N Engl J Med 293:152. https://doi.org/10.1056/nejm197507172930317

Ducker GS, Rabinowitz JD (2017) One-carbon metabolism in health and disease. Cell Metab 25:27–42. https://doi.org/10.1016/j.cmet.2016.08.009

Eisen SF, Brown HA (2002) Selective estrogen receptor (ER) modulators differentially regulate phospholipase D catalytic activity in ER-negative breast cancer cells. Mol Pharmacol 62:911–920. https://doi.org/10.1124/mol.62.4.911

Fischer LM et al (2005) Ad libitum choline intake in healthy individuals meets or exceeds the proposed adequate intake level. J Nutr 135:826–829. https://doi.org/10.1093/jn/135.4.826

Gadiya M et al (2014) Phospholipase D1 and choline kinase-alpha are interactive targets in breast cancer. Cancer Biol Ther 15:593–601. https://doi.org/10.4161/cbt.28165

Gibellini F, Smith TK (2010) The Kennedy pathway – de novo synthesis of phosphatidylethanolamine and phosphatidylcholine. IUBMB Life 62:414–428. https://doi.org/10.1002/iub.337

Glunde K, Bhujwalla ZM, Ronen SM (2011) Choline metabolism in malignant transformation. Nat Rev Cancer 11:835–848. https://doi.org/10.1038/nrc3162

Glunde K, Penet MF, Jiang L, Jacobs MA, Bhujwalla ZM (2015) Choline metabolism-based molecular diagnosis of cancer: an update. Expert Rev Mol Diagn 15:735–747. https://doi.org/10.1586/14737159.2015.1039515

Growdon JH, Hirsch MJ, Wurtman RJ, Wiener W (1977) Oral choline administration to patients with tardive dyskinesia. N Engl J Med 297:524–527. https://doi.org/10.1056/nejm197709082971002

Hamza M, Lloveras J, Ribbes G, Soula G, Douste-Blazy L (1983) An in vitro study of hemicholinium-3 on phospholipid metabolism of Krebs II ascites cells. Biochem Pharmacol 32:1893–1897. https://doi.org/10.1016/0006-2952(83)90055-2

Hanley MP, Kadaveru K, Perret C, Giardina C, Rosenberg DW (2016) Dietary methyl donor depletion suppresses intestinal adenoma development. Cancer Prevent Res 9:812–820. https://doi.org/10.1158/1940-6207.capr-16-0042

Henkels KM, Boivin GP, Dudley ES, Berberich SJ, Gomez-Cambronero J (2013) Phospholipase D (PLD) drives cell invasion, tumor growth and metastasis in a human breast cancer xenograph model. Oncogene 32:5551–5562. https://doi.org/10.1038/onc.2013.207

Hernandez-Alcoceba R, Fernandez F, Lacal JC (1999) In vivo antitumor activity of choline kinase inhibitors: a novel target for anticancer drug discovery. Cancer Res 59:3112–3118

Institute of Medicine (US) Standing Committee on the Scientific Evaluation of Dietary Reference Intakes and its Panel on Folate, Other B Vitamins, and Choline (1998) Dietary reference intakes for thiamin, riboflavin, niacin, vitamin B6, folate, vitamin B12, pantothenic acid, biotin, and choline. National Academies Press (US) National Academy of Sciences, Washington

Kadaveru K, Protiva P, Greenspan EJ, Kim YI, Rosenberg DW (2012) Dietary methyl donor depletion protects against intestinal tumorigenesis in Apc(Min/+) mice. Cancer Prevent Res 5:911–920. https://doi.org/10.1158/1940-6207.capr-11-0544

Kennedy EP, Weiss SB (1956) The function of cytidine coenzymes in the biosynthesis of phospholipids. J Biol Chem 222:193–214

Lacal JC (2001) Choline kinase: a novel target for antitumor drugs. IDrugs 4:419–426

Lacal JC, Campos JM (2015) Preclinical characterization of RSM-932A, a novel anticancer drug targeting the human choline kinase alpha, an enzyme involved in increased lipid metabolism of cancer cells. Mol Cancer Ther 14:31–39. https://doi.org/10.1158/1535-7163.Mct-14-0531

Lamming DW et al (2015) Restriction of dietary protein decreases mTORC1 in tumors and somatic tissues of a tumor-bearing mouse xenograft model. Oncotarget 6:31233–31240. https://doi.org/10.18632/oncotarget.5180

Lavieri RR et al (2010) Design, synthesis, and biological evaluation of halogenated N-(2-(4-oxo-1-phenyl-1,3,8-triazaspiro[4.5]decan-8-yl)ethyl)benzamides: discovery of an isoform-selective small molecule phospholipase D2 inhibitor. J Med Chem 53:6706–6719. https://doi.org/10.1021/jm100814g

Lawrence CM, Millac P, Stout GS, Ward JW (1980) The use of choline chloride in ataxic disorders. J Neurol Neurosurg Psychiatry 43:452–454. https://doi.org/10.1136/jnnp.43.5.452

Lewis JA et al (2009) Design and synthesis of isoform-selective phospholipase D (PLD) inhibitors. Part I: impact of alternative halogenated privileged structures for PLD1 specificity. Bioorg Med Chem Lett 19:1916–1920. https://doi.org/10.1016/j.bmcl.2009.02.057

Li Z, Vance DE (2008) Phosphatidylcholine and choline homeostasis. J Lipid Res 49:1187–1194. https://doi.org/10.1194/jlr.R700019-JLR200

Lykidis A (2007) Comparative genomics and evolution of eukaryotic phospholipid biosynthesis. Prog Lipid Res 46:171–199. https://doi.org/10.1016/j.plipres.2007.03.003

Marjon K et al (2016) MTAP deletions in cancer create vulnerability to targeting of the MAT2A/PRMT5/RIOK1 axis. Cell Rep 15:574–587. https://doi.org/10.1016/j.celrep.2016.03.043

McDermott M, Wakelam MJ, Morris AJ (2004) Phospholipase D. Biochem Cell Biol 82:225–253. https://doi.org/10.1139/o03-079

McGuire S (2016) Scientific report of the 2015 Dietary Guidelines Advisory Committee. Washington, DC: US Departments of Agriculture and Health and Human Services, 2015. Adv Nutr 7:202–204. https://doi.org/10.3945/an.115.011684

Meacham CE, Morrison SJ (2013) Tumour heterogeneity and cancer cell plasticity. Nature 501:328–337. https://doi.org/10.1038/nature12624

Mehendale HM, Dauterman WC, Hodgson E (1966) Phosphatidyl carnitine: a possible intermediate in the biosynthesis of phosphatidyl beta-methylcholine in Phormia regina (Meigen). Nature 211:759–761. https://doi.org/10.1038/211759b0

Mentch SJ, Locasale JW (2016) One-carbon metabolism and epigenetics: understanding the specificity. Ann N Y Acad Sci 1363:91–98. https://doi.org/10.1111/nyas.12956

Min DS et al (2001) Neoplastic transformation and tumorigenesis associated with overexpression of phospholipase D isozymes in cultured murine fibroblasts. Carcinogenesis 22:1641–1647. https://doi.org/10.1093/carcin/22.10.1641

Monovich L et al (2007) Optimization of halopemide for phospholipase D2 inhibition. Bioorg Med Chem Lett 17:2310–2311. https://doi.org/10.1016/j.bmcl.2007.01.059

Morris AJ (2007) Regulation of phospholipase D activity, membrane targeting and intracellular trafficking by phosphoinositides. Biochem Soc Symp 74:247–257. https://doi.org/10.1042/bss0740247

Nanjundan M, Possmayer F (2003) Pulmonary phosphatidic acid phosphatase and lipid phosphate phosphohydrolase. Am J Physiol Lung Cell Mol Physiol 284:L1–L23. https://doi.org/10.1152/ajplung.00029.2002

O'Reilly MC et al (2013) Development of dual PLD1/2 and PLD2 selective inhibitors from a common 1,3,8-triazaspiro[4.5]decane core: discovery of Ml298 and Ml299 that decrease invasive migration in U87-MG glioblastoma cells. J Med Chem 56:2695–2699. https://doi.org/10.1021/jm301782e

Pajares MA, Perez-Sala D (2006) Betaine homocysteine S-methyltransferase: just a regulator of homocysteine metabolism? Cell Mol Life Sci 63:2792–2803. https://doi.org/10.1007/s00018-006-6249-6

Pettitt TR, McDermott M, Saqib KM, Shimwell N, Wakelam MJ (2001) Phospholipase D1b and D2a generate structurally identical phosphatidic acid species in mammalian cells. Biochem J 360:707–715. https://doi.org/10.1042/0264-6021:3600707

Quinlan CL et al (2017) Targeting S-adenosylmethionine biosynthesis with a novel allosteric inhibitor of Mat2A. Nat Chem Biol 13:785–792. https://doi.org/10.1038/nchembio.2384

Ramirez de Molina A et al (2002a) Increased choline kinase activity in human breast carcinomas: clinical evidence for a potential novel antitumor strategy. Oncogene 21:4317–4322. https://doi.org/10.1038/sj.onc.1205556

Ramirez de Molina A et al (2002b) Overexpression of choline kinase is a frequent feature in human tumor-derived cell lines and in lung, prostate, and colorectal human cancers. Biochem Biophys Res Commun 296:580–583

Schrager TF, Newberne PM, Pikul AH, Groopman JD (1990) Aflatoxin-DNA adduct formation in chronically dosed rats fed a choline-deficient diet. Carcinogenesis 11:177–180. https://doi.org/10.1093/carcin/11.1.177

Scott SA et al (2009) Design of isoform-selective phospholipase D inhibitors that modulate cancer cell invasiveness. Nat Chem Biol 5:108–117. https://doi.org/10.1038/nchembio.140

Scott SA et al (2015) Discovery of desketoraloxifene analogues as inhibitors of mammalian, Pseudomonas aeruginosa, and NAPE phospholipase D enzymes. ACS Chem Biol 10:421–432. https://doi.org/10.1021/cb500828m

Selvy PE, Lavieri RR, Lindsley CW, Brown HA (2011) Phospholipase D: enzymology, functionality, and chemical modulation. Chem Rev 111:6064–6119. https://doi.org/10.1021/cr200296t

Shane B, Stokstad EL (1985) Vitamin B12-folate interrelationships. Annu Rev Nutr 5:115–141. https://doi.org/10.1146/annurev.nu.05.070185.000555

Sherriff JL, O'Sullivan TA, Properzi C, Oddo JL, Adams LA (2016) Choline, its potential role in nonalcoholic fatty liver disease, and the case for human and bacterial genes. Adv Nutr 7:5–13. https://doi.org/10.3945/an.114.007955

Stead LM, Brosnan JT, Brosnan ME, Vance DE, Jacobs RL (2006) Is it time to reevaluate methyl balance in humans? Am J Clin Nutr 83:5–10. https://doi.org/10.1093/ajcn/83.1.5

Stipanuk MH (2004) Sulfur amino acid metabolism: pathways for production and removal of homocysteine and cysteine. Annu Rev Nutr 24:539–577. https://doi.org/10.1146/annurev.nutr.24.012003.132418

Stover PJ (2004) Physiology of folate and vitamin B12 in health and disease. Nutr Rev 62:S3–S12. Discussion S13. https://doi.org/10.1111/j.1753-4887.2004.tb00070.x

Su W et al (2009) 5-Fluoro-2-indolyl des-chlorohalopemide (FIPI), a phospholipase D pharmacological inhibitor that alters cell spreading and inhibits chemotaxis. Mol Pharmacol 75:437–446. https://doi.org/10.1124/mol.108.053298

Su X, Wellen KE, Rabinowitz JD (2016) Metabolic control of methylation and acetylation. Curr Opin Chem Biol 30:52–60. https://doi.org/10.1016/j.cbpa.2015.10.030

Sundler R, Akesson B (1975) Regulation of phospholipid biosynthesis in isolated rat hepatocytes. Effect of different substrates. J Biol Chem 250:3359–3367

Ueland PM (2011) Choline and betaine in health and disease. J Inherit Metab Dis 34:3–15. https://doi.org/10.1007/s10545-010-9088-4

Van Horn L (2010) Development of the 2010 US Dietary Guidelines Advisory Committee Report: perspectives from a registered dietitian. J Am Diet Assoc 110:1638–1645. https://doi.org/10.1016/j.jada.2010.08.018

Wang Z et al (2011) Gut flora metabolism of phosphatidylcholine promotes cardiovascular disease. Nature 472:57–63. https://doi.org/10.1038/nature09922

Wood JL, Allison RG (1982) Effects of consumption of choline and lecithin on neurological and cardiovascular systems. Fed Proc 41:3015–3021

Yamada Y et al (2003) Association of a polymorphism of the phospholipase D2 gene with the prevalence of colorectal cancer. J Mol Med 81:126–131. https://doi.org/10.1007/s00109-002-0411-x

Zeisel SH (2009) Importance of methyl donors during reproduction. Am J Clin Nutr 89:673s–677s. https://doi.org/10.3945/ajcn.2008.26811D

Zeisel SH (2012a) A brief history of choline. Ann Nutr Metab 61:254–258. https://doi.org/10.1159/000343120

Zeisel SH (2012b) Dietary choline deficiency causes DNA strand breaks and alters epigenetic marks on DNA and histones. Mutat Res 733:34–38. https://doi.org/10.1016/j.mrfmmm.2011.10.008

Zeisel SH, Blusztajn JK (1994) Choline and human nutrition. Annu Rev Nutr 14:269–296. https://doi.org/10.1146/annurev.nu.14.070194.001413

Zeisel SH, da Costa KA (2009) Choline: an essential nutrient for public health. Nutr Rev 67:615–623. https://doi.org/10.1111/j.1753-4887.2009.00246.x

Zeisel SH, Mar MH, Howe JC, Holden JM (2003) Concentrations of choline-containing compounds and betaine in common foods. J Nutr 133:1302–1307. https://doi.org/10.1093/jn/133.5.1302

Zhang Y, Frohman MA (2014) Cellular and physiological roles for phospholipase D1 in cancer. J Biol Chem 289:22567–22574. https://doi.org/10.1074/jbc.R114.576876

Zhang W et al (2013) Fluorinated N,N-dialkylaminostilbenes repress colon cancer by targeting methionine S-adenosyltransferase 2A. ACS Chem Biol 8:796–803. https://doi.org/10.1021/cb3005353

Zhao C, Du G, Skowronek K, Frohman MA, Bar-Sagi D (2007) Phospholipase D2-generated phosphatidic acid couples EGFR stimulation to Ras activation by Sos. Nat Cell Biol 9:706–712. https://doi.org/10.1038/ncb1594

Part V

Lipids and Membrane Microdomains

Regulation of Inositol Biosynthesis: Balancing Health and Pathophysiology

Kendall C. Case, Michael Salsaa, Wenxi Yu, and Miriam L. Greenberg

Contents

Abstract

Inositol is the precursor for all inositol compounds and is essential for viability of eukaryotic cells. Numerous cellular processes and signaling functions are dependent on inositol compounds, and perturbation of their synthesis leads to a wide

Kendall C. Case, Michael Salsaa and Wenxi Yu contributed equally.

K. C. Case · M. Salsaa · M. L. Greenberg (✉)
Department of Biological Sciences, Wayne State University, Detroit, MI, USA
e-mail: mgreenberg@wayne.edu

W. Yu
Department of Biological Sciences, Wayne State University, Detroit, MI, USA

Department of Pharmacology, University of Michigan Medical School, Ann Arbor, MI, USA

J. Gomez-Cambronero, M. A. Frohman (eds.), *Lipid Signaling in Human Diseases*, Handbook of Experimental Pharmacology 259, https://doi.org/10.1007/164_2018_181

range of human diseases. Although considerable research has been directed at understanding the function of inositol compounds, especially phosphoinositides and inositol phosphates, a focus on regulatory and homeostatic mechanisms controlling inositol biosynthesis has been largely neglected. Consequently, little is known about how synthesis of inositol is regulated in human cells. Identifying physiological regulators of inositol synthesis and elucidating the molecular mechanisms that regulate inositol synthesis will contribute fundamental insight into cellular processes that are mediated by inositol compounds and will provide a foundation to understand numerous disease processes that result from perturbation of inositol homeostasis. In addition, elucidating the mechanisms of action of inositol-depleting drugs may suggest new strategies for the design of second-generation pharmaceuticals to treat psychiatric disorders and other illnesses.

Keywords
Energy metabolism · *INO1* · Inositol · Inositol synthesis · *myo*-inositol-3-phosphate synthase

1 Introduction

Inositol is a ubiquitous six-carbon cyclitol that is essential for viability of eukaryotic cells. *Myo*-inositol, physiologically the most important inositol stereoisomer, is the precursor of all inositol compounds, including phosphoinositides, inositol polyphosphates and pyrophosphates, inositol sphingolipids, and glycosylphosphatidylinositols (Fig. 1a). Inositol compounds play pivotal roles in osmoregulation, membrane biogenesis, cytoskeletal organization, membrane trafficking, signal transduction, gene expression, DNA repair, energy metabolism, and autophagy (Fig. 1b) (Czech 2003; Di Paolo and De Camilli 2006; Fisher et al. 2002; Shears 2015; Wilson et al. 2013). Thus, it is not surprising that perturbation of inositol homeostasis leads to a wide range of human illnesses, including neurological, psychiatric, and cardiovascular disorders, among others (Fisher et al. 2002; Piatkevich et al. 1984).

Elucidating the mechanisms underlying the control of inositol homeostasis would contribute greatly to understanding the pathologies underlying these illnesses. In this light, it is remarkable that very little is known regarding the mechanisms that control inositol synthesis in human cells. In contrast, many elegant studies have identified genetic regulators of inositol synthesis in the yeast model, largely due to the genetic tractability of this organism. Guided by insights from the yeast model, regulatory mechanisms of inositol biosynthesis in mammalian cells are being revealed. In the current review, we discuss: (1) mechanisms that regulate inositol synthesis in yeast and mammalian cells; (2) the function of inositol in the brain, including the potential role of inositol depletion as a therapeutic mechanism for treating mood disorders; (3) the relationship between inositol, energy metabolism, and insulin resistance; and (4) the link between inositol, autophagy, and disorders associated with perturbation of autophagy, including Parkinson's disease and Huntington's disease. Finally, we highlight important unanswered questions for further exploration.

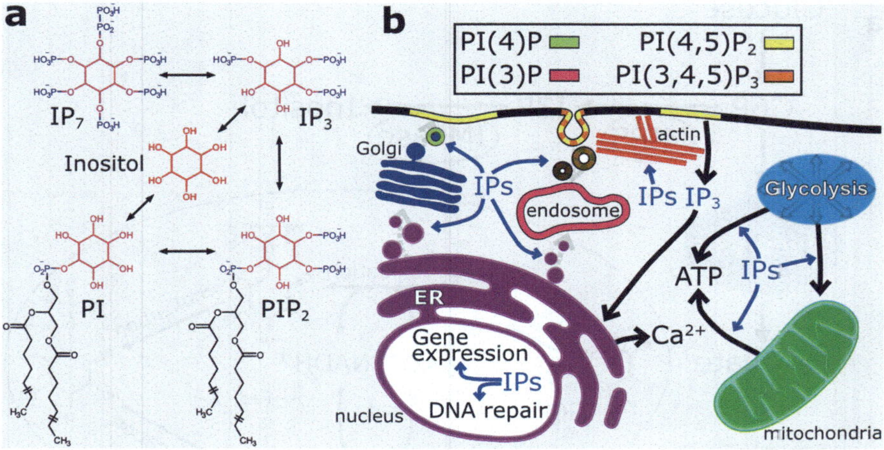

Fig. 1 Inositol metabolites and inositol function within the cell. (**a**) Inositol (red) is the precursor to phosphatidylinositol (PI) and inositol phosphates (IPs, e.g., IP_3). PI can be phosphorylated (blue) to form phosphatidylinositol phosphate (PIP, e.g., PIP_2). PIPs can be cleaved by a lipase to produce diacylglycerol (not shown) and IPs. IPs can be further phosphorylated to produce inositol pyrophosphates (e.g., IP_7) which have two phosphates bound to a carbon residue. Inositol sphingolipids and glycosylphosphatidylinositols are not shown. (**b**) Inositol-containing compounds are essential for many cellular processes. PIPs regulate endo- and exocytosis and label membrane domains for vesicle trafficking. PI(4,5)P_2 can be hydrolyzed, forming IP_3 which stimulates Ca^{2+} release from the ER. Other IP compounds (including inositol phosphates and inositol pyrophosphates) regulate vesicle trafficking, cytoskeleton organization, energy metabolism, gene expression, and DNA repair, among others

2 Regulation of Inositol Biosynthesis

Myo-inositol-3-phosphate synthase (MIPS), first purified from yeast (Donahue and Henry 1981), is the rate-limiting enzyme of inositol synthesis. MIPS catalyzes the conversion of glucose-6-phosphate (G6P) to inositol-3-phosphate (I3P) (Geiger and Jin 2006) (Fig. 2). I3P is dephosphorylated by inositol monophosphatase (IMPase) to form inositol (Fig. 2) (Chen and Charalampous 1966). Both inositol synthesis and glycolysis utilize G6P, and partitioning of this substrate in response to the energy and inositol needs of the cell is likely pivotal. In yeast, several mechanisms that regulate MIPS have been identified, including transcriptional control of the MIPS structural gene *INO1* and regulation of MIPS catalytic activity. We suggest that cross talk between inositol synthesis and cellular energy metabolism likely contributes to these (and other) mechanisms of regulation.

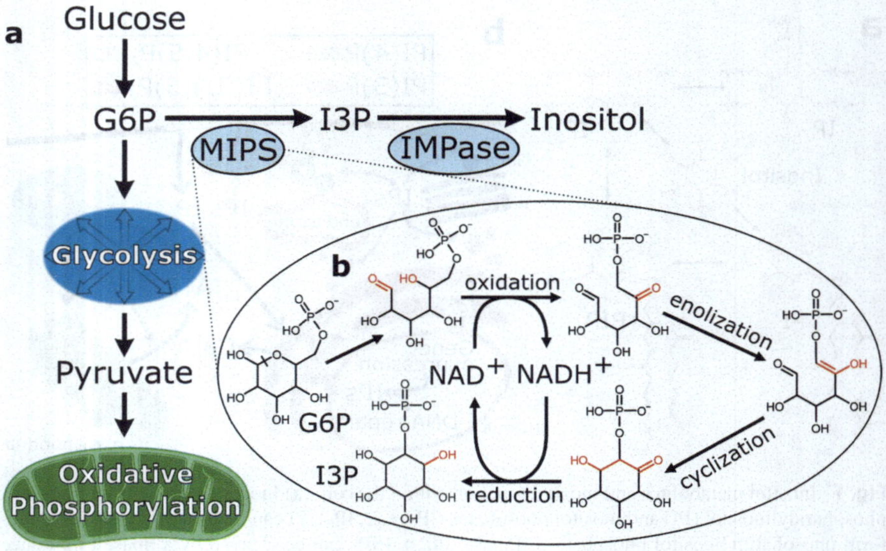

Fig. 2 Inositol biosynthesis. (**a**) Inositol synthesis and glycolysis utilize the common substrate glucose-6-phosphate (G6P). Myo-inositol-3-phosphate synthase (MIPS) converts G6P to inositol-3-phosphate (I3P), which is dephosphorylated to inositol by inositol monophosphatase (IMPase). G6P is the initial substrate that is utilized in glycolysis. (**b**) Catalytic reaction of MIPS. The five-step reaction that converts G6P to I3P utilizes the redox potential of $NADH^+/NAD^+$. NAD^+ is not consumed, as the same molecule is used in both oxidation and reduction steps. Catalytically modified residues are highlighted in red (Geiger and Jin 2006)

2.1 Transcriptional Regulation of *INO1*

2.1.1 The Henry Regulatory Circuit (Ino2-Ino4-Opi1) Controls Yeast *INO1* Expression in Response to Phospholipid Precursors, Inositol and Choline

Inositol synthesis in yeast is regulated in response to the availability of phospholipid precursors, inositol and choline. Transcriptional control is mediated by three regulatory proteins, Ino2, Ino4, and Opi1, which form what has been termed the Henry regulatory circuit, describing the studies of the Susan Henry laboratory (Carman and Han 2011; Qiu et al. 2016; Salsaa et al. 2017). When inositol is limiting, transcriptional activation is initiated by the Ino2-Ino4 activator complex bound at the UAS_{INO} sequence in the promoter of *INO1* (coding for MIPS), as well as genes encoding phospholipid biosynthetic enzymes. When inositol is abundant, transcriptional activation is repressed by binding of the negative regulator, Opi1, to Ino2.

The UAS_{INO} Element

The upstream activating sequence (UAS_{INO}) in the regulatory region of *INO1* is located within the coding sequence (Klig and Henry 1984) upstream of the TATA element (Lopes et al. 1991). A similar regulatory region is found in the promoters of at least 33 other genes involved in phospholipid biosynthesis, all of which are similarly regulated in response to inositol and choline, (Greenberg and Lopes 1996). The UAS_{INO} is thus also referred to as the inositol/choline-responsive element (ICRE). The UAS_{INO} contains the consensus sequence CATGTGAAAT, which includes the canonical basic helix-loop-helix (bHLH) binding site CANNTG (Lopes et al. 1991). Flanking regions of the UAS_{INO} are important for regulating expression, but the core element is required for both repression and derepression of *INO1* in response to inositol and choline (Bachhawat et al. 1995).

Transcriptional Activators Ino2-Ino4

Transcriptional activator proteins, Ino2 and Ino4, interact with the bHLH binding domain of the canonical UAS_{INO} sequence to derepress transcription of *INO1* (Ashburner and Lopes 1995; Bailis et al. 1987; Lai and McGraw 1994; Loewy and Henry 1984; Lopes and Henry 1991; Lopes et al. 1991). Ino2 and Ino4 interact with the UAS_{INO} as a heterodimer formed by the interaction of the bHLH domains in both proteins (Ambroziak and Henry 1994; Hoshizaki et al. 1990; Lopes and Henry 1991; Nikoloff et al. 1992; Schwank et al. 1995). Perturbation of *INO2* or *INO4* expression leads to reduced Ino2-Ino4 complexes, resulting in the inability to derepress *INO1* and, thus, inositol auxotrophy (Loewy and Henry 1984; Lopes and Henry 1991; Nikoloff and Henry 1994).

Interestingly, the *INO2* and *INO4* regulatory sequences themselves contain the UAS_{INO} element (or a variation of the sequence) and are, therefore, autoregulated (Ashburner and Lopes 1995). However, while activation of the UAS_{INO} of *INO2* requires the Ino2-Ino4 heterodimer (similar to *INO1*), activation of the *INO4* UAS_{INO} does not require Ino2. As binding of bHLH proteins is generally dependent on dimerization to localize and interact with DNA, a likely explanation is that Ino4 dimerizes with other bHLH proteins to activate *INO4*. Unlike *INO2*, *INO4* appears to be regulated to a much lower extent in response to inositol and choline (Ashburner and Lopes 1995; Schwank et al. 1997). Thus, autoregulation of *INO2*, but not *INO4*, appears to affect the magnitude of the regulatory response but is not necessary for *INO1* regulation (Ashburner and Lopes 1995).

Ino4 is constitutively localized to the nucleus, likely due to the basic amino acid nuclear localization sequence in the protein (Kumme et al. 2008). In contrast, the basic amino acid sequence is absent from Ino2, which requires Ino4 for nuclear localization, presumably reflecting the need to heterodimerize with Ino4 (Kumme et al. 2008). It is tempting to speculate that regulation of *INO1* can be achieved by breaking the Ino2-Ino4 heterodimer complex (Kumme et al. 2008). However, this does not appear to be a significant mechanism of *INO1* regulation, as Ino2-Ino4 heterodimers are constitutively associated with the UAS_{INO} element of *INO1*, even in repressing conditions (Brickner and Walter 2004; Dasgupta et al. 2005). This suggests that the mechanism of repression of *INO1* is sufficient to inhibit transcription, even in the presence of bound activators.

Transcriptional Repressor Opi1

OPI1 encodes a repressor of expression of *INO1* and other UAS_{INO}-containing genes. This repressor was discovered by the identification of an inositol-excreting mutant and named after the phenotype, **o**ver**p**roduction of **i**nositol (Greenberg et al. 1982). Mutating the *OPI1* locus resulted in unregulated expression of *INO1* and constitutive synthesis of inositol (Greenberg et al. 1982; White et al. 1991). Opi1 localizes to the UAS_{INO} element by interaction with Ino2 (Dietz et al. 2003; Heyken et al. 2005; Wagner et al. 2001), thus repressing genes with the canonical UAS_{INO} sequence. A repressor interaction domain (RID) within Ino2 was determined to be necessary and sufficient for binding by Opi1 (Dietz et al. 2003). Notably, RID partially overlaps one of the transcriptional activation domains (TAD2) of Ino2, which may contribute to Opi1-mediated repression (Dietz et al. 2003; Heyken et al. 2005).

Genes containing UAS_{INO} sequences that vary from the consensus sequence, such as *INO4*, are not repressed by Opi1 (Ashburner and Lopes 1995; Bachhawat et al. 1995; Bailis et al. 1987; Klig et al. 1985; Lai and McGraw 1994). Interestingly, overexpressing *INO2*, but not *INO4*, leads to strong activation of UAS_{INO}-containing genes even during repressing conditions (Schwank et al. 1997). Excess Ino2 may act as an Opi1 "sink" to reduce the available Opi1 for interaction with the Ino2-Ino4-DNA complex. In addition to this repression mechanism, Opi1-mediated repression occurs through recruitment of other inhibitory machinery (discussed below).

The *OPI1* gene contains sequences that encode the classical leucine-zipper DNA interaction domain as well as polyglutamine stretches that have been shown to interact with DNA in yeast (Wagner et al. 1999; White et al. 1991). Interestingly, however, there is no evidence that Opi1 interacts directly with DNA (Bachhawat et al. 1995), which instead relies on the interaction with Ino2 for localization to the UAS_{INO} element (Dietz et al. 2003; Heyken et al. 2005; Wagner et al. 2001). *INO4* contains a variation of the UAS_{INO} consensus sequence and is not repressed by Opi1, as Ino2 does not interact with its regulatory region (Ashburner and Lopes 1995; Klig et al. 1985).

OPI1 does not contain a UAS_{INO} element, and there is no evidence that *OPI1* expression is affected by inositol or choline (Ashburner and Lopes 1995; Kumme et al. 2008). Nevertheless, Opi1 is highly regulated, primarily by cellular localization and by phosphorylation of the protein. When inositol is limiting, Opi1 is tethered to the endoplasmic reticulum (ER) by interaction with the integral ER protein, Scs2, and the lipid phosphatidic acid (PA) (Loewen et al. 2003; Nikawa et al. 1995). When inositol levels are high, PA is consumed in PI synthesis, subsequently decreasing PA levels and freeing Opi1 to translocate to the nucleus (Gaspar et al. 2017; Salsaa et al. 2017). Interestingly, Opi1 preferentially binds to PA with C16 fatty acids over C18 fatty acids (Hofbauer et al. 2014). Regulating the fatty acid length may thus be a mechanism to fine tune Opi1-mediated repression. The C16/C18 ratio is maintained by acetyl-CoA carboxylase (Acc1), which is controlled by the metabolic regulatory kinase Snf1, the yeast homolog of AMP-activated protein kinase (AMPK). Acc1 activity, which decreases the C16/C18 ratio, is reduced by Snf1-dependent phosphorylation (Hofbauer et al. 2014). Therefore, inhibition of Acc1 by Snf1 may increase the availability of C16 PA for binding of Opi1, increasing retention of Opi1 in the ER. Snf1 also functions in the nucleus as a chromatin remodeler and transcriptional regulator of *INO1*. Consistent with both of these mechanisms, the *snf1*Δ mutant exhibits decreased *INO1* expression and is an inositol auxotroph (Lo et al. 2001; Shirra et al. 2001, 2005). Finally, Opi1 activity is also regulated posttranslationally by PKC, which inactivates Opi1 by phosphorylation of Ser 26, resulting in increased expression of *INO1* (Fig. 3a) (Sreenivas et al. 2001). The metabolic significance of regulation by PKC is not clear. In summary, Opi1 is regulated by subcellular localization in response to metabolic control of phospholipid synthesis and energy metabolism.

2.1.2 Regulation of the General Transcriptional Machinery at the *INO1* Locus

The general transcription factor TFIIB and the TATA-binding protein (TBP) are required for formation of the preinitiation complex (Luse 2014). TFIIB is recruited to the *INO1* promoter by the interaction between the TFIIB subunit Sua7 and the Ino2 TAD domains, especially TAD1 (Dietz et al. 2003). The Sua7 interaction domain of Ino2 partially overlaps with the bHLH domain. Therefore, the Ino2-Sua7 interaction may displace Ino4, leading to dissociation of Ino2 from UAS_{INO}. This may explain how the remodeling complex INO80, which is recruited to *INO1* by Ino2, dissociates from the promotor region shortly after transcription initiation (discussed below) (Ford et al. 2008). However, a trimeric complex, Ino2-Ino4-Sua7, may still be possible and requires further elucidation at the level of molecular interaction.

Disruption of TBP-DNA binding by Mot1 and Sit4 contributes to *INO1* repression. Mot1 disrupts TBP-DNA interactions via ATP hydrolysis (Dasgupta et al. 2005), facilitating *INO1* repression. The ceramide-activated phosphatase, Sit4, indirectly reduces the interaction of TBP at the *INO1* locus by antagonizing Snf1, the activity of which induces TBP binding (Shirra et al. 2005) (discussed further below). Interestingly, the TOR complex, inactivates Sit4, potentially modulating inositol synthesis (Fig. 3a) (Shirra et al. 2005). It remains to be determined if Opi1 is required for Mot1 and Sit4 regulation of *INO1*.

2.1.3 Regulation of *INO1* by Chromatin Remodeling

Repression by HDACs

In addition to the UAS_{INO} element, the *INO1* promotor also contains an upstream repressor sequence (URS1), which represses UAS_{INO}-driven expression (Lopes et al. 1993; Slekar and Henry 1995). Interestingly, both URS1 and UAS_{INO} indirectly recruit histone deacetylase complexes (HDACs) to *INO1*. URS1 binds to Ume6, a subunit of Rpd3 HDAC which then recruits the pleiotropic repressor, Sin3 (Dasgupta et al. 2005; Kadosh and Struhl 1997). Sin3 is also partially recruited to UAS_{INO}, mediated by interaction with the Opi1-Ino2 complex (Jaschke et al. 2011; Lopes et al. 1993; Slekar and Henry 1995). The paired amphipathic helix domain (PAH1) of Sin3 directly interacts with Opi1 at the Opi1-Sin3 interaction

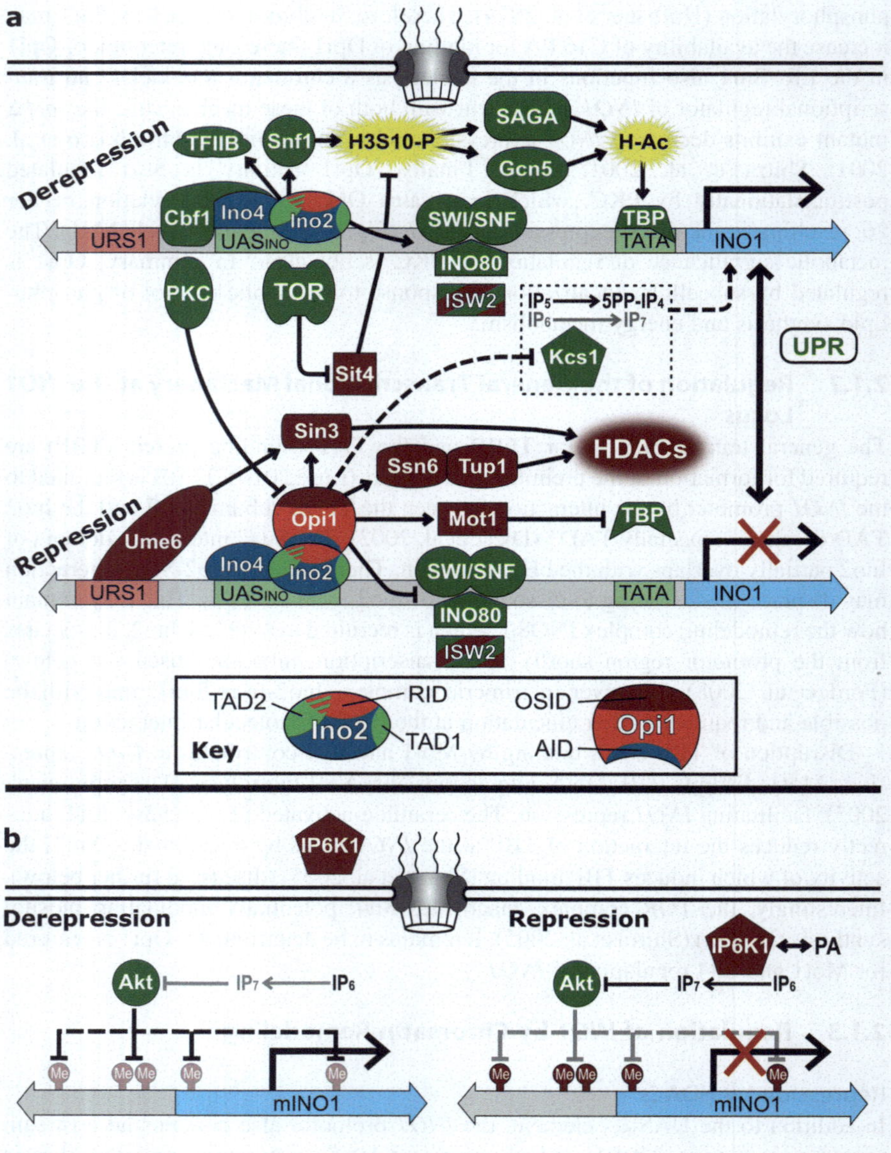

Fig. 3 Model for regulation of *INO1* in yeast (**a**) and mammalian (**b**) cells. See Sect. 2.1.6 for more details. Red proteins denote an inhibitory effect on transcription of *INO1*, whereas green proteins are activating. For simplicity, the gene recruitment sequences (GRS I and II) are not shown but are required for nuclear periphery localization. Kcs1 is contained within a dotted box because it is unknown if the catalytic reaction occurs in the nucleus, unlike all the other reactions depicted

domain (OSID) (Wagner et al. 2001). In contrast, recruitment to URS1 is not dependent on Ino2 (Lopes et al. 1993). Recruitment of Sin3 to URS1 and UAS_{INO} localizes the HDAC Rpd3, putting it in close proximity to the promotor (Kadosh and Struhl 1997). Sin3 likely recruits additional HDACs, as some of the histone modifications cannot be explained by Rpd3 alone (Rundlett et al. 1998). Although Sin3-Rpd3 recruitment contributes to *INO1* repression, it is not required for repression. However, the Opi1-Sin3 interaction domain of Opi1, OSID, is required for repression of *INO1*, suggesting that this domain plays a larger role than just the recruitment of Sin3 (Graves and Henry 2000; Jaschke et al. 2011; Wagner et al. 2001). Indeed, the OSID also recruits and binds the pleiotropic repressor Ssn6, which interacts with the HDAC recruiter Tup1 (Jaschke et al. 2011). Overall, the recruitment of HDACs is expected to reduce histone acetylation, resulting in the inaccessible heterochromatin structure of *INO1* during repressing conditions (Ford et al. 2007; Jaschke et al. 2011; Rundlett et al. 1998).

Activation by Chromatin Remodeling

Displacement of repressing machinery and chromosome remodeling at the *INO1* promotor make it more accessible to transcription factors (Ford et al. 2007). One element of derepression is Ino2-Ino4 recruitment of centromere-binding factor 1 (Cbf1), which further enhances the interaction of Ino2-Ino4 with the UAS_{INO} and is required for complete derepression (Shetty and Lopes 2010). Cbf1 interacts with an unknown binding sequence upstream of the UAS_{INO} region. The enhanced binding of Ino2-Ino4 more efficiently recruits the chromatin remodeling complex ISW2 (Shetty and Lopes 2010). Shetty and Lopes demonstrated that ISW2 contributes to derepression of *INO1* transcription, while other studies report that ISW complexes act as transcriptional repressors of *INO1* (Gelbart et al. 2005; Goldmark et al. 2000; Mellor and Morillon 2004; Shetty and Lopes 2010; Yadon et al. 2013). These conflicting conclusions warrant further investigation to clarify the role of ISW2 in *INO1* transcriptional regulation.

The remodeling complexes SWI/SNF and INO80, which generally enhance transcription, are recruited to the *INO1* promoter by Ino2 (Ford et al. 2008). Both SWI/SNF and INO80 are required to promote *INO1* transcription (Ford et al. 2007; Lo et al. 2001; Peterson et al. 1991; Pollard and Peterson 1997; Shirra et al. 2001, 2005). Chromatin remodeling of *INO1* by these complexes is linked to displacement of the repressor complex Ume6-Sin3-Rpd3. Similar to Ino2-Ino4, INO80 and SWI/SNF are constitutively associated with the *INO1* promotor during repressing conditions (Ford et al. 2008), although remodeling activity is attenuated under these conditions. As discussed earlier, INO80 departs from the promotor region shortly after transcriptional initiation, whereas low levels of SWI/SNF remain (Ford et al. 2008). INO80 may be required for initial remodeling of the chromatin structure prior to transcription, and SWI/SNF may remain after transcription initiation to maintain the euchromatin structure.

The protein kinase Snf1 and acetyltransferase Gcn5 enhance the transcription of *INO1* by histone activating modifications, including phosphorylation of the Ser 10 residue of histone 3 (H3S10) and acetylation of Lys 14 of H3 (Lo et al. 2001,

2005; Weaver 2012). Recruitment of Gcn5 is dependent on H3S10 phosphorylation by Snf1, which is recruited to *INO1* by the TAD of Ino2 (Dietz et al. 2003; Lo et al. 2005), linking Ino2-Ino4-Opi1 regulation to histone modification. Snf1-mediated H3S10 phosphorylation also recruits the histone acetyltransferase SAGA complex to *INO1*, which is required for maximal *INO1* expression (Dietz et al. 2003; Lo et al. 2005). The SAGA complex recruits TBP, required for transcription of *INO1* (Dasgupta et al. 2005; Lo et al. 2005; Shirra et al. 2005). This mechanism opposes the effects of Sit4 and Mot1, discussed earlier. Interestingly, Snf1 promotes transcription of *INO1* by facilitating histone activation and also contributes to localization of Opi1 to the ER (Hofbauer et al. 2014), which leads to *INO1* derepression. Therefore, *INO1* expression can be controlled and fine-tuned by regulating Snf1 activity and localization.

2.1.4 Regulation by the Unfolded Protein Response (UPR) and Nuclear Localization

Derepression of *INO1* is dependent on components of the UPR. Ire1, a transmembrane kinase that transmits the signal for UPR activation, and Hac1, a transcription factor that activates UPR target genes, are both required for efficient transcription of *INO1* (Cox et al. 1997). Hac1 appears to promote Opi1 dissociation from Ino2-Ino4 (Brickner and Walter 2004) and is only detectable with activation of the UPR (Cox and Walter 1996). Some evidence suggests that the UPR must be activated in order for yeast cells to effectively produce MIPS protein at a concentration that permits growth (Cox et al. 1997). The mechanism linking the UPR to *INO1* activation requires further investigation. However, its role may lie in regulation of chromatin localization.

Although the nuclear periphery is generally associated with repression of genes and tightly packaged, transcriptionally inactive chromatin (Weaver 2012), transcriptional activation of *INO1* (and other genes induced by the UPR) is facilitated by localization to the nuclear periphery (Ahmed et al. 2010; Brickner and Walter 2004). Two gene recruitment sequences (GRS I and II) mediate localization of *INO1* to the nuclear periphery at the nuclear pore complexes (Ahmed et al. 2010). Interestingly, GRS sequences are also enriched in genes that respond to protein folding stress (UPR-induced genes). Localizing the *INO1* promotor may be the mechanism by which UPR activates *INO1* expression.

2.1.5 Synthesis of Inositol Pyrophosphate by Inositol Hexakisphosphate Kinase Regulates *INO1* Expression Differently in Yeast and Mammalian Cells

Activation of Yeast *INO1* by Kcs1

Inositol pyrophosphates are high energy metabolic signaling molecules that are regulated in response to perturbations in energy homeostasis (Choi et al. 2008; Shears 2009). The first indication that inositol pyrophosphates regulate inositol synthesis was the finding that yeast cells lacking the inositol hexakisphosphate kinase Kcs1 are inositol auxotrophs (Ye et al. 2013). The Kcs1-catalyzed synthesis of the inositol pyrophosphate 5PP-IP_5 (IP_7) from IP_6 is essential for activation of *INO1*. Both the kinase and bZIP domains of Kcs1 are required for activation. Interestingly, the bZIP domains of Kcs1 and Opi1 share sequence homology, and Opi1 regulates Kcs1 protein levels, suggesting that these proteins may regulate *INO1* antagonistically by competing for a common binding site (Ye et al. 2013).

Repression of Mouse *INO1* by IP6K1

ISYNA1 is the mammalian homolog of yeast *INO1*, which we refer to as *mINO1* for simplicity in this review. Transcription of *mINO1* in mouse cells was shown to be regulated by inositol hexakisphosphate kinase IP6K1, the functional homolog of yeast Kcs1 (Yu et al. 2016). However, in striking contrast to yeast, IP6K1 *negatively* regulates *mINO1*. Deletion of IP6K1 leads to altered DNA methylation and upregulated expression of *mINO1* (Yu et al. 2016). Low IP6K1 activity decreases IP_7 levels, which leads to increased Akt signaling (Chakraborty et al. 2010), resulting in decreased DNA methylation (Popkie et al. 2010). Therefore, IP6K1-mediated DNA methylation acts through Akt signaling (Fig. 3b). Other studies have shown that IP6K1 regulates histone modification and indirectly alters DNA methylation (Burton et al. 2013; Tamaru and Selker 2001; Tamaru et al. 2003). Thus, with respect to regulation of *mINO1*, IP6K1 is more similar to the yeast negative regulator Opi1 than to yeast Kcs1. Both IP6K1 and Opi1 translocate to the nucleus to repress transcription of *INO1*. Interestingly, both regulators bind specifically to PA. However, binding of IP6K1 to PA is required for nuclear localization, while binding of Opi1 to PA anchors the protein in the ER. As both regulatory mechanisms are mediated by the concentration of PA, it is interesting to speculate that MIPS expression in response to PA is a conserved mechanism of regulation of *INO1* transcription (Salsaa et al. 2017; Yu et al. 2016).

2.1.6 Summary: Transcriptional Control of *INO1* Expression (Fig. 3)

In yeast, activation of *INO1* transcription occurs when the master negative regulator, Opi1, is sequestered in the ER. This is facilitated by the presence of Scs2 and high PA levels in the ER during derepressing conditions (low inositol and choline). When Opi1 is absent from the nucleus, the activators Ino2 and Ino4, which are constitutively bound to UAS_{INO}, recruit factors that enhance transcription. Among these, Cbf1 reinforces the Ino2-Ino4-DNA interaction, enhancing the recruitment of other activation factors, including transcription factor TFIIB, histone kinase Snf1, and chromatin remodelers ISW2, INO80, and SWI/SNF. Phosphorylation of H3S10 by Snf1 leads to recruitment of acetyltransferases Gcn5 and SAGA complex, which acetylate histones and induce euchromatin formation. Relaxation of the chromatin structure promotes corepressor dissociation from the *INO1* promotor and allows TBP and TFIIB to access the *INO1* promotor, recruit other transcription factors, and form the preinitiation complex. Transcription of *INO1* is further enhanced by the UPR, which likely mediates localization to the nuclear periphery where its euchromatin structure is maintained. Furthermore, yeast *INO1* transcription is also activated by Kcs1 and inositol pyrophosphates, the mechanism of which may include antagonism to Opi1.

Most of the activating machinery appears to be constitutively present at the *INO1* promotor. Some activation components are also required for recruitment of repressing machinery, while activation by others, including SWI/SNF and INO80, is attenuated by the presence of repression machinery. During repressing conditions, when cellular inositol and choline levels are high and PA levels are reduced, Opi1 translocates to the nucleus and interacts with Ino2. Opi1-Ino2 interaction partially covers one of the TADs, likely contributing to Opi1-mediated repression. The URS elements interact with Ume6 which, along with Opi1, recruits the pleiotropic repressor Sin3 and known HDAC associate, Rpd3. Opi1 additionally recruits the pleiotropic repressor Ssn6, which interacts with the HDAC recruiter Tup1. The combined recruitment of all the HDACs initiates the formation of transcriptionally inactive heterochromatin and results in localization of INO1 away from the nuclear periphery. In addition to HDAC-facilitated repression of *INO1*, Opi1 also recruits Mot1 and Sit4. Mot1 inhibits TBP from interacting with the TATA element, whereas Sit4 phosphatase antagonizes Snf1-mediated activation. Figure 3a summarizes the yeast model of transcriptional regulation.

In mammalian cells, the only regulator of *INO1* transcription that has been described is IP6K1. In contrast to the yeast homolog Kcs1, which activates *INO1* transcription, IP6K1 negatively regulates *mINO1* expression. IP_7, the product of IP6K1, inhibits Akt activity, likely accounting for *mINO1* methylation. When IP6K1 binds to PA, it translocates into the nucleus, leading to decreased *mINO1* methylation and increased expression. Figure 3b summarizes what is known about *mINO1* transcriptional regulation.

2.2 Regulation of MIPS Catalytic Activity

2.2.1 Phosphorylation of Conserved Sites Regulates MIPS Activity

Both yeast and mammalian MIPS are phosphorylated in vivo (Deranieh et al. 2013; Parthasarathy et al. 2013). While the regulatory role of MIPS phosphorylation has not been determined, in vitro studies indicate that enzymatic activity of MIPS is regulated by at least three conserved phosphosites in yeast and human MIPS (Deranieh et al. 2013). Phosphomimetic mutations of two of the three conserved sites (yeast S184/S374 and human S279/S357) decrease enzymatic activity (Deranieh et al. 2013). Physiological relevance is supported by in vivo studies in yeast indicating that the inositol-depleting drug valproate (VPA) increases phosphorylation of the enzyme and reduces growth. Consistent with a role for phosphoregulation, phosphodeficient yeast mutants of these sites exhibit rescued growth in the presence of VPA. In addition to these sites, Ser 524 near the C-terminus of rat brain and testis MIPS were shown to be phosphorylated (Parthasarathy et al. 2013), although the functional significance of this modification is not known. It was suggested that phosphorylation may play a role in vivo (Parthasarathy et al. 2013), possibly by recruitment of modifier proteins.

2.2.2 Regulation by GSK3

GSK3 is required for optimal de novo inositol synthesis in yeast. MIPS activity is significantly reduced in yeast cells lacking the four GSK3 homologs, resulting in decreased intracellular inositol and defective growth in inositol-deficient medium (Azab et al. 2007). Mck1 was identified as the yeast GSK3 homolog required for optimal synthesis of inositol (Yu et al. 2017). Although wild-type cells exhibit decreased MIPS activity in the presence of VPA, the drug does not inhibit MIPS in *mck1*Δ cells, suggesting that inhibition of MIPS by VPA is Mck1-dependent. The mechanism whereby Mck1 regulates yeast MIPS is not known. Mck1 does not affect *INO1* expression levels. While Mck1 does not directly phosphorylate MIPS, phosphorylation of the protein by the GSK3 signaling cascade remains a possibility (Yu et al. 2017).

While there is no direct evidence that GSK3 regulates inositol synthesis in mammalian cells, indirect evidence suggests mechanisms whereby this may occur. IP6K1, which negatively regulates MIPS expression (discussed above), activates GSK3 by at least two mechanisms. First, IP6K1 directly binds to and activates GSK3, and IP6K1 KO mice have significantly reduced GSK3 activity (Chakraborty et al. 2014). Second, the product of IP6K1, IP_7, inhibits the kinase AKT, which catalyzes the inhibitory phosphorylation of GSK3 (Chakraborty et al. 2010). Thus, in addition to negatively regulating transcription of the mammalian *INO1* gene, IP6K1 may indirectly regulate MIPS enzymatic activity by activating GSK3.

3 Inositol and the Brain

3.1 *Myo*-Inositol Levels in the Brain

3.1.1 Inositol Synthesis

Myo-inositol is maintained at high (mM) levels in the brain in many species, including humans (Shimon et al. 1997; Stokes et al. 1983; Stokes and Hawthorne 1987). Inositol has important osmoregulatory and protective functions in the brain, especially during chronic tonicity changes (Strange 1992; Yancey 2005). The synthesis of inositol in mammals was once thought to be nonessential because MIPS activity is low in most animal tissues (Whiting et al. 1979). However, de novo synthesis in the brain contributes approximately 50% of inositol, with the remainder being transported from the blood (Spector 1976). When dietary intake of inositol is low, inositol levels decrease in most tissues but are maintained in the brain (Burton et al. 1976).

MIPS is highly conserved from yeast to humans, and expression of the recombinant human enzyme complements the inositol deficiency of yeast cells lacking the enzyme (Ju and Greenberg 2003). In addition, enzyme activity is similarly affected by mutation of conserved phosphosites in yeast and human MIPS (as discussed above) (Deranieh et al. 2013). The essential role of inositol synthesis in neuronal cells was demonstrated by the finding that exogenous inositol was dispensable for proliferation of SK-N-SH human neuroblastoma cells and that inhibition of inositol synthesis by siRNA-mediated knockdown of *INO1* inhibited cell proliferation and neurite outgrowth (Ye and Greenberg 2015). Taken together, these findings indicate that inositol synthesis in the mammalian brain plays a significant role in maintaining inositol levels and normal cell function.

3.1.2 Inositol Uptake

About half of the free inositol in the mammalian brain is transported from the blood (Spector 1976). This is accomplished by two groups of inositol active transporters: the high-affinity, sodium-dependent inositol transporters (SMIT1/2) and the low-affinity, hydrogen/*myo*-inositol symporter (HMIT). SMIT transporters function by co-transporting two sodium ions down the concentration gradient to generate enough energy to actively transport inositol (Bourgeois et al. 2005). SMIT activity is regulated by several factors, including pH (Hager et al. 1995), osmotic stress (Ibsen and Strange 1996; Strange et al. 1991), inositol levels (Lubrich et al. 2000), and PKA and PKC activity (which suggests posttranslational modification) (Preston et al. 1995), as well as by glucose (Haneda et al. 1990). Interestingly, physiological concentrations of glucose have been shown to inhibit inositol uptake (Kollros et al. 1990). HMIT transporters, which cotransport H^+ with inositol, are present almost exclusively in the central nervous system (Uldry et al. 2001). Important differences exist between the two transporter groups. For example, HMIT is insensitive to glucose. Moreover, inositol uptake by HMIT is decreased at higher pH levels (Uldry et al. 2001), in contrast to uptake by SMIT (Matskevitch et al. 1998). Fu and coworkers determined that in astrocytes (glial cells), HMIT accounts for at least half of total inositol uptake at physiologically relevant plasma concentrations of inositol (Fu et al. 2012). The authors argue that because bipolar medications increase pH in astrocytes (Song et al. 2008) and inhibit inositol uptake at high extracellular concentrations of inositol (Wolfson et al. 2000), HMIT is the transporter that is primarily inhibited by chronic treatment with mood-stabilizing drugs (Fu et al. 2012).

3.2 Inositol and Bipolar Disorder

Bipolar disorder (BD) is a severe psychiatric illness characterized by extreme mood changes that include manic and depressive episodes. It has a high prevalence rate of 1–2% worldwide (Merikangas et al. 2011) and the highest suicide rate of all psychiatric disorders (Chesney et al. 2014). Patients with the disorder are at a higher risk of death from natural causes than the general population (Mansur and Brietzke 2012), especially from cardiovascular disease (Hayes et al. 2015), which is likely caused by the increased incidence of obesity, diabetes, and hyperlipidemia (Blanco et al. 2017; Leboyer et al. 2012). Despite extensive study, the pathogenesis underlying BD is not known. A genetic component is suggested by the concordance rate (40–70%) of BD in monozygotic twins; however, concordance of less than 100% indicates that other factors modify phenotypic expression (Craddock and Sklar 2013). Environmental factors are known contributors to BD development (Aldinger

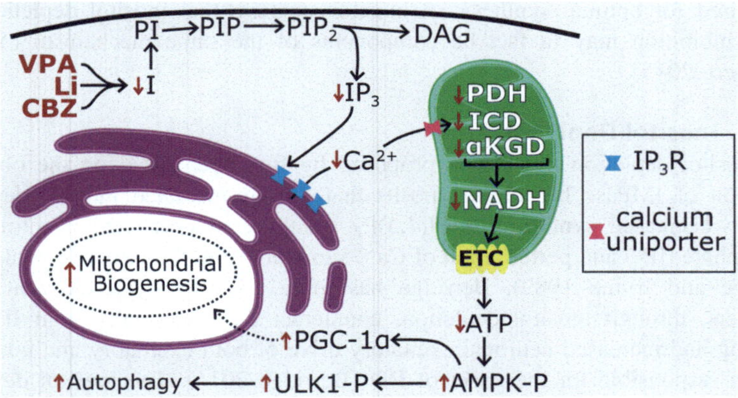

Fig. 4 Three mood-stabilizing medications, lithium (Li^+), VPA, and carbamazepine (CBZ), decrease inositol levels leading to decreased Ca^{2+} release through the IP_3R channel. Ca^{2+} is important for the activity of key mitochondrial enzymes, pyruvate dehydrogenase (PDH), isocitrate dehydrogenase (ICD), and α-ketoglutarate dehydrogenase (α-KGD), which produce NADH, used by oxidative phosphorylation complexes of the electron transport chain (ETC). Therefore, the decreased Ca^{2+} uptake by mitochondria impairs ATP production by limiting the ETC activity. An increased AMP/ATP ratio activates the energy sensor, AMPK, by phosphorylation. AMPK phosphorylates and activates the transcription of PGC1-α, a master regulator of mitochondrial biogenesis, as well as ULK1, a general activator of autophagy. We hypothesize that the combined activity of increased autophagy, which recycles defective mitochondria, and activated mitochondrial biogenesis may increase the proportion of healthy mitochondria in BD patients

and Schulze 2017). The pathophysiology of BD is complex, involving a decrease in neuronal generation and plasticity (Soeiro-de-Souza et al. 2012) as well as volumetric abnormalities in specific brain regions (Hajek et al. 2005). Other pathophysiological features include altered phosphoinositide signaling (Brown et al. 1993; Jope et al. 1996) and impaired mitochondrial activity (Kato and Kato 2000; Kato et al. 2000, 2001; Murashita et al. 2000), both of which are proposed to lead to impaired regulation of Ca^{2+} signaling (Fig. 4) (Berridge 2014; Kato 2008; Machado-Vieira et al. 2011).

Lithium and VPA have been used for decades to treat BD (Koch-Weser et al. 1980; Shorter 2009). Other medications used in treatment include carbamazepine, lamotrigine (Ng et al. 2007), and olanzapine (Mitchell and Malhi 2002). However, the therapeutic mechanisms of action of the drugs are not understood. The observation of Berridge that lithium inhibits the synthesis of inositol led to the inositol depletion hypothesis to explain the therapeutic mechanism of action (Berridge et al. 1982; Berridge and Irvine 1989). This hypothesis stimulated decades of research to explore the role of inositol in the pathology and treatment of BD. A hypothesis that seemed to contradict inositol depletion as a therapeutic mechanism was suggested by the finding of Klein and Melton that the effects of lithium on the development of *Xenopus* embryos could be explained by inhibition of GSK3β, and not by inhibition of inositol synthesis (Klein and Melton 1996). The demonstration in yeast that GSK3 is required for optimal synthesis of inositol suggests that inositol depletion and GSK3 inhibition may in fact be components of the same mechanism (Ye and Greenberg 2015).

3.2.1 Inositol Depletion

The inositol depletion hypothesis proposed by Berridge, based on the observed inhibition of IMPase by lithium, posits that lithium-mediated inositol depletion leads to decreased synthesis of PI(4,5)P_2, resulting in decreased inositol-1,4,5-triphosphate (IP_3) and perturbation of Ca^{2+} signaling (Fig. 4) (Berridge et al. 1982; Berridge and Irvine 1989). Berridge has more recently suggested that mood stabilizers, through inositol depletion, counteract the abnormally high IP_3/Ca^{2+} signaling and increased neuronal excitatory drive of both excitatory and inhibitory neurons responsible for the onset of BD (Berridge 2014). The inositol depletion hypothesis was supported by the finding that other mood-stabilizing drugs, including VPA and carbamazepine, also lead to inositol depletion, albeit by different mechanisms (Lubrich and van Calker 1999; Vaden et al. 2001; Wolfson et al. 2000). In behavioral studies, the IMPase inhibitor and lithium mimetic, ebselen, was shown to affect mouse behavior similar to lithium (Singh et al. 2013), and inositol was shown to reverse the behavioral effects of lithium (Agam et al. 2009; Belmaker et al. 1996; Kofman and Belmaker 1990). Furthermore, inositol reversed the increase in growth cone area caused by lithium, VPA, and carbamazepine (Williams et al. 2002), lending further support to the inositol depletion hypothesis.

An important cellular consequence of inositol depletion is the activation of AMPK and autophagy. This effect is mediated through decreased Ca^{2+} transfer to the mitochondria, which is important for the function of several key enzymes (e.g., pyruvate dehydrogenase, isocitrate dehydrogenase, and α-ketoglutarate dehydrogenase) involved in energy metabolism (Tarasov et al. 2012). When IP_3 binds the inositol triphosphate receptor (IP_3R), Ca^{2+} is released from the ER and transferred to mitochondria to support normal mitochondrial function (Cardenas et al. 2010). Decreased IP_3R signaling and Ca^{2+} release result in decreased oxygen consumption and ATP production, which activates AMPK. Inhibition of IP_3R signaling by CBZ-mediated depletion of inositol and, consequently, IP_3 leads to decreased mitochondrial Ca^{2+} uptake, decreased ATP levels, activation of AMPK, and increased autophagy (Schiebler et al. 2015) (Fig. 4). This effect of inositol depletion on cellular bioenergetics has not been studied in relation to BD and may provide important insights in the future.

Although supported by many studies, some findings cast doubt on the inositol depletion hypothesis (Azab et al. 2008; Yu and Greenberg 2016). For example, decreased inositol levels were not observed after acute or chronic lithium treatment (Shapiro et al. 2000; Silverstone et al. 2002). These findings do not conclusively argue against the hypothesis, as mammalian cells may compensate for inositol depletion by upregulating inositol synthesis, a regulatory phenomenon that is well-characterized in yeast (as discussed above). Nevertheless, *SMIT1+/−* heterozygote mice did exhibit decreased brain inositol levels; however, this was not associated with mood improvement, as measured by decreased immobility time in the forced swim test model of depression (Can et al. 2012), in contrast to the reaction of lithium-treated mice (Shaldubina et al. 2006, 2007). Furthermore, *SMIT1−/−* mice exhibited decreased brain inositol but did not have decreased levels of PI (Berry et al. 2003, 2004). An understanding of the molecular mechanisms that control inositol homeostasis in human cells is essential to clarify the role of inositol depletion in the therapeutic effects of mood-stabilizing drugs.

3.2.2 GSK3 Inhibition, Neurogenesis, and Cellular Plasticity

Increased neurogenesis and cellular plasticity are proposed mechanisms of action of mood-stabilizing drugs (Berridge 2014; Soeiro-de-Souza et al. 2012). Several studies have linked mood disorders to dysfunctional signaling mechanisms regulating neurogenesis (Machado-Vieira et al. 2009; Martinowich et al. 2009). Interestingly, GSK3 is an intermediary in numerous signaling pathways and an important regulator of neurogenesis (Doble and Woodgett 2003; Jope 2003; Jope and Johnson 2004; Valvezan and Klein 2012). GSK3 is an inhibitor of the transcription factors CREB and β-catenin (Hur and Zhou 2010; Rowe et al. 2007). Activation of CREB supports neurogenesis by increasing the expression of brain-derived neurotrophic factor (BDNF) and Bcl-2, an anti-apoptotic protein (Berridge 2014). Overexpression of β-catenin, an important regulator of neuronal connectivity (Ciani and Salinas 2005), decreased hyperactivity in mouse models of mania and decreased immobility time in the forced swim test (Gould et al. 2007). Therefore, mood-stabilizing drugs may exert therapeutic effects by promoting neurogenesis through inhibition of GSK3 signaling.

Lithium has been shown to inhibit GSK3-β in *Xenopus*, *Drosophila*, cultured mammalian cells, and rat brain (Lovestone et al. 1999; Munoz-Montano et al. 1997; Stambolic et al. 1996). Decreasing levels of GSK3 in mice, in heterozygous GSK3 null animals (O'Brien et al. 2004) or in response to GSK3 inhibitors (Gould et al. 2004; Kaidanovich-Beilin et al. 2004), replicated the observed lithium-induced decreased immobility time in the forced swim test (Cryan et al. 2002). Moreover, inhibition of GSK3 decreased hyperactivity in mouse models of mania (Beaulieu et al. 2004; Gould et al. 2004). Similar to lithium, some studies have shown that VPA also inhibits GSK3 (Chen et al. 1999; Hall et al. 2002; Kim et al. 2005), although other studies contradicted this finding (Jonathan Ryves et al. 2005; Phiel et al. 2001). Whether GSK3 inhibition is a common target of BD drugs requires further investigation.

3.2.3 Unifying Hypothesis of GSK3 Inhibition and Inositol Depletion

Studies in yeast and mammalian cells suggest that inositol depletion and GSK3 inhibition by mood-stabilizing drugs may be components of a single mechanism. As discussed earlier, GSK3 is a positive regulator of inositol biosynthesis in yeast (Azab et al. 2007; Yu et al. 2017). Yeast *mck1*Δ cells exhibit several aspects of inositol depletion, including decreased levels of intracellular inositol and MIPS enzymatic activity and decreased rates of inositol de novo synthesis in vivo (Yu et al. 2017). The mechanism underlying regulation of MIPS by Mck1 is not understood. One possibility is that MIPS is regulated directly or indirectly by a GSK3 phosphorylation cascade. Interestingly, a potential GSK3 phosphorylation site exists in both human and yeast MIPS, and mutation of this site affects activity of both human and yeast enzymes to a similar extent (Deranieh et al. 2013).

GSK3 may also control inositol synthesis by regulating the availability of the MIPS substrate, G6P. In yeast, GSK3 homologues are required for the expression of phosphoglucomutase, which catalyzes the interconversion of G1P and G6P (Dey et al. 1994; Hirata et al. 2003). Consistent with this, lithium, which inhibits GSK3, inhibits yeast and human phosphoglucomutase (Masuda et al. 2001). Yeast cells grown in the presence of lithium exhibited increased accumulation of G1P and decreased levels of G6P due to the inhibition of phosphoglucomutase activity. In hepatoma cells, decreased GSK3 activity reduces the expression of a key gluconeogenesis gene encoding phosphoenolpyruvate carboxykinase and reduces glucose production (Bosch et al. 1992; Lochhead et al. 2001). Together, these findings suggest that GSK3 inhibition induced by lithium, VPA, and other drugs may decrease the availability of G6P for the de novo synthesis of inositol, thereby contributing to inositol depletion.

Interestingly, while GSK3 affects inositol synthesis in yeast, inositol synthesis was shown to affect GSK3 activity in the neuronal cell line, SK-N-SH, as knockdown of MIPS in this cell line promotes the inhibitory phosphorylation of GSK3α on S21 (Ye and Greenberg 2015). It is tempting to speculate that a feedback loop may exist in which GSK3 activation and inositol synthesis are coordinately regulated.

A model that unifies the inositol depletion and GSK3 inhibition hypotheses was proposed (Yu and Greenberg 2016). Accordingly, because GSK3 is required for optimal activity of MIPS, inhibition of GSK3 causes inositol depletion. Perturbation of inositol homeostasis alters IP_3/Ca^{2+} and PI signaling (Shi et al. 2006; Simonsen et al. 2001; Toker 2002). Among numerous cellular consequences induced by inositol depletion are those that are beneficial for mood stabilization (Deranieh and Greenberg 2009; Jesch et al. 2005). Furthermore, GSK3 inhibition may reduce loss of neuronal cells by downregulating apoptosis, thereby effecting mood stabilization.

3.2.4 Energy Metabolism and AMPK (AMP-Activated Protein Kinase)

Many studies have shown that the pathophysiology of BD involves altered energy metabolism. The prevalence of metabolic disorders, including obesity, cardiovascular disease, and diabetes, is higher in BD patients than in the general population (Mansur and Brietzke 2012). Energy production and glucose utilization are altered in BD patient neurons (Li et al. 2015). Magnetic resonance spectroscopy of BD patient brains identified a decrease in intracellular pH resulting from an increase in lactate production (Dager et al. 2004; Hamakawa et al. 2004; Kato et al. 1998), and a decrease in the high energy compound phosphocreatine (Kato et al. 1994, 1995), which acts as a reservoir for the generation of ATP (Modica-Napolitano and Renshaw 2004). In addition, studies have found a decrease in N-acetylaspartate, a marker for neuronal mitochondrial health (Clark 1998; De Stefano et al. 1995) in BD patient brains. Furthermore, a finding of dysfunctional mitochondria has been reported in BD patient cells (Cataldo et al. 2010). Taken together, these findings suggest that the brain in BD displays an increase in glycolysis as a result of impaired mitochondrial function (Stork and Renshaw 2005).

If mitochondrial function is decreased in BD, activating mitochondrial biogenesis may be a therapeutic mechanism for the treatment of the disorder. Studies of the effects of lithium on mitochondrial function are inconclusive (Cataldo et al. 2010; Maurer et al. 2009; Mertens et al. 2015; Struewing et al. 2007). However, VPA was shown to increase mitochondrial biogenesis in human fibroblasts, possibly by upregulating the transcription of PGC-1α (peroxisome proliferator-activated receptor γ coactivator 1α) (Sitarz et al. 2014), the master regulator of mitochondrial biogenesis (Fernandez-Marcos and Auwerx 2011). VPA was shown to activate AMPK (Avery and Bumpus 2014), which upregulates PGC-1α transcription in muscles (Avery and Bumpus 2014; Bergeron et al. 2001; Chaube et al. 2015; Marin et al. 2017). AMPK also activates autophagy through phosphorylation of ULK1 protein kinase (Egan et al. 2011). However, several studies also indicate that VPA inhibits mitochondrial metabolism (Aires et al. 2008; Komulainen et al. 2015; Ponchaut et al. 1992; Silva et al. 2008), which may be a cause of VPA-induced hepatotoxicity (Lee et al. 2007; Lewis et al. 1982).

In light of the observed mitochondrial dysfunction in BD, it is interesting to speculate that inositol-depleting drugs alleviate some of this dysfunction through activating autophagy and mitochondrial biogenesis. Toker and Agam suggested that mitochondrial dysfunction in psychiatric disorders may be a consequence of impaired autophagy (Toker and Agam 2015). Activation of autophagy may help recycle defective mitochondria (Lionaki et al. 2015). Moreover, activation of AMPK may upregulate PGC-1α transcription, leading to mitochondrial biogenesis (Fig. 4).

3.2.5 The Unfolded Protein Response (UPR)

A potential link between BD and the UPR is suggested by several studies in yeast and mammals. The UPR is a signal transduction pathway that is activated in response to the accumulation of unfolded proteins (Ron and Walter 2007). Activation of the UPR results in increased transcription of chaperone proteins, protein degradation, decreased protein synthesis, and the induction of apoptosis (Lai et al. 2007). The UPR in mammals consists of three parallel branches that are defined by ER transmembrane signaling proteins, which initiate the signal (Walter and Ron 2011). Activation through IRE1 (inositol requiring enzyme 1) is the most conserved branch and the only branch of the UPR found in yeast (Mori 2009). Upon UPR activation, IRE1 forms oligomers that activate the ribonuclease function of the enzyme (Korennykh et al. 2009). Active IRE1 splices XBP1 mRNA, producing an active transcription factor (Yoshida et al. 2001). XBP1 then induces its own transcription as well as that of chaperone proteins. A polymorphism (C to G) in the promoter of XBP1, which decreases the expression of XBP1 protein, was shown to be genetically associated with BD and is a potential genetic risk factor for the disorder (Kakiuchi et al. 2003). Activation of the UPR in the presence of the XBP1 polymorphism can be rescued by VPA-mediated induction of ATF6, the gene upstream of XBP1 (Kakiuchi et al. 2003). Additional evidence for involvement of the UPR in BD comes from the finding that lymphoblasts derived from BD patients have lower levels of total and active XBP1 and an impaired UPR stress response (Hayashi et al. 2009; So et al. 2007). Both Li and VPA increase expression of ER stress response proteins by a mechanism not yet determined (Bown et al. 2002; Shao et al. 2006). A clue regarding this mechanism comes from studies in yeast indicating that VPA induces the UPR as a result of increasing ceramide levels (Jadhav et al. 2016). Interestingly, the increase in ceramide and induction of the UPR were replicated by genetically depleting inositol (Jadhav et al. 2016). Whether drug-mediated inositol depletion is linked to UPR activation in mammals is not known and an interesting topic for future research.

3.3 Inositol and Depression

Depression is characterized by feelings of sadness, reduced energy, anhedonia, pessimistic thinking, and insomnia and is prevalent in over 4% of the population (Blazer et al. 1994; Jenkins et al. 1997). Depression is a leading cause of disability worldwide (Whiteford et al. 2013). However, less than 50% of patients reach remission after 8 weeks of antidepressant therapy (Saveanu et al. 2015). The characterization of depression is complicated by comorbidity with other disorders; thus, the identification of reliable biomarkers would aid in diagnosis. Inositol levels have been investigated as a potential biomarker for depression. Some studies indicate that inositol levels are decreased in the prefrontal and anterior cingulate cortex in brains of depressed, suicidal, and bipolar patients (Chen et al. 2014; Coupland et al. 2005; Frey et al. 1998; Shimon et al. 1997). Glial cells have high levels of inositol (Brand et al. 1993; Griffin et al. 2002), and it has been suggested that decreased inositol levels result from glial loss or altered glial metabolism in depression (Chen et al. 2014; Coupland et al. 2005).

A positive clinical outcome in depression has been associated with increased supplementation of inositol (Chen et al. 2014; Chiappelli et al. 2015; Zheng et al. 2010), which is well-tolerated with no serious side effects and results in increased inositol levels in the brain and cerebrospinal fluid (Bizzarri et al. 2016; Levine 1997; Levine et al. 1993, 1995; Moore et al. 1999; Papaleo et al. 2009). One study suggests that decreased inositol levels is a reliable biomarker of depression in schizophrenic patients (Chiappelli et al. 2015). However, contrasting studies have reported increased inositol levels in depressed patients (Caetano et al. 2005; Lirng et al. 2015). In addition, a meta-analysis of studies that have used inositol supplementation in the treatment of depression found no significant effect of inositol in the course of treatment (Mukai et al. 2014). Thus, the role of inositol in depression has yet to be clarified.

4 Inositol and Insulin Resistance

4.1 Inositol and Insulin Signaling

There are nine possible stereoisomers of inositol. Eight isomers, including *myo*-, *scyllo*-, *epi*-, *muco*-, *neo*-, *allo*-, D-*chiro*-, and L-*chiro*-inositol, have been found in biological systems. A ninth isomer, *cis*-inositol, is not naturally occurring (Thomas et al. 2016). Among these, *myo*-inositol is the most physiologically relevant isomer. D-*chiro*-inositol and *myo*-inositol are interconverted by epimerase (Larner 2002). Recent studies suggest that *myo*-inositol and D-*chiro*-inositol are involved in insulin resistance. Increased urinary excretion of *myo*-inositol and decreased excretion of D-*chiro*-inositol were reported in multiple studies in human subjects, rats, and monkeys with type 2 diabetes (Kennington et al. 1990; Ortmeyer et al. 1993; Sun et al. 2002). Biopsied muscles from type 2 diabetic subjects contain dramatically reduced levels of D-*chiro*-inositol and increased levels of *myo*-inositol (Kennington et al. 1990). An altered *myo*-/D-*chiro*-inositol ratio was also reported in type 1 and nondiabetic relatives of diabetic patients (Larner et al. 2010; Larner and Craig 1996). Based on these findings, the increased urinary *myo*-/D-*chiro*-inositol ratio has been proposed as a biomarker for insulin resistance in diabetes diagnosis (Larner and Craig 1996). The increased *myo*-/D-*chiro*-inositol ratio suggests that diabetic patients may have impaired synthesis of D-*chiro*-inositol. A severe defect in the conversion of *myo*-inositol to D-*chiro*-inositol was observed in type 2 diabetic rats (Pak et al. 1998). Decreased epimerase activity was also observed in cytosolic extracts from various tissues of type 2 diabetic rats (Sun et al. 2002). In addition, insulin treatment increased D-*chiro*-inositol in control subjects but not in diabetic patients (Kennington et al. 1990). These studies suggest that a deficiency of D-*chiro*-inositol is directly associated with the progression of insulin resistance (Ortmeyer et al. 1993).

Myo-inositol and D-*chiro*-inositol can be incorporated into inositol phosphoglycans (IPGs) to act as insulin second messengers (Larner et al. 2010). *Myo*-inositol and D-*chiro*-inositol-containing IPGs have insulin-mimetic effects, demonstrated by dose-dependent reduction of hyperglycemia and promotion of glycogenesis when administrated in vivo in rats (Huang et al. 1993; Larner 2002). A decrease in D-*chiro*-inositol-containing IPG was found in type 2 diabetic patients (Kennington et al. 1990). In addition, insulin stimulates the release of D-*chiro*-inositol-IPG in normal subjects but not in insulin-resistant patients (Baillargeon et al. 2010). Overall, alterations in the availability of inositol may affect insulin signaling directly or indirectly by altering inositol-containing IPG levels. Supplementation of inositol to restore inositol levels or the balance of *myo*-/D-*chiro*-inositol in vivo may be beneficial for treating insulin resistance.

4.2 Inositol in the Treatment of Polycystic Ovary Syndrome (PCOS)

Abnormal inositol metabolism is associated with polycystic ovary syndrome (PCOS). PCOS, one of the most common causes of infertility, is an endocrine and metabolic disorder that affects 9–12% of women of reproductive age (March et al. 2010). Although the direct cause of PCOS is not clear (Orio and Palomba 2014), the disorder is usually accompanied by insulin resistance and compensatory hyperinsulinemia (Croze and Soulage 2013; Genazzani 2016), which increases the risk of developing type 2 diabetes (Celik et al. 2014; Hudecova et al. 2011). A decrease in plasma levels of D-*chiro*-inositol was reported in PCOS patients compared to normal subjects (Baillargeon et al. 2006). In a glucose tolerance test, PCOS patients also exhibited a reduced D-*chiro*-inositol-containing IPG to insulin ratio (Baillargeon et al. 2006). In addition, diabetic patients and PCOS patients with familial predisposition to diabetes may have decreased availability of D-*chiro*-inositol due to abnormal epimerase activity (Larner et al. 2010; Larner and Craig 1996). These findings suggest that the decreased D-*chiro*-inositol levels are correlated with insulin resistance in PCOS. *Myo*-inositol also plays an important role in regulating ovarian function, and increased *myo*-inositol in the follicular fluid was shown to positively affect oocyte maturation (Carlomagno et al. 2011; Chiu et al. 2002).

Both *myo*-inositol and D-*chiro*-inositol have been shown to have beneficial effects in the treatment of PCOS. In multiple studies, PCOS patients receiving *myo*-inositol treatment exhibited improved insulin sensitivity (Genazzani et al. 2008, 2012; Unfer et al. 2012). *Myo*-inositol supplementation also improved ovarian activity and hormonal parameters and, thereby, restored fertility in PCOS patients (Artini et al. 2013; Genazzani et al. 2008; Gerli et al. 2003, 2007; Papaleo et al. 2007; Unfer et al. 2012). D-*chiro*-inositol supplementation also exhibited beneficial effects in the treatment of PCOS. D-*chiro*-inositol increased insulin sensitivity in obese patients (Genazzani et al. 2014; Iuorno et al. 2002; La Marca et al. 2015; Nestler et al. 1999). Treating PCOS patients with D-*chiro*-inositol and folic acid together significantly improved insulin sensitivity and metabolic parameters (Lagana et al. 2015). Combining *myo*-inositol and D-*chiro*-inositol supplementation was more effective than *myo*-inositol alone when administrated to PCOS patients (Nordio and Proietti 2012). The combined treatment with *myo*-inositol and D-*chiro*-inositol exhibited promising effects in improving insulin resistance and ovarian activities (Benelli et al. 2016; Monastra et al. 2017). Accumulating evidence suggests that an optimal ratio of *myo*-inositol/D-*chiro*-inositol is critical for improving ovarian function and achieving insulin-sensitizing effects simultaneously (Dinicola et al. 2014). A 40:1 ratio of *myo*-inositol/D-*chiro*-inositol, which matches the *myo*-/D-*chiro*-inositol ratio in the plasma of healthy subjects, has been proposed as a first-line approach to treat PCOS (Facchinetti et al. 2015; Nordio and Proietti 2012).

5 Inositol and Autophagy

Inositol is essential for regulation of autophagy, the selective and nonselective degradation of cytoplasmic components and organelles. Cellular autophagy events fall into three categories: microautophagy, macroautophagy, and chaperone-mediated autophagy. Macroautophagy is the most well-characterized category and is the subject of this section (Mizushima et al. 2008). Autophagy is critical for cell survival and health, and malfunction of autophagy leads to many disease conditions (Sarkar and Rubinsztein 2006). Under nutrient deficient and/or growth factor deprivation conditions, autophagy non-selectively degrades cellular components into building blocks to maintain synthesis of proteins that are critical for cell survival until conditions improve (Levine and Klionsky 2004). A constitutive basal level of autophagy leads to removal of damaged or old organelles, reducing reactive oxygen species (ROS) production and promoting longevity (Mizushima et al. 2008). Basal autophagy also prevents the accumulation of protein aggregates. These functions are critical for the homeostasis of a variety of cells, especially neurons (Hara et al. 2006; Komatsu et al. 2006). Perturbation of autophagy has been reported in the pathogenesis of many neurodegenerative diseases, including Alzheimer's disease (AZ), Huntington's diseases (HD), and Parkinson's diseases (PD) (Menzies et al. 2017).

Autophagy was shown to be negatively regulated by IP_3, which inhibits autophagy by activating the IP_3R (Criollo et al. 2007; Sarkar et al. 2005; Sarkar and Rubinsztein 2006). Consistent with this, autophagy is increased in response to IP_3R antagonist and by knockdown of the IP_3R (Criollo et al. 2007). Inhibition of IMPase by lithium or L-690,330 was shown to induce autophagy by reducing IP_3 levels (Sarkar et al. 2005). Together, these findings suggest that IP_3 is a critical regulator of autophagy that may function through the AMPK activating mechanism described in Fig. 4.

5.1 Parkinson's Disease

Parkinson's disease (PD) is a neurodegenerative disease that mainly affects the motor system, resulting in tremor, motor impairment, and muscle rigidity (Sveinbjornsdottir 2016). The pathogenesis of PD is associated with reduced dopamine levels due to the loss of dopaminergic neurons in the substantia nigra (Chinta and Andersen 2005; Groger et al. 2014). Significantly increased levels of IP_3 were observed in the cerebral cortex of PD rats (Nandhu et al. 2011). Elevated IP_3 levels stimulate excessive release of Ca^{2+} from the ER, which stresses mitochondria and prompts ROS production. This leads to induction of apoptosis by upregulating expression of the pro-apoptotic regulator, BAX (Li et al. 2014). The expression of BAX is increased in PD rats, leading to cytosolic release of apoptotic factors followed by cell death. These effects together may contribute, at least in part, to neurodegeneration in PD patients. In a mouse model of PD (induced by 1-methyl-4-phenyl-1,2,3,6-tetrahydropyridine), lithium combined with VPA treatment increased the number of dopaminergic neurons in the substantia nigra and improved motor functions by promoting autophagy (Li et al. 2013). The neuroprotective effects of lithium and VPA may result from reduction of the abnormally elevated IP_3 levels as a consequence of inositol depletion by the drugs.

Another consequence of IMPase inhibition pertains to enhanced clearance of α-synuclein. Aggregates of α-synuclein in Lewy bodies constitute hallmark lesions in neurons of PD patients (Spillantini et al. 1997). Lithium as well as L-690,330 enhanced clearance of α-synuclein by inducing autophagy (Sarkar et al. 2005). The α-synuclein clearance-enhancing effect of L-690,330 was abrogated when autophagy was blocked (Atack et al. 1993). Taken together, these findings suggest that IP_3 may be a potential therapeutic target for the treatment of PD.

5.2 Huntington's Disease

Huntington's disease (HD) is a progressive neurodegenerative disorder characterized by loss of motor ability and dementia (Warby et al. 1993). HD is caused by the expansion of CAG repeats in the autosomal gene *huntingtin* (Walker 2007). The mutant huntingtin (mHTT) protein can be cleaved by different proteases, generating protein fragments that aggregate in neurons and cause progressive neuron loss (Dayalu and Albin 2015). As discussed above, a basal level of autophagy is critical for purging intracellular misfolded proteins and protein aggregates, especially in neurons (Hara et al. 2006; Komatsu et al. 2006). Inhibition of IMPase by lithium has been shown to induce autophagy leading to enhanced clearance of mHTT (Sarkar et al. 2005).

Recent studies suggest that abnormal IP_3R functions are associated with the progression of HD. mHTT was shown to bind directly to the IC10 domain in the C-terminal tail of type 1 IP_3R (IP_3R1) in medium spiny striatal neurons (Tang et al. 2009), and mHTT was able to activate IP_3R1 in vitro and in vivo (Tang et al. 2003). mHTT-induced IP_3R1 activation promotes Ca^{2+} release from the ER and results in mitochondrial Ca^{2+} overload, which in turn leads to mitochondrial cytochrome c release and subsequent neuronal cell death from apoptosis (Tang et al. 2005). The IP_3R1 blocker, 2-APB, exhibited neuroprotective effects against glutamate-induced apoptosis. Furthermore, expression of the IC10 fragment in the HD mouse improved motor impairment and reduced the loss of medium spiny striatal neurons by disrupting mHTT-IP_3R associations (Tang et al. 2009). Interestingly, lithium and VPA exhibited beneficial effects in the treatment of HD (Linares et al. 2016; Scheuing et al. 2014). As described previously, inositol depletion leads to decreased intracellular IP_3 levels and reduced IP_3R activation. Reduced IP_3R activation enhances the clearance of mutant protein aggregates by promoting autophagy and decreases abnormal Ca^{2+} signaling-induced neuronal cell death. Therefore, therapeutic effects of lithium and VPA in treating HD may result, at least in part, from inositol depletion and IP_3 reduction. These studies suggest that reducing IP_3R activity in HD patients is a potential therapeutic strategy.

6 Unanswered Questions

Our understanding of the essential cellular processes that require inositol and the cellular consequences of perturbation of inositol metabolism will benefit from elucidating the molecular mechanisms that control inositol homeostasis. In this area, molecular characterization of inositol synthesis in the yeast model provides a strong foundation for studies in mammalian cells. The following questions will be interesting to explore in this regard:

1. As discussed above, IP6K1 promotes the methylation of *mINO1* and negatively regulates *mINO1* by a mechanism not yet determined (Yu et al. 2016). In mammalian cells, IP6K1 potentiates GSK3 in two ways – It directly activates GSK3 upon binding, and its product, IP_7, inhibits Akt, which catalyzes the

inhibitory phosphorylation of GSK3 (Chakraborty et al. 2014). Does GSK3 regulate inositol synthesis in mammalian cells, as it does in yeast (Yu et al. 2017)? What are the physiological stimuli affecting regulation by inositol pyrophosphate and GSK3?

2. Inositol pyrophosphates play a key role in responding to and regulating cellular energy metabolism and regulating ATP synthesis by altering the ratio of glycolysis to mitochondrial energy metabolism (Szijgyarto et al. 2011). As G6P is both the essential substrate for inositol synthesis and the control point for glycolysis, is the commitment to inositol synthesis affected by the energy needs of the cell? Intriguingly, the inositol-depleting drugs VPA and carbamazepine activate the energy sensor AMPK (Avery and Bumpus 2014; Schiebler et al. 2015), which has been shown to increase mitochondrial biogenesis in muscle tissue (Jager et al. 2007). What is the link between regulation of inositol synthesis and mitochondrial energy metabolism?
3. PA plays a key role in the negative regulation of *INO1* expression in yeast and mammalian cells. Binding of PA to the yeast repressor Opi1 *inhibits* repression of *yINO1* by tethering the repressor to the ER. In contrast, PA binding to the repressor IP6K1 *promotes* repression of *mINO1* by facilitating entry to the nucleus. Does PA act as a sensor of phospholipid metabolism, coordinating synthesis of phospholipid and inositol metabolic pathways?
4. MIPS phosphorylation is conserved from yeast to humans, but the physiological signals that regulate phosphorylation are not yet known. Eliminating two inhibitory phosphorylation sites from yeast MIPS results in a protein that confers increased growth and, importantly, resistance to growth inhibition by VPA. What are the signals that initiate phosphorylation of MIPS?
5. What is the relationship between inositol depletion, UPR activation, and BD? Impaired UPR activation has been linked to BD (Hayashi et al. 2009; So et al. 2007), and polymorphisms in UPR genes are suggested genetic risk factors for the disorder (Kakiuchi et al. 2003). Consistent with this, both lithium and VPA have been shown to increase UPR activation and expression of ER stress response genes (Bown et al. 2002; Shao et al. 2006). In yeast, increased ceramide levels resulting from inositol depletion lead to activation of the UPR (Jadhav et al. 2016). What is the mechanism linking inositol depletion to activation of the UPR in mammalian cells?

Acknowledgments The Greenberg lab gratefully acknowledges support from grant R01 GM 125082 from the National Institutes of Health.

References

Agam G, Bersudsky Y, Berry GT, Moechars D, Lavi-Avnon Y, Belmaker RH (2009) Knockout mice in understanding the mechanism of action of lithium. Biochem Soc Trans 37:1121–1125

Ahmed S, Brickner DG, Light WH, Cajigas I, McDonough M, Froyshteter AB, Volpe T, Brickner JH (2010) DNA zip codes control an ancient mechanism for gene targeting to the nuclear periphery. Nat Cell Biol 12:111–118

Aires CC, Soveral G, Luis PB, ten Brink HJ, de Almeida IT, Duran M, Wanders RJ, Silva MF (2008) Pyruvate uptake is inhibited by valproic acid and metabolites in mitochondrial membranes. FEBS Lett 582:3359–3366

Aldinger F, Schulze TG (2017) Environmental factors, life events, and trauma in the course of bipolar disorder. Psychiatry Clin Neurosci 71:6–17

Ambroziak J, Henry SA (1994) INO2 and INO4 gene products, positive regulators of phospholipid biosynthesis in Saccharomyces cerevisiae, form a complex that binds to the INO1 promoter. J Biol Chem 269:15344–15349

Artini PG, Di Berardino OM, Papini F, Genazzani AD, Simi G, Ruggiero M, Cela V (2013) Endocrine and clinical effects of myo-inositol administration in polycystic ovary syndrome. A randomized study. Gynecol Endocrinol 29:375–379

Ashburner BP, Lopes JM (1995) Autoregulated expression of the yeast INO2 and INO4 helix-loop-helix activator genes effects cooperative regulation on their target genes. Mol Cell Biol 15:1709–1715

Atack JR, Cook SM, Watt AP, Fletcher SR, Ragan CI (1993) In vitro and in vivo inhibition of inositol monophosphatase by the bisphosphonate L-690,330. J Neurochem 60:652–658

Avery LB, Bumpus NN (2014) Valproic acid is a novel activator of AMP-activated protein kinase and decreases liver mass, hepatic fat accumulation, and serum glucose in obese mice. Mol Pharmacol 85:1–10

Azab AN, He Q, Ju S, Li G, Greenberg ML (2007) Glycogen synthase kinase-3 is required for optimal de novo synthesis of inositol. Mol Microbiol 63:1248–1258

Azab A, Agam G, Kaplanski J, Delbar V, Greenberg ML (2008) Inositol depletion: a good or bad outcome of valproate treatment? Future Neurol 3:275–286

Bachhawat N, Ouyang Q, Henry SA (1995) Functional characterization of an inositol-sensitive upstream activation sequence in yeast. A cis-regulatory element responsible for inositol-choline mediated regulation of phospholipid biosynthesis. J Biol Chem 270:25087–25095

Bailis AM, Poole MA, Carman GM, Henry SA (1987) The membrane-associated enzyme phosphatidylserine synthase is regulated at the level of mRNA abundance. Mol Cell Biol 7:167–176

Baillargeon JP, Diamanti-Kandarakis E, Ostlund RE Jr, Apridonidze T, Iuorno MJ, Nestler JE (2006) Altered D-chiro-inositol urinary clearance in women with polycystic ovary syndrome. Diabetes Care 29:300–305

Baillargeon JP, Iuorno MJ, Apridonidze T, Nestler JE (2010) Uncoupling between insulin and release of a D-chiro-inositol-containing inositolphosphoglycan mediator of insulin action in obese women with polycystic ovary syndrome. Metab Syndr Relat Disord 8:127–136

Beaulieu JM, Sotnikova TD, Yao WD, Kockeritz L, Woodgett JR, Gainetdinov RR, Caron MG (2004) Lithium antagonizes dopamine-dependent behaviors mediated by an AKT/glycogen synthase kinase 3 signaling cascade. Proc Natl Acad Sci U S A 101:5099–5104

Belmaker RH, Bersudsky Y, Agam G, Levine J, Kofman O (1996) How does lithium work on manic depression? Clinical and psychological correlates of the inositol theory. Annu Rev Med 47:47–56

Benelli E, Del Ghianda S, Di Cosmo C, Tonacchera M (2016) A combined therapy with myo-inositol and D-chiro-inositol improves endocrine parameters and insulin resistance in PCOS young overweight women. Int J Endocrinol 2016:3204083

Bergeron R, Ren JM, Cadman KS, Moore IK, Perret P, Pypaert M, Young LH, Semenkovich CF, Shulman GI (2001) Chronic activation of AMP kinase results in NRF-1 activation and mitochondrial biogenesis. Am J Physiol Endocrinol Metab 281:E1340–E1346

Berridge MJ (2014) Calcium signalling and psychiatric disease: bipolar disorder and schizophrenia. Cell Tissue Res 357:477–492

Berridge MJ, Irvine RF (1989) Inositol phosphates and cell signalling. Nature 341:197–205

Berridge MJ, Downes CP, Hanley MR (1982) Lithium amplifies agonist-dependent phosphatidylinositol responses in brain and salivary glands. Biochem J 206:587–595

Berry GT, Wu S, Buccafusca R, Ren J, Gonzales LW, Ballard PL, Golden JA, Stevens MJ, Greer JJ (2003) Loss of murine Na+/myo-inositol cotransporter leads to brain myo-inositol depletion and central apnea. J Biol Chem 278:18297–18302
Berry GT, Buccafusca R, Greer JJ, Eccleston E (2004) Phosphoinositide deficiency due to inositol depletion is not a mechanism of lithium action in brain. Mol Genet Metab 82:87–92
Bizzarri M, Fuso A, Dinicola S, Cucina A, Bevilacqua A (2016) Pharmacodynamics and pharmacokinetics of inositol(s) in health and disease. Expert Opin Drug Metab Toxicol 12:1181–1196
Blanco C, Compton WM, Saha TD, Goldstein BI, Ruan WJ, Huang B, Grant BF (2017) Epidemiology of DSM-5 bipolar I disorder: results from the National Epidemiologic Survey on alcohol and related conditions-III. J Psychiatr Res 84:310–317
Blazer DG, Kessler RC, McGonagle KA, Swartz MS (1994) The prevalence and distribution of major depression in a national community sample: the National Comorbidity Survey. Am J Psychiatry 151:979–986
Bosch F, Rodriguez-Gil JE, Hatzoglou M, Gomez-Foix AM, Hanson RW (1992) Lithium inhibits hepatic gluconeogenesis and phosphoenolpyruvate carboxykinase gene expression. J Biol Chem 267:2888–2893
Bourgeois F, Coady MJ, Lapointe JY (2005) Determination of transport stoichiometry for two cation-coupled myo-inositol cotransporters: SMIT2 and HMIT. J Physiol 563:333–343
Bown CD, Wang JF, Chen B, Young LT (2002) Regulation of ER stress proteins by valproate: therapeutic implications. Bipolar Disord 4:145–151
Brand A, Richter-Landsberg C, Leibfritz D (1993) Multinuclear NMR studies on the energy metabolism of glial and neuronal cells. Dev Neurosci 15:289–298
Brickner JH, Walter P (2004) Gene recruitment of the activated INO1 locus to the nuclear membrane. PLoS Biol 2:e342
Brown AS, Mallinger AG, Renbaum LC (1993) Elevated platelet membrane phosphatidylinositol-4,5-bisphosphate in bipolar mania. Am J Psychiatry 150:1252–1254
Burton LE, Ray RE, Bradford JR, Orr JP, Nickerson JA, Wells WW (1976) Myo-inositol metabolism in the neonatal and developing rat fed a myo-inositol-free diet. J Nutr 106:1610–1616
Burton A, Azevedo C, Andreassi C, Riccio A, Saiardi A (2013) Inositol pyrophosphates regulate JMJD2C-dependent histone demethylation. Proc Natl Acad Sci U S A 110:18970–18975
Caetano SC, Fonseca M, Olvera RL, Nicoletti M, Hatch JP, Stanley JA, Hunter K, Lafer B, Pliszka SR, Soares JC (2005) Proton spectroscopy study of the left dorsolateral prefrontal cortex in pediatric depressed patients. Neurosci Lett 384:321–326
Can A, Dao DT, Arad M, Terrillion CE, Piantadosi SC, Gould TD (2012) The mouse forced swim test. J Vis Exp 59:e3638
Cardenas C, Miller RA, Smith I, Bui T, Molgo J, Muller M, Vais H, Cheung KH, Yang J, Parker I, Thompson CB, Birnbaum MJ, Hallows KR, Foskett JK (2010) Essential regulation of cell bioenergetics by constitutive InsP3 receptor Ca2+ transfer to mitochondria. Cell 142:270–283
Carlomagno G, Nordio M, Chiu TT, Unfer V (2011) Contribution of myo-inositol and melatonin to human reproduction. Eur J Obstet Gynecol Reprod Biol 159:267–272
Carman GM, Han G-S (2011) Regulation of phospholipid synthesis in the yeast Saccharomyces cerevisiae. Annu Rev Biochem 80:859–883
Cataldo AM, McPhie DL, Lange NT, Punzell S, Elmiligy S, Ye NZ, Froimowitz MP, Hassinger LC, Menesale EB, Sargent LW, Logan DJ, Carpenter AE, Cohen BM (2010) Abnormalities in mitochondrial structure in cells from patients with bipolar disorder. Am J Pathol 177:575–585
Celik C, Tasdemir N, Abali R, Bastu E, Yilmaz M (2014) Progression to impaired glucose tolerance or type 2 diabetes mellitus in polycystic ovary syndrome: a controlled follow-up study. Fertil Steril 101:1123–1128.e1
Chakraborty A, Koldobskiy MA, Bello NT, Maxwell M, Potter JJ, Juluri KR, Maag D, Kim S, Huang AS, Dailey MJ, Saleh M, Snowman AM, Moran TH, Mezey E, Snyder SH (2010) Inositol pyrophosphates inhibit Akt signaling, thereby regulating insulin sensitivity and weight gain. Cell 143:897–910

Chakraborty A, Latapy C, Xu J, Snyder SH, Beaulieu JM (2014) Inositol hexakisphosphate kinase-1 regulates behavioral responses via GSK3 signaling pathways. Mol Psychiatry 19:284–293

Chaube B, Malvi P, Singh SV, Mohammad N, Viollet B, Bhat MK (2015) AMPK maintains energy homeostasis and survival in cancer cells via regulating p38/PGC-1alpha-mediated mitochondrial biogenesis. Cell Death Discovery 1:15063

Chen I-W, Charalampous FC (1966) Biochemical studies on inositol IX. D-inositol 1-phosphate as intermediate in the biosynthesis of inositol from glucose 6-phosphate, and characteristics of two reactions in this biosynthesis. J Biol Chem 241:2194–2199

Chen G, Huang LD, Jiang YM, Manji HK (1999) The mood-stabilizing agent valproate inhibits the activity of glycogen synthase kinase-3. J Neurochem 72:1327–1330

Chen LP, Dai HY, Dai ZZ, Xu CT, Wu RH (2014) Anterior cingulate cortex and cerebellar hemisphere neurometabolite changes in depression treatment: a 1H magnetic resonance spectroscopy study. Psychiatry Clin Neurosci 68:357–364

Chesney E, Goodwin GM, Fazel S (2014) Risks of all-cause and suicide mortality in mental disorders: a meta-review. World Psychiatry 13:153–160

Chiappelli J, Rowland LM, Wijtenburg SA, Muellerklein F, Tagamets M, McMahon RP, Gaston F, Kochunov P, Hong LE (2015) Evaluation of myo-inositol as a potential biomarker for depression in schizophrenia. Neuropsychopharmacology 40:2157–2164

Chinta SJ, Andersen JK (2005) Dopaminergic neurons. Int J Biochem Cell Biol 37:942–946

Chiu TT, Rogers MS, Law EL, Briton-Jones CM, Cheung LP, Haines CJ (2002) Follicular fluid and serum concentrations of myo-inositol in patients undergoing IVF: relationship with oocyte quality. Hum Reprod 17:1591–1596

Choi K, Mollapour E, Choi JH, Shears SB (2008) Cellular energetic status supervises the synthesis of bis-diphosphoinositol tetrakisphosphate independently of AMP-activated protein kinase. Mol Pharmacol 74:527–536

Ciani L, Salinas PC (2005) WNTs in the vertebrate nervous system: from patterning to neuronal connectivity. Nat Rev Neurosci 6:351–362

Clark JB (1998) N-acetyl aspartate: a marker for neuronal loss or mitochondrial dysfunction. Dev Neurosci 20:271–276

Coupland NJ, Ogilvie CJ, Hegadoren KM, Seres P, Hanstock CC, Allen PS (2005) Decreased prefrontal myo-inositol in major depressive disorder. Biol Psychiatry 57:1526–1534

Cox JS, Walter P (1996) A novel mechanism for regulating activity of a transcription factor that controls the unfolded protein response. Cell 87:391–404

Cox JS, Chapman RE, Walter P (1997) The unfolded protein response coordinates the production of endoplasmic reticulum protein and endoplasmic reticulum membrane. Mol Biol Cell 8:1805–1814

Craddock N, Sklar P (2013) Genetics of bipolar disorder. Lancet 381:1654–1662

Criollo A, Maiuri MC, Tasdemir E, Vitale I, Fiebig AA, Andrews D, Molgo J, Diaz J, Lavandero S, Harper F, Pierron G, di Stefano D, Rizzuto R, Szabadkai G, Kroemer G (2007) Regulation of autophagy by the inositol trisphosphate receptor. Cell Death Differ 14:1029–1039

Croze ML, Soulage CO (2013) Potential role and therapeutic interests of myo-inositol in metabolic diseases. Biochimie 95:1811–1827

Cryan JF, Markou A, Lucki I (2002) Assessing antidepressant activity in rodents: recent developments and future needs. Trends Pharmacol Sci 23:238–245

Czech MP (2003) Dynamics of phosphoinositides in membrane retrieval and insertion. Annu Rev Physiol 65:791–815

Dager SR, Friedman SD, Parow A, Demopulos C, Stoll AL, Lyoo IK, Dunner DL, Renshaw PF (2004) Brain metabolic alterations in medication-free patients with bipolar disorder. Arch Gen Psychiatry 61:450–458

Dasgupta A, Juedes SA, Sprouse RO, Auble DT (2005) Mot1-mediated control of transcription complex assembly and activity. EMBO J 24:1717–1729

Dayalu P, Albin RL (2015) Huntington disease: pathogenesis and treatment. Neurol Clin 33:101–114

De Stefano N, Matthews PM, Arnold DL (1995) Reversible decreases in N-acetylaspartate after acute brain injury. Magn Reson Med 34:721–727

Deranieh RM, Greenberg ML (2009) Cellular consequences of inositol depletion. Biochem Soc Trans 37:1099–1103

Deranieh RM, He Q, Caruso JA, Greenberg ML (2013) Phosphorylation regulates myo-inositol-3-phosphate synthase: a novel regulatory mechanism of inositol biosynthesis. J Biol Chem 288:26822–26833

Dey NB, Bounelis P, Fritz TA, Bedwell DM, Marchase RB (1994) The glycosylation of phosphoglucomutase is modulated by carbon source and heat shock in Saccharomyces cerevisiae. J Biol Chem 269:27143–27148

Di Paolo G, De Camilli P (2006) Phosphoinositides in cell regulation and membrane dynamics. Nature 443:651–657

Dietz M, Heyken WT, Hoppen J, Geburtig S, Schuller HJ (2003) TFIIB and subunits of the SAGA complex are involved in transcriptional activation of phospholipid biosynthetic genes by the regulatory protein Ino2 in the yeast Saccharomyces cerevisiae. Mol Microbiol 48:1119–1130

Dinicola S, Chiu TT, Unfer V, Carlomagno G, Bizzarri M (2014) The rationale of the myo-inositol and D-chiro-inositol combined treatment for polycystic ovary syndrome. J Clin Pharmacol 54:1079–1092

Doble BW, Woodgett JR (2003) GSK-3: tricks of the trade for a multi-tasking kinase. J Cell Sci 116:1175–1186

Donahue TF, Henry SA (1981) Myo-inositol-1-phosphate synthase. Characteristics of the enzyme and identification of its structural gene in yeast. J Biol Chem 256:7077–7085

Egan DF, Shackelford DB, Mihaylova MM, Gelino S, Kohnz RA, Mair W, Vasquez DS, Joshi A, Gwinn DM, Taylor R, Asara JM, Fitzpatrick J, Dillin A, Viollet B, Kundu M, Hansen M, Shaw RJ (2011) Phosphorylation of ULK1 (hATG1) by AMP-activated protein kinase connects energy sensing to mitophagy. Science 331:456–461

Facchinetti F, Bizzarri M, Benvenga S, D'Anna R, Lanzone A, Soulage C, Di Renzo GC, Hod M, Cavalli P, Chiu TT, Kamenov ZA, Bevilacqua A, Carlomagno G, Gerli S, Oliva MM, Devroey P (2015) Results from the international consensus conference on myo-inositol and D-chiro-inositol in obstetrics and gynecology: the link between metabolic syndrome and PCOS. Eur J Obstet Gynecol Reprod Biol 195:72–76

Fernandez-Marcos PJ, Auwerx J (2011) Regulation of PGC-1alpha, a nodal regulator of mitochondrial biogenesis. Am J Clin Nutr 93:884S–890S

Fisher SK, Novak JE, Agranoff BW (2002) Inositol and higher inositol phosphates in neural tissues: homeostasis, metabolism and functional significance. J Neurochem 82:736–754

Ford J, Odeyale O, Eskandar A, Kouba N, Shen C-H (2007) A SWI/SNF-and INO80-dependent nucleosome movement at the INO1 promoter. Biochem Biophys Res Commun 361:974–979

Ford J, Odeyale O, Shen C-H (2008) Activator-dependent recruitment of SWI/SNF and INO80 during INO1 activation. Biochem Biophys Res Commun 373:602–606

Frey R, Metzler D, Fischer P, Heiden A, Scharfetter J, Moser E, Kasper S (1998) Myo-inositol in depressive and healthy subjects determined by frontal 1H-magnetic resonance spectroscopy at 1.5 tesla. J Psychiatr Res 32:411–420

Fu H, Li B, Hertz L, Peng L (2012) Contributions in astrocytes of SMIT1/2 and HMIT to myo-inositol uptake at different concentrations and pH. Neurochem Int 61:187–194

Gaspar ML, Chang Y-F, Jesch SA, Aregullin M, Henry SA (2017) Interaction between repressor Opi1p and ER membrane protein Scs2p facilitates transit of phosphatidic acid from the ER to mitochondria and is essential for INO1 gene expression in the presence of choline. J Biol Chem M117:809970

Geiger JH, Jin X (2006) The structure and mechanism of myo-inositol-1-phosphate synthase. Subcell Biochem 39:157

Gelbart ME, Bachman N, Delrow J, Boeke JD, Tsukiyama T (2005) Genome-wide identification of Isw2 chromatin-remodeling targets by localization of a catalytically inactive mutant. Genes Dev 19:942–954

Genazzani AD (2016) Inositol as putative integrative treatment for PCOS. Reprod Biomed Online 33:770–780

Genazzani AD, Lanzoni C, Ricchieri F, Jasonni VM (2008) Myo-inositol administration positively affects hyperinsulinemia and hormonal parameters in overweight patients with polycystic ovary syndrome. Gynecol Endocrinol 24:139–144

Genazzani AD, Prati A, Santagni S, Ricchieri F, Chierchia E, Rattighieri E, Campedelli A, Simoncini T, Artini PG (2012) Differential insulin response to myo-inositol administration in obese polycystic ovary syndrome patients. Gynecol Endocrinol 28:969–973

Genazzani AD, Santagni S, Rattighieri E, Chierchia E, Despini G, Marini G, Prati A, Simoncini T (2014) Modulatory role of D-chiro-inositol (DCI) on LH and insulin secretion in obese PCOS patients. Gynecol Endocrinol 30:438–443

Gerli S, Mignosa M, Di Renzo GC (2003) Effects of inositol on ovarian function and metabolic factors in women with PCOS: a randomized double blind placebo-controlled trial. Eur Rev Med Pharmacol Sci 7:151–159

Gerli S, Papaleo E, Ferrari A, Di Renzo GC (2007) Randomized, double blind placebo-controlled trial: effects of myo-inositol on ovarian function and metabolic factors in women with PCOS. Eur Rev Med Pharmacol Sci 11:347–354

Goldmark JP, Fazzio TG, Estep PW, Church GM, Tsukiyama T (2000) The Isw2 chromatin remodeling complex represses early meiotic genes upon recruitment by Ume6p. Cell 103:423–433

Gould TD, Einat H, Bhat R, Manji HK (2004) AR-A014418, a selective GSK-3 inhibitor, produces antidepressant-like effects in the forced swim test. Int J Neuropsychopharmacol 7:387–390

Gould TD, Einat H, O'Donnell KC, Picchini AM, Schloesser RJ, Manji HK (2007) Beta-catenin overexpression in the mouse brain phenocopies lithium-sensitive behaviors. Neuropsychopharmacology 32:2173–2183

Graves JA, Henry SA (2000) Regulation of the yeast INO1 gene. The products of the INO2, INO4 and OPI1 regulatory genes are not required for repression in response to inositol. Genetics 154:1485–1495

Greenberg ML, Lopes JM (1996) Genetic regulation of phospholipid biosynthesis in Saccharomyces cerevisiae. Microbiol Rev 60:1

Greenberg ML, Goldwasser P, Henry SA (1982) Characterization of a yeast regulatory mutant constitutive for synthesis of inositol-1-phosphate synthase. Mol Gen Genet 186:157–163

Griffin JL, Bollard M, Nicholson JK, Bhakoo K (2002) Spectral profiles of cultured neuronal and glial cells derived from HRMAS (1)H NMR spectroscopy. NMR Biomed 15:375–384

Groger A, Kolb R, Schafer R, Klose U (2014) Dopamine reduction in the substantia nigra of Parkinson's disease patients confirmed by in vivo magnetic resonance spectroscopic imaging. PLoS One 9:e84081

Hager K, Hazama A, Kwon HM, Loo DD, Handler JS, Wright EM (1995) Kinetics and specificity of the renal Na+/myo-inositol cotransporter expressed in Xenopus oocytes. J Membr Biol 143:103–113

Hajek T, Carrey N, Alda M (2005) Neuroanatomical abnormalities as risk factors for bipolar disorder. Bipolar Disord 7:393–403

Hall AC, Brennan A, Goold RG, Cleverley K, Lucas FR, Gordon-Weeks PR, Salinas PC (2002) Valproate regulates GSK-3-mediated axonal remodeling and synapsin I clustering in developing neurons. Mol Cell Neurosci 20:257–270

Hamakawa H, Murashita J, Yamada N, Inubushi T, Kato N, Kato T (2004) Reduced intracellular pH in the basal ganglia and whole brain measured by 31P-MRS in bipolar disorder. Psychiatry Clin Neurosci 58:82–88

Haneda M, Kikkawa R, Arimura T, Ebata K, Togawa M, Maeda S, Sawada T, Horide N, Shigeta Y (1990) Glucose inhibits myo-inositol uptake and reduces myo-inositol content in cultured rat glomerular mesangial cells. Metabolism 39:40–45

Hara T, Nakamura K, Matsui M, Yamamoto A, Nakahara Y, Suzuki-Migishima R, Yokoyama M, Mishima K, Saito I, Okano H, Mizushima N (2006) Suppression of basal autophagy in neural cells causes neurodegenerative disease in mice. Nature 441:885–889

Hayashi A, Kasahara T, Kametani M, Toyota T, Yoshikawa T, Kato T (2009) Aberrant endoplasmic reticulum stress response in lymphoblastoid cells from patients with bipolar disorder. Int J Neuropsychopharmacol 12:33–43

Hayes JF, Miles J, Walters K, King M, Osborn DP (2015) A systematic review and meta-analysis of premature mortality in bipolar affective disorder. Acta Psychiatr Scand 131:417–425

Heyken WT, Repenning A, Kumme J, Schuller HJ (2005) Constitutive expression of yeast phospholipid biosynthetic genes by variants of Ino2 activator defective for interaction with Opi1 repressor. Mol Microbiol 56:696–707

Hirata Y, Andoh T, Asahara T, Kikuchi A (2003) Yeast glycogen synthase kinase-3 activates Msn2p-dependent transcription of stress responsive genes. Mol Biol Cell 14:302–312

Hofbauer HF, Schopf FH, Schleifer H, Knittelfelder OL, Pieber B, Rechberger GN, Wolinski H, Gaspar ML, Kappe CO, Stadlmann J, Mechtler K, Zenz A, Lohner K, Tehlivets O, Henry SA, Kohlwein SD (2014) Regulation of gene expression through a transcriptional repressor that senses acyl-chain length in membrane phospholipids. Dev Cell 29:729–739

Hoshizaki DK, Hill JE, Henry SA (1990) The Saccharomyces cerevisiae INO4 gene encodes a small, highly basic protein required for derepression of phospholipid biosynthetic enzymes. J Biol Chem 265:4736–4745

Huang LC, Fonteles MC, Houston DB, Zhang C, Larner J (1993) Chiroinositol deficiency and insulin resistance. III. Acute glycogenic and hypoglycemic effects of two inositol phosphoglycan insulin mediators in normal and streptozotocin-diabetic rats in vivo. Endocrinology 132:652–657

Hudecova M, Holte J, Olovsson M, Larsson A, Berne C, Poromaa IS (2011) Diabetes and impaired glucose tolerance in patients with polycystic ovary syndrome – a long term follow-up. Hum Reprod 26:1462–1468

Hur EM, Zhou FQ (2010) GSK3 signalling in neural development. Nat Rev Neurosci 11:539–551

Ibsen L, Strange K (1996) In situ localization and osmotic regulation of the Na(+)-myo-inositol cotransporter in rat brain. Am J Phys 271:F877–F885

Iuorno MJ, Jakubowicz DJ, Baillargeon JP, Dillon P, Gunn RD, Allan G, Nestler JE (2002) Effects of D-chiro-inositol in lean women with the polycystic ovary syndrome. Endocr Pract 8:417–423

Jadhav S, Russo S, Cottier S, Schneiter R, Cowart A, Greenberg ML (2016) Valproate induces the unfolded protein response by increasing ceramide levels. J Biol Chem 291:22253–22261

Jager S, Handschin C, St-Pierre J, Spiegelman BM (2007) AMP-activated protein kinase (AMPK) action in skeletal muscle via direct phosphorylation of PGC-1alpha. Proc Natl Acad Sci U S A 104:12017–12022

Jaschke Y, Schwarz J, Clausnitzer D, Muller C, Schuller HJ (2011) Pleiotropic corepressors Sin3 and Ssn6 interact with repressor Opi1 and negatively regulate transcription of genes required for phospholipid biosynthesis in the yeast Saccharomyces cerevisiae. Mol Gen Genomics 285:91–100

Jenkins R, Lewis G, Bebbington P, Brugha T, Farrell M, Gill B, Meltzer H (1997) The National Psychiatric Morbidity surveys of Great Britain – initial findings from the household survey. Psychol Med 27:775–789

Jesch SA, Zhao X, Wells MT, Henry SA (2005) Genome-wide analysis reveals inositol, not choline, as the major effector of Ino2p-Ino4p and unfolded protein response target gene expression in yeast. J Biol Chem 280:9106–9118

Jonathan Ryves W, Dalton EC, Harwood AJ, Williams RS (2005) GSK-3 activity in neocortical cells is inhibited by lithium but not carbamazepine or valproic acid. Bipolar Disord 7:260–265

Jope RS (2003) Lithium and GSK-3: one inhibitor, two inhibitory actions, multiple outcomes. Trends Pharmacol Sci 24:441–443

Jope RS, Johnson GV (2004) The glamour and gloom of glycogen synthase kinase-3. Trends Biochem Sci 29:95–102

Jope RS, Song L, Li PP, Young LT, Kish SJ, Pacheco MA, Warsh JJ (1996) The phosphoinositide signal transduction system is impaired in bipolar affective disorder brain. J Neurochem 66:2402–2409

Ju S, Greenberg ML (2003) Valproate disrupts regulation of inositol responsive genes and alters regulation of phospholipid biosynthesis. Mol Microbiol 49:1595–1603

Kadosh D, Struhl K (1997) Repression by Ume6 involves recruitment of a complex containing Sin3 corepressor and Rpd3 histone deacetylase to target promoters. Cell 89:365–371

Kaidanovich-Beilin O, Milman A, Weizman A, Pick CG, Eldar-Finkelman H (2004) Rapid antidepressive-like activity of specific glycogen synthase kinase-3 inhibitor and its effect on beta-catenin in mouse hippocampus. Biol Psychiatry 55:781–784

Kakiuchi C, Iwamoto K, Ishiwata M, Bundo M, Kasahara T, Kusumi I, Tsujita T, Okazaki Y, Nanko S, Kunugi H, Sasaki T, Kato T (2003) Impaired feedback regulation of XBP1 as a genetic risk factor for bipolar disorder. Nat Genet 35:171–175

Kato T (2008) Role of mitochondrial DNA in calcium signaling abnormality in bipolar disorder. Cell Calcium 44:92–102

Kato T, Kato N (2000) Mitochondrial dysfunction in bipolar disorder. Bipolar Disord 2:180–190

Kato T, Shioiri T, Murashita J, Hamakawa H, Inubushi T, Takahashi S (1994) Phosphorus-31 magnetic resonance spectroscopy and ventricular enlargement in bipolar disorder. Psychiatry Res 55:41–50

Kato T, Shioiri T, Murashita J, Hamakawa H, Takahashi Y, Inubushi T, Takahashi S (1995) Lateralized abnormality of high energy phosphate metabolism in the frontal lobes of patients with bipolar disorder detected by phase-encoded 31P-MRS. Psychol Med 25:557–566

Kato T, Murashita J, Kamiya A, Shioiri T, Kato N, Inubushi T (1998) Decreased brain intracellular pH measured by 31P-MRS in bipolar disorder: a confirmation in drug-free patients and correlation with white matter hyperintensity. Eur Arch Psychiatry Clin Neurosci 248:301–306

Kato T, Kunugi H, Nanko S, Kato N (2000) Association of bipolar disorder with the 5178 polymorphism in mitochondrial DNA. Am J Med Genet 96:182–186

Kato T, Kunugi H, Nanko S, Kato N (2001) Mitochondrial DNA polymorphisms in bipolar disorder. J Affect Disord 62:151–164

Kennington AS, Hill CR, Craig J, Bogardus C, Raz I, Ortmeyer HK, Hansen BC, Romero G, Larner J (1990) Low urinary chiro-inositol excretion in non-insulin-dependent diabetes mellitus. N Engl J Med 323:373–378

Kim AJ, Shi Y, Austin RC, Werstuck GH (2005) Valproate protects cells from ER stress-induced lipid accumulation and apoptosis by inhibiting glycogen synthase kinase-3. J Cell Sci 118:89–99

Klein PS, Melton DA (1996) A molecular mechanism for the effect of lithium on development. Proc Natl Acad Sci U S A 93:8455–8459

Klig LS, Henry SA (1984) Isolation of the yeast INO1 gene: located on an autonomously replicating plasmid, the gene is fully regulated. Proc Natl Acad Sci U S A 81:3816–3820

Klig LS, Homann MJ, Carman GM, Henry SA (1985) Coordinate regulation of phospholipid biosynthesis in Saccharomyces cerevisiae: pleiotropically constitutive opi1 mutant. J Bacteriol 162:1135–1141

Koch-Weser J, O'Malley K, O'Brien E (1980) Drug therapy: management of hypertension in the elderly. N Engl J Med 302:1397–1401

Kofman O, Belmaker RH (1990) Intracerebroventricular myo-inositol antagonizes lithium-induced suppression of rearing behaviour in rats. Brain Res 534:345–347

Kollros PE, Goldstein GW, Betz AL (1990) Myo-inositol transport into endothelial cells derived from nervous system microvessels. Brain Res 511:259–264

Komatsu M, Waguri S, Chiba T, Murata S, Iwata J, Tanida I, Ueno T, Koike M, Uchiyama Y, Kominami E, Tanaka K (2006) Loss of autophagy in the central nervous system causes neurodegeneration in mice. Nature 441:880–884

Komulainen T, Lodge T, Hinttala R, Bolszak M, Pietila M, Koivunen P, Hakkola J, Poulton J, Morten KJ, Uusimaa J (2015) Sodium valproate induces mitochondrial respiration dysfunction in HepG2 in vitro cell model. Toxicology 331:47–56

Korennykh AV, Egea PF, Korostelev AA, Finer-Moore J, Zhang C, Shokat KM, Stroud RM, Walter P (2009) The unfolded protein response signals through high-order assembly of Ire1. Nature 457:687–693

Kumme J, Dietz M, Wagner C, Schuller HJ (2008) Dimerization of yeast transcription factors Ino2 and Ino4 is regulated by precursors of phospholipid biosynthesis mediated by Opi1 repressor. Curr Genet 54:35–45

La Marca A, Grisendi V, Dondi G, Sighinolfi G, Cianci A (2015) The menstrual cycle regularization following D-chiro-inositol treatment in PCOS women: a retrospective study. Gynecol Endocrinol 31:52–56

Lagana AS, Barbaro L, Pizzo A (2015) Evaluation of ovarian function and metabolic factors in women affected by polycystic ovary syndrome after treatment with D-chiro-inositol. Arch Gynecol Obstet 291:1181–1186

Lai K, McGraw P (1994) Dual control of inositol transport in Saccharomyces cerevisiae by irreversible inactivation of permease and regulation of permease synthesis by INO2, INO4, and OPI1. J Biol Chem 269:2245–2251

Lai E, Teodoro T, Volchuk A (2007) Endoplasmic reticulum stress: signaling the unfolded protein response. Physiology (Bethesda) 22:193–201

Larner J (2002) D-chiro-inositol – its functional role in insulin action and its deficit in insulin resistance. Int J Exp Diabetes Res 3:47–60

Larner J, Craig JW (1996) Urinary myo-inositol-to-chiro-inositol ratios and insulin resistance. Diabetes Care 19:76–78

Larner J, Brautigan DL, Thorner MO (2010) D-chiro-inositol glycans in insulin signaling and insulin resistance. Mol Med 16:543–552

Leboyer M, Soreca I, Scott J, Frye M, Henry C, Tamouza R, Kupfer DJ (2012) Can bipolar disorder be viewed as a multi-system inflammatory disease? J Affect Disord 141:1–10

Lee MH, Hong I, Kim M, Lee BH, Kim JH, Kang KS, Kim HL, Yoon BI, Chung H, Kong G, Lee MO (2007) Gene expression profiles of murine fatty liver induced by the administration of valproic acid. Toxicol Appl Pharmacol 220:45–59

Levine J (1997) Controlled trials of inositol in psychiatry. Eur Neuropsychopharmacol 7:147–155

Levine B, Klionsky DJ (2004) Development by self-digestion: molecular mechanisms and biological functions of autophagy. Dev Cell 6:463–477

Levine J, Rapaport A, Lev L, Bersudsky Y, Kofman O, Belmaker RH, Shapiro J, Agam G (1993) Inositol treatment raises CSF inositol levels. Brain Res 627:168–170

Levine J, Barak Y, Gonzalves M, Szor H, Elizur A, Kofman O, Belmaker RH (1995) Double-blind, controlled trial of inositol treatment of depression. Am J Psychiatry 152:792–794

Lewis JH, Zimmerman HJ, Garrett CT, Rosenberg E (1982) Valproate-induced hepatic steatogenesis in rats. Hepatology 2:870–873

Li XZ, Chen XP, Zhao K, Bai LM, Zhang H, Zhou XP (2013) Therapeutic effects of valproate combined with lithium carbonate on MPTP-induced parkinsonism in mice: possible mediation through enhanced autophagy. Int J Neurosci 123:73–79

Li L, Gu Z, Liu Z, Su L (2014) The effect of reactive oxygen species regulation of expression of Bcl-2 and Bax in apoptosis of human umbilical vein endothelial cell induced by heat stress. Zhonghua Wei Zhong Bing Ji Jiu Yi Xue 26:458–463

Li CT, Bai YM, Hsieh JC, Lee HC, Yang BH, Chen MH, Lin WC, Tsai CF, Tu PC, Wang SJ, Su TP (2015) Peripheral and central glucose utilizations modulated by mitochondrial DNA 10398A in bipolar disorder. Psychoneuroendocrinology 55:72–80

Linares GR, Chiu CT, Scheuing L, Leng Y, Liao HM, Maric D, Chuang DM (2016) Preconditioning mesenchymal stem cells with the mood stabilizers lithium and valproic acid enhances therapeutic efficacy in a mouse model of Huntington's disease. Exp Neurol 281:81–92

Lionaki E, Markaki M, Palikaras K, Tavernarakis N (2015) Mitochondria, autophagy and age-associated neurodegenerative diseases: new insights into a complex interplay. Biochim Biophys Acta 1847:1412–1423

Lirng JF, Chen HC, Fuh JL, Tsai CF, Liang JF, Wang SJ (2015) Increased myo-inositol level in dorsolateral prefrontal cortex in migraine patients with major depression. Cephalalgia 35:702–709

Lo WS, Duggan L, Emre NC, Belotserkovskya R, Lane WS, Shiekhattar R, Berger SL (2001) Snf1 – a histone kinase that works in concert with the histone acetyltransferase Gcn5 to regulate transcription. Science 293:1142–1146

Lo WS, Gamache ER, Henry KW, Yang D, Pillus L, Berger SL (2005) Histone H3 phosphorylation can promote TBP recruitment through distinct promoter-specific mechanisms. EMBO J 24:997–1008

Lochhead PA, Coghlan M, Rice SQ, Sutherland C (2001) Inhibition of GSK-3 selectively reduces glucose-6-phosphatase and phosphatase and phosphoenolypyruvate carboxykinase gene expression. Diabetes 50:937–946

Loewen CJ, Roy A, Levine TP (2003) A conserved ER targeting motif in three families of lipid binding proteins and in Opi1p binds VAP. EMBO J 22:2025–2035

Loewy BS, Henry SA (1984) The INO2 and INO4 loci of Saccharomyces cerevisiae are pleiotropic regulatory genes. Mol Cell Biol 4:2479–2485

Lopes JM, Henry SA (1991) Interaction of trans and cis regulatory elements in the INO1 promoter of Saccharomyces cerevisiae. Nucleic Acids Res 19:3987–3994

Lopes JM, Hirsch JP, Chorgo PA, Schulze KL, Henry SA (1991) Analysis of sequences in the INO1 promoter that are involved in its regulation by phospholipid precursors. Nucleic Acids Res 19:1687–1693

Lopes J, Schulze K, Yates J, Hirsch J, Henry S (1993) The INO1 promoter of Saccharomyces cerevisiae includes an upstream repressor sequence (URS1) common to a diverse set of yeast genes. J Bacteriol 175:4235–4238

Lovestone S, Davis DR, Webster MT, Kaech S, Brion JP, Matus A, Anderton BH (1999) Lithium reduces tau phosphorylation: effects in living cells and in neurons at therapeutic concentrations. Biol Psychiatry 45:995–1003

Lubrich B, van Calker D (1999) Inhibition of the high affinity myo-inositol transport system: a common mechanism of action of antibipolar drugs? Neuropsychopharmacology 21:519–529

Lubrich B, Spleiss O, Gebicke-Haerter PJ, van Calker D (2000) Differential expression, activity and regulation of the sodium/myo-inositol cotransporter in astrocyte cultures from different regions of the rat brain. Neuropharmacology 39:680–690

Luse DS (2014) The RNA polymerase II preinitiation complex. Through what pathway is the complex assembled? Transcription 5:e27050

Machado-Vieira R, Manji HK, Zarate CA Jr (2009) The role of lithium in the treatment of bipolar disorder: convergent evidence for neurotrophic effects as a unifying hypothesis. Bipolar Disord 11(Suppl 2):92–109

Machado-Vieira R, Pivovarova NB, Stanika RI, Yuan P, Wang Y, Zhou R, Zarate CA Jr, Drevets WC, Brantner CA, Baum A, Laje G, McMahon FJ, Chen G, Du J, Manji HK, Andrews SB (2011) The Bcl-2 gene polymorphism rs956572AA increases inositol 1,4,5-trisphosphate receptor-mediated endoplasmic reticulum calcium release in subjects with bipolar disorder. Biol Psychiatry 69:344–352

Mansur RB, Brietzke E (2012) The "selfish brain" hypothesis for metabolic abnormalities in bipolar disorder and schizophrenia. Trends Psychiatry Psychother 34:121–128

March WA, Moore VM, Willson KJ, Phillips DI, Norman RJ, Davies MJ (2010) The prevalence of polycystic ovary syndrome in a community sample assessed under contrasting diagnostic criteria. Hum Reprod 25:544–551

Marin TL, Gongol B, Zhang F, Martin M, Johnson DA, Xiao H, Wang Y, Subramaniam S, Chien S, Shyy JY (2017) AMPK promotes mitochondrial biogenesis and function by phosphorylating the epigenetic factors DNMT1, RBBP7, and HAT1. Sci Signal 10:eaaf7478

Martinowich K, Schloesser RJ, Manji HK (2009) Bipolar disorder: from genes to behavior pathways. J Clin Invest 119:726–736
Masuda CA, Xavier MA, Mattos KA, Galina A, Montero-Lomeli M (2001) Phosphoglucomutase is an in vivo lithium target in yeast. J Biol Chem 276:37794–37801
Matskevitch J, Wagner CA, Risler T, Kwon HM, Handler JS, Waldegger S, Busch AE, Lang F (1998) Effect of extracellular pH on the myo-inositol transporter SMIT expressed in Xenopus oocytes. Pflugers Arch 436:854–857
Maurer IC, Schippel P, Volz HP (2009) Lithium-induced enhancement of mitochondrial oxidative phosphorylation in human brain tissue. Bipolar Disord 11:515–522
Mellor J, Morillon A (2004) ISWI complexes in Saccharomyces cerevisiae. Biochim Biophys Acta 1677:100–112
Menzies FM, Fleming A, Caricasole A, Bento CF, Andrews SP, Ashkenazi A, Fullgrabe J, Jackson A, Jimenez Sanchez M, Karabiyik C, Licitra F, Lopez Ramirez A, Pavel M, Puri C, Renna M, Ricketts T, Schlotawa L, Vicinanza M, Won H, Zhu Y, Skidmore J, Rubinsztein DC (2017) Autophagy and neurodegeneration: pathogenic mechanisms and therapeutic opportunities. Neuron 93:1015–1034
Merikangas KR, Jin R, He JP, Kessler RC, Lee S, Sampson NA, Viana MC, Andrade LH, Hu C, Karam EG, Ladea M, Medina-Mora ME, Ono Y, Posada-Villa J, Sagar R, Wells JE, Zarkov Z (2011) Prevalence and correlates of bipolar spectrum disorder in the world mental health survey initiative. Arch Gen Psychiatry 68:241–251
Mertens J, Wang QW, Kim Y, Yu DX, Pham S, Yang B, Zheng Y, Diffenderfer KE, Zhang J, Soltani S, Eames T, Schafer ST, Boyer L, Marchetto MC, Nurnberger JI, Calabrese JR, Odegaard KJ, McCarthy MJ, Zandi PP, Alda M, Nievergelt CM, The Pharmacogenomics of Bipolar Disorder Study, Mi S, Brennand KJ, Kelsoe JR, Gage FH, Yao J (2015) Differential responses to lithium in hyperexcitable neurons from patients with bipolar disorder. Nature 527:95–99
Mitchell PB, Malhi GS (2002) The expanding pharmacopoeia for bipolar disorder. Annu Rev Med 53:173–188
Mizushima N, Levine B, Cuervo AM, Klionsky DJ (2008) Autophagy fights disease through cellular self-digestion. Nature 451:1069–1075
Modica-Napolitano JS, Renshaw PF (2004) Ethanolamine and phosphoethanolamine inhibit mitochondrial function in vitro: implications for mitochondrial dysfunction hypothesis in depression and bipolar disorder. Biol Psychiatry 55:273–277
Monastra G, Unfer V, Harrath AH, Bizzarri M (2017) Combining treatment with myo-inositol and D-chiro-inositol (40:1) is effective in restoring ovary function and metabolic balance in PCOS patients. Gynecol Endocrinol 33:1–9
Moore CM, Breeze JL, Kukes TJ, Rose SL, Dager SR, Cohen BM, Renshaw PF (1999) Effects of myo-inositol ingestion on human brain myo-inositol levels: a proton magnetic resonance spectroscopic imaging study. Biol Psychiatry 45:1197–1202
Mori K (2009) Signalling pathways in the unfolded protein response: development from yeast to mammals. J Biochem 146:743–750
Mukai T, Kishi T, Matsuda Y, Iwata N (2014) A meta-analysis of inositol for depression and anxiety disorders. Hum Psychopharmacol 29:55–63
Munoz-Montano JR, Moreno FJ, Avila J, Diaz-Nido J (1997) Lithium inhibits Alzheimer's disease-like tau protein phosphorylation in neurons. FEBS Lett 411:183–188
Murashita J, Kato T, Shioiri T, Inubushi T, Kato N (2000) Altered brain energy metabolism in lithium-resistant bipolar disorder detected by photic stimulated 31P-MR spectroscopy. Psychol Med 30:107–115
Nandhu MS, Paul J, Kuruvilla KP, Malat A, Romeo C, Paulose CS (2011) Enhanced glutamate, IP3 and cAMP activity in the cerebral cortex of unilateral 6-hydroxydopamine induced Parkinson's rats: effect of 5-HT, GABA and bone marrow cell supplementation. J Biomed Sci 18:5
Nestler JE, Jakubowicz DJ, Reamer P, Gunn RD, Allan G (1999) Ovulatory and metabolic effects of D-chiro-inositol in the polycystic ovary syndrome. N Engl J Med 340:1314–1320
Ng F, Hallam K, Lucas N, Berk M (2007) The role of lamotrigine in the management of bipolar disorder. Neuropsychiatr Dis Treat 3:463–474

Nikawa J, Murakami A, Esumi E, Hosaka K (1995) Cloning and sequence of the SCS2 gene, which can suppress the defect of INO1 expression in an inositol auxotrophic mutant of Saccharomyces cerevisiae. J Biochem 118:39–45

Nikoloff DM, Henry SA (1994) Functional characterization of the INO2 gene of Saccharomyces cerevisiae. A positive regulator of phospholipid biosynthesis. J Biol Chem 269:7402–7411

Nikoloff DM, McGraw P, Henry SA (1992) The INO2 gene of Saccharomyces cerevisiae encodes a helix-loop-helix protein that is required for activation of phospholipid synthesis. Nucleic Acids Res 20:3253

Nordio M, Proietti E (2012) The combined therapy with myo-inositol and D-chiro-inositol reduces the risk of metabolic disease in PCOS overweight patients compared to myo-inositol supplementation alone. Eur Rev Med Pharmacol Sci 16:575–581

O'Brien WT, Harper AD, Jove F, Woodgett JR, Maretto S, Piccolo S, Klein PS (2004) Glycogen synthase kinase-3beta haploinsufficiency mimics the behavioral and molecular effects of lithium. J Neurosci 24:6791–6798

Orio F, Palomba S (2014) Reproductive endocrinology: new guidelines for the diagnosis and treatment of PCOS. Nat Rev Endocrinol 10:130–132

Ortmeyer HK, Bodkin NL, Lilley K, Larner J, Hansen BC (1993) Chiroinositol deficiency and insulin resistance. I. Urinary excretion rate of chiroinositol is directly associated with insulin resistance in spontaneously diabetic rhesus monkeys. Endocrinology 132:640–645

Pak Y, Hong Y, Kim S, Piccariello T, Farese RV, Larner J (1998) In vivo chiro-inositol metabolism in the rat: a defect in chiro-inositol synthesis from myo-inositol and an increased incorporation of chiro-[3H]inositol into phospholipid in the Goto-Kakizaki (G.K) rat. Mol Cells 8:301–309

Papaleo E, Unfer V, Baillargeon JP, De Santis L, Fusi F, Brigante C, Marelli G, Cino I, Redaelli A, Ferrari A (2007) Myo-inositol in patients with polycystic ovary syndrome: a novel method for ovulation induction. Gynecol Endocrinol 23:700–703

Papaleo E, Unfer V, Baillargeon JP, Fusi F, Occhi F, De Santis L (2009) Myo-inositol may improve oocyte quality in intracytoplasmic sperm injection cycles. A prospective, controlled, randomized trial. Fertil Steril 91:1750–1754

Parthasarathy RN, Lakshmanan J, Thangavel M, Seelan RS, Stagner JI, Janckila AJ, Vadnal RE, Casanova MF, Parthasarathy LK (2013) Rat brain myo-inositol 3-phosphate synthase is a phosphoprotein. Mol Cell Biochem 378:83–89

Peterson CL, Kruger W, Herskowitz I (1991) A functional interaction between the C-terminal domain of RNA polymerase II and the negative regulator SIN1. Cell 64:1135–1143

Phiel CJ, Zhang F, Huang EY, Guenther MG, Lazar MA, Klein PS (2001) Histone deacetylase is a direct target of valproic acid, a potent anticonvulsant, mood stabilizer, and teratogen. J Biol Chem 276:36734–36741

Piatkevich MM, Lisakovich MV, Efimov LA (1984) Method of identifying persons by their skulls using the photomatching technic. Sud Med Ekspert 27:31–33

Pollard KJ, Peterson CL (1997) Role for ADA/GCN5 products in antagonizing chromatin-mediated transcriptional repression. Mol Cell Biol 17:6212–6222

Ponchaut S, van Hoof F, Veitch K (1992) Cytochrome aa3 depletion is the cause of the deficient mitochondrial respiration induced by chronic valproate administration. Biochem Pharmacol 43:644–647

Popkie AP, Zeidner LC, Albrecht AM, D'Ippolito A, Eckardt S, Newsom DE, Groden J, Doble BW, Aronow B, McLaughlin KJ, White P, Phiel CJ (2010) Phosphatidylinositol 3-kinase (PI3K) signaling via glycogen synthase kinase-3 (Gsk-3) regulates DNA methylation of imprinted loci. J Biol Chem 285:41337–41347

Preston AS, Yamauchi A, Kwon HM, Handler JS (1995) Activators of protein kinase A and of protein kinase C inhibit MDCK cell myo-inositol and betaine uptake. J Am Soc Nephrol 6:1559–1564

Qiu Y, Hassaninasab A, Han G-S, Carman GM (2016) Phosphorylation of Dgk1 diacylglycerol kinase by casein kinase II regulates phosphatidic acid production in Saccharomyces cerevisiae. J Biol Chem 291:26455–26467

Ron D, Walter P (2007) Signal integration in the endoplasmic reticulum unfolded protein response. Nat Rev Mol Cell Biol 8:519–529

Rowe MK, Wiest C, Chuang DM (2007) GSK-3 is a viable potential target for therapeutic intervention in bipolar disorder. Neurosci Biobehav Rev 31:920–931

Rundlett SE, Carmen AA, Suka N, Turner BM, Grunstein M (1998) Transcriptional repression by UME6 involves deacetylation of lysine 5 of histone H4 by RPD3. Nature 392:831–835

Salsaa M, Case K, Greenberg ML (2017) Orchestrating phospholipid biosynthesis: phosphatidic acid conducts and Opi1p performs. J Biol Chem 292:18729–18730

Sarkar S, Rubinsztein DC (2006) Inositol and IP3 levels regulate autophagy: biology and therapeutic speculations. Autophagy 2:132–134

Sarkar S, Floto RA, Berger Z, Imarisio S, Cordenier A, Pasco M, Cook LJ, Rubinsztein DC (2005) Lithium induces autophagy by inhibiting inositol monophosphatase. J Cell Biol 170:1101–1111

Saveanu R, Etkin A, Duchemin AM, Goldstein-Piekarski A, Gyurak A, Debattista C, Schatzberg AF, Sood S, Day CV, Palmer DM, Rekshan WR, Gordon E, Rush AJ, Williams LM (2015) The international Study to Predict Optimized Treatment in Depression (iSPOT-D): outcomes from the acute phase of antidepressant treatment. J Psychiatr Res 61:1–12

Scheuing L, Chiu CT, Liao HM, Linares GR, Chuang DM (2014) Preclinical and clinical investigations of mood stabilizers for Huntington's disease: what have we learned? Int J Biol Sci 10:1024–1038

Schiebler M, Brown K, Hegyi K, Newton SM, Renna M, Hepburn L, Klapholz C, Coulter S, Obregon-Henao A, Henao Tamayo M, Basaraba R, Kampmann B, Henry KM, Burgon J, Renshaw SA, Fleming A, Kay RR, Anderson KE, Hawkins PT, Ordway DJ, Rubinsztein DC, Floto RA (2015) Functional drug screening reveals anticonvulsants as enhancers of mTOR-independent autophagic killing of Mycobacterium tuberculosis through inositol depletion. EMBO Mol Med 7:127–139

Schwank S, Ebbert R, Rautenstrauss K, Schweizer E, Schuller HJ (1995) Yeast transcriptional activator INO2 interacts as an Ino2p/Ino4p basic helix-loop-helix heteromeric complex with the inositol/choline-responsive element necessary for expression of phospholipid biosynthetic genes in Saccharomyces cerevisiae. Nucleic Acids Res 23:230–237

Schwank S, Hoffmann B, Sch-uller HJ (1997) Influence of gene dosage and autoregulation of the regulatory genes INO2 and INO4 on inositol/choline-repressible gene transcription in the yeast Saccharomyces cerevisiae. Curr Genet 31:462–468

Shaldubina A, Johanson RA, O'Brien WT, Buccafusca R, Agam G, Belmaker RH, Klein PS, Bersudsky Y, Berry GT (2006) SMIT1 haploinsufficiency causes brain inositol deficiency without affecting lithium-sensitive behavior. Mol Genet Metab 88:384–388

Shaldubina A, Buccafusca R, Johanson RA, Agam G, Belmaker RH, Berry GT, Bersudsky Y (2007) Behavioural phenotyping of sodium-myo-inositol cotransporter heterozygous knockout mice with reduced brain inositol. Genes Brain Behav 6:253–259

Shao L, Sun X, Xu L, Young LT, Wang JF (2006) Mood stabilizing drug lithium increases expression of endoplasmic reticulum stress proteins in primary cultured rat cerebral cortical cells. Life Sci 78:1317–1323

Shapiro J, Belmaker RH, Biegon A, Seker A, Agam G (2000) Scyllo-inositol in post-mortem brain of bipolar, unipolar and schizophrenic patients. J Neural Transm (Vienna) 107:603–607

Shears SB (2009) Diphosphoinositol polyphosphates: metabolic messengers? Mol Pharmacol 76:236–252

Shears SB (2015) Inositol pyrophosphates: why so many phosphates? Adv Biol Regul 57:203–216

Shetty A, Lopes JM (2010) Derepression of INO1 transcription requires cooperation between the Ino2p-Ino4p heterodimer and Cbf1p and recruitment of the ISW2 chromatin-remodeling complex. Eukaryot Cell 9:1845–1855

Shi Y, Azab AN, Thompson MN, Greenberg ML (2006) Inositol phosphates and phosphoinositides in health and disease. Subcell Biochem 39:265–292

Shimon H, Agam G, Belmaker RH, Hyde TM, Kleinman JE (1997) Reduced frontal cortex inositol levels in postmortem brain of suicide victims and patients with bipolar disorder. Am J Psychiatry 154:1148–1150

Shirra MK, Patton-Vogt J, Ulrich A, Liuta-Tehlivets O, Kohlwein SD, Henry SA, Arndt KM (2001) Inhibition of acetyl coenzyme A carboxylase activity restores expression of the INO1 gene in a snf1 mutant strain of Saccharomyces cerevisiae. Mol Cell Biol 21:5710–5722

Shirra MK, Rogers SE, Alexander DE, Arndt KM (2005) The Snf1 protein kinase and Sit4 protein phosphatase have opposing functions in regulating TATA-binding protein association with the Saccharomyces cerevisiae INO1 promoter. Genetics 169:1957–1972

Shorter E (2009) The history of lithium therapy. Bipolar Disord 11(Suppl 2):4–9

Silva MF, Aires CC, Luis PB, Ruiter JP, IJlst L, Duran M, Wanders RJ, de Almeida IT (2008) Valproic acid metabolism and its effects on mitochondrial fatty acid oxidation: a review. J Inherit Metab Dis 31:205–216

Silverstone PH, Wu RH, O'Donnell T, Ulrich M, Asghar SJ, Hanstock CC (2002) Chronic treatment with both lithium and sodium valproate may normalize phosphoinositol cycle activity in bipolar patients. Hum Psychopharmacol 17:321–327

Simonsen A, Wurmser AE, Emr SD, Stenmark H (2001) The role of phosphoinositides in membrane transport. Curr Opin Cell Biol 13:485–492

Singh N, Halliday AC, Thomas JM, Kuznetsova OV, Baldwin R, Woon EC, Aley PK, Antoniadou I, Sharp T, Vasudevan SR, Churchill GC (2013) A safe lithium mimetic for bipolar disorder. Nat Commun 4:1332

Sitarz KS, Elliott HR, Karaman BS, Relton C, Chinnery PF, Horvath R (2014) Valproic acid triggers increased mitochondrial biogenesis in POLG-deficient fibroblasts. Mol Genet Metab 112:57–63

Slekar KH, Henry SA (1995) SIN3 works through two different promoter elements to regulate INO1 gene expression in yeast. Nucleic Acids Res 23:1964–1969

So J, Warsh JJ, Li PP (2007) Impaired endoplasmic reticulum stress response in B-lymphoblasts from patients with bipolar-I disorder. Biol Psychiatry 62:141–147

Soeiro-de-Souza MG, Dias VV, Figueira ML, Forlenza OV, Gattaz WF, Zarate CA Jr, Machado-Vieira R (2012) Translating neurotrophic and cellular plasticity: from pathophysiology to improved therapeutics for bipolar disorder. Acta Psychiatr Scand 126:332–341

Song D, Du T, Li B, Cai L, Gu L, Li H, Chen Y, Hertz L, Peng L (2008) Astrocytic alkalinization by therapeutically relevant lithium concentrations: implications for myo-inositol depletion. Psychopharmacology 200:187–195

Spector R (1976) Inositol accumulation by brain slices in vitro. J Neurochem 27:1273–1276

Spillantini MG, Schmidt ML, Lee VM, Trojanowski JQ, Jakes R, Goedert M (1997) Alpha-synuclein in Lewy bodies. Nature 388:839–840

Sreenivas A, Villa-Garcia MJ, Henry SA, Carman GM (2001) Phosphorylation of the yeast phospholipid synthesis regulatory protein Opi1p by protein kinase C. J Biol Chem 276:29915–29923

Stambolic V, Ruel L, Woodgett JR (1996) Lithium inhibits glycogen synthase kinase-3 activity and mimics wingless signalling in intact cells. Curr Biol 6:1664–1668

Stokes CE, Hawthorne JN (1987) Reduced phosphoinositide concentrations in anterior temporal cortex of Alzheimer-diseased brains. J Neurochem 48:1018–1021

Stokes CE, Gillon KR, Hawthorne JN (1983) Free and total lipid myo-inositol concentrations decrease with age in human brain. Biochim Biophys Acta 753:136–138

Stork C, Renshaw PF (2005) Mitochondrial dysfunction in bipolar disorder: evidence from magnetic resonance spectroscopy research. Mol Psychiatry 10:900–919

Strange K (1992) Regulation of solute and water balance and cell volume in the central nervous system. J Am Soc Nephrol 3:12–27

Strange K, Morrison R, Heilig CW, DiPietro S, Gullans SR (1991) Upregulation of inositol transport mediates inositol accumulation in hyperosmolar brain cells. Am J Phys 260: C784–C790

Struewing IT, Barnett CD, Tang T, Mao CD (2007) Lithium increases PGC-1alpha expression and mitochondrial biogenesis in primary bovine aortic endothelial cells. FEBS J 274:2749–2765

Sun TH, Heimark DB, Nguygen T, Nadler JL, Larner J (2002) Both myo-inositol to chiro-inositol epimerase activities and chiro-inositol to myo-inositol ratios are decreased in tissues of GK type 2 diabetic rats compared to Wistar controls. Biochem Biophys Res Commun 293:1092–1098
Sveinbjornsdottir S (2016) The clinical symptoms of Parkinson's disease. J Neurochem 139 (Suppl 1):318–324
Szijgyarto Z, Garedew A, Azevedo C, Saiardi A (2011) Influence of inositol pyrophosphates on cellular energy dynamics. Science 334:802–805
Tamaru H, Selker EU (2001) A histone H3 methyltransferase controls DNA methylation in Neurospora crassa. Nature 414:277–283
Tamaru H, Zhang X, McMillen D, Singh PB, Nakayama J, Grewal SI, Allis CD, Cheng X, Selker EU (2003) Trimethylated lysine 9 of histone H3 is a mark for DNA methylation in Neurospora crassa. Nat Genet 34:75–79
Tang TS, Tu H, Chan EY, Maximov A, Wang Z, Wellington CL, Hayden MR, Bezprozvanny I (2003) Huntingtin and huntingtin-associated protein 1 influence neuronal calcium signaling mediated by inositol-(1,4,5) triphosphate receptor type 1. Neuron 39:227–239
Tang TS, Slow E, Lupu V, Stavrovskaya IG, Sugimori M, Llinas R, Kristal BS, Hayden MR, Bezprozvanny I (2005) Disturbed Ca2+ signaling and apoptosis of medium spiny neurons in Huntington's disease. Proc Natl Acad Sci U S A 102:2602–2607
Tang TS, Guo C, Wang H, Chen X, Bezprozvanny I (2009) Neuroprotective effects of inositol 1,4,5-trisphosphate receptor C-terminal fragment in a Huntington's disease mouse model. J Neurosci 29:1257–1266
Tarasov AI, Griffiths EJ, Rutter GA (2012) Regulation of ATP production by mitochondrial Ca(2+). Cell Calcium 52:28–35
Thomas MP, Mills SJ, Potter BV (2016) The "other" inositols and their phosphates: synthesis, biology, and medicine (with recent advances in myo-inositol chemistry). Angew Chem Int Ed Engl 55:1614–1650
Toker A (2002) Phosphoinositides and signal transduction. Cell Mol Life Sci 59:761–779
Toker L, Agam G (2015) Mitochondrial dysfunction in psychiatric morbidity: current evidence and therapeutic prospects. Neuropsychiatr Dis Treat 11:2441–2447
Uldry M, Ibberson M, Horisberger JD, Chatton JY, Riederer BM, Thorens B (2001) Identification of a mammalian H(+)-myo-inositol symporter expressed predominantly in the brain. EMBO J 20:4467–4477
Unfer V, Carlomagno G, Dante G, Facchinetti F (2012) Effects of myo-inositol in women with PCOS: a systematic review of randomized controlled trials. Gynecol Endocrinol 28:509–515
Vaden DL, Ding D, Peterson B, Greenberg ML (2001) Lithium and valproate decrease inositol mass and increase expression of the yeast INO1 and INO2 genes for inositol biosynthesis. J Biol Chem 276:15466–15471
Valvezan AJ, Klein PS (2012) GSK-3 and Wnt signaling in neurogenesis and bipolar disorder. Front Mol Neurosci 5:1
Wagner C, Blank M, Strohmann B, Schuller HJ (1999) Overproduction of the Opi1 repressor inhibits transcriptional activation of structural genes required for phospholipid biosynthesis in the yeast Saccharomyces cerevisiae. Yeast 15:843–854
Wagner C, Dietz M, Wittmann J, Albrecht A, Schuller HJ (2001) The negative regulator Opi1 of phospholipid biosynthesis in yeast contacts the pleiotropic repressor Sin3 and the transcriptional activator Ino2. Mol Microbiol 41:155–166
Walker FO (2007) Huntington's disease. Semin Neurol 27:143–150
Walter P, Ron D (2011) The unfolded protein response: from stress pathway to homeostatic regulation. Science 334:1081–1086
Warby SC, Graham RK, Hayden MR (1993) Huntington disease. In: Adam MP, Ardinger HH, Pagon RA, Wallace SE, Bean LJH, Mefford HC, Stephens K, Amemiya A, Ledbetter N (eds) GeneReviews(R). University of Washington, Seattle
Weaver R (2012) Molecular biology. McGraw-Hill, New York
White MJ, Hirsch JP, Henry SA (1991) The OPI1 gene of Saccharomyces cerevisiae, a negative regulator of phospholipid biosynthesis, encodes a protein containing polyglutamine tracts and a leucine zipper. J Biol Chem 266:863–872

Whiteford HA, Degenhardt L, Rehm J, Baxter AJ, Ferrari AJ, Erskine HE, Charlson FJ, Norman RE, Flaxman AD, Johns N, Burstein R, Murray CJ, Vos T (2013) Global burden of disease attributable to mental and substance use disorders: findings from the Global Burden of Disease Study 2010. Lancet 382:1575–1586

Whiting PH, Palmano KP, Hawthorne JN (1979) Enzymes of myo-inositol and inositol lipid metabolism in rats with streptozotocin-induced diabetes. Biochem J 179:549–553

Williams RS, Cheng L, Mudge AW, Harwood AJ (2002) A common mechanism of action for three mood-stabilizing drugs. Nature 417:292–295

Wilson MS, Livermore TM, Saiardi A (2013) Inositol pyrophosphates: between signalling and metabolism. Biochem J 452:369–379

Wolfson M, Bersudsky Y, Zinger E, Simkin M, Belmaker RH, Hertz L (2000) Chronic treatment of human astrocytoma cells with lithium, carbamazepine or valproic acid decreases inositol uptake at high inositol concentrations but increases it at low inositol concentrations. Brain Res 855:158–161

Yadon AN, Singh BN, Hampsey M, Tsukiyama T (2013) DNA looping facilitates targeting of a chromatin remodeling enzyme. Mol Cell 50:93–103

Yancey PH (2005) Organic osmolytes as compatible, metabolic and counteracting cytoprotectants in high osmolarity and other stresses. J Exp Biol 208:2819–2830

Ye C, Greenberg ML (2015) Inositol synthesis regulates the activation of GSK-3alpha in neuronal cells. J Neurochem 133:273–283

Ye C, Bandara WM, Greenberg ML (2013) Regulation of inositol metabolism is fine-tuned by inositol pyrophosphates in Saccharomyces cerevisiae. J Biol Chem 288:24898–24908

Yoshida H, Matsui T, Yamamoto A, Okada T, Mori K (2001) XBP1 mRNA is induced by ATF6 and spliced by IRE1 in response to ER stress to produce a highly active transcription factor. Cell 107:881–891

Yu W, Greenberg ML (2016) Inositol depletion, GSK3 inhibition and bipolar disorder. Future Neurol 11:135–148

Yu W, Ye C, Greenberg ML (2016) Inositol hexakisphosphate kinase 1 (IP6K1) regulates inositol synthesis in mammalian cells. J Biol Chem 291:10437–10444

Yu W, Daniel J, Mehta D, Maddipati KR, Greenberg ML (2017) MCK1 is a novel regulator of myo-inositol phosphate synthase (MIPS) that is required for inhibition of inositol synthesis by the mood stabilizer valproate. PLoS One 12:e0182534

Zheng H, Zhang L, Li L, Liu P, Gao J, Liu X, Zou J, Zhang Y, Liu J, Zhang Z, Li Z, Men W (2010) High-frequency rTMS treatment increases left prefrontal myo-inositol in young patients with treatment-resistant depression. Prog Neuro-Psychopharmacol Biol Psychiatry 34:1189–1195

Lipids and Membrane Microdomains: The Glycerolipid and Alkylphosphocholine Class of Cancer Chemotherapeutic Drugs

Vanina Zaremberg, Suriakarthiga Ganesan, and Mark Mahadeo

Contents

Abstract

Synthetic antitumor lipids are metabolically stable lysophosphatidylcholine derivatives, encompassing a class of non-mutagenic drugs that selectively target cancerous cells. In this chapter we review the literature as relates to the clinical efficacy of these antitumor lipid drugs and how our understanding of their mode of action has evolved alongside key advances in our knowledge of membrane structure, organization, and function. First, the history of the development of this class of drugs is described, providing a summary of clinical outcomes of key members including edelfosine, miltefosine, perifosine, erufosine, and erucylphosphocholine. A detailed description of the biophysical properties of

V. Zaremberg (✉) · S. Ganesan · M. Mahadeo
University of Calgary, Calgary, AB, Canada
e-mail: vzarembe@ucalgary.ca

J. Gomez-Cambronero, M. A. Frohman (eds.), *Lipid Signaling in Human Diseases*, Handbook of Experimental Pharmacology 259, https://doi.org/10.1007/164_2019_222

these drugs and specific drug–lipid interactions which may contribute to the selectivity of the antitumor lipids for cancer cells follows. An updated model on the mode of action of these lipid drugs as membrane disorganizing agents is presented. Membrane domain organization as opposed to targeting specific proteins on membranes is discussed. By altering membranes, these antitumor lipids inhibit many survival pathways while activating pro-apoptotic signals leading to cell demise.

Keywords
Antitumor lipids · Lateral membrane organization · Lipid rafts · Lysophosphatidylcholine analogues · Membrane microdomains · Non-mutagenic

1 Introduction

The toolbox of effective chemotherapeutic agents currently used to treat cancer predominantly targets proteins and nucleic acids. In the majority of cases, their mode of action is well known. For example, taxanes and vinca alkaloids inhibit microtubule dynamics, bleomycin interacts with DNA to cause strand scission at the binding site, and etoposide inhibits topoisomerases. These drugs were discovered from the late 1960s to the early 1970s and affect both normal and cancer cells indiscriminately. In parallel, a new class of synthetic lipid drugs emerged, so-called synthetic antitumor lipids (ATLs), which showed selective toxicity toward cancer cells while sparing normal ones. It was immediately accepted that ATLs do not act on nucleic acids and therefore are non-mutagenic, while investigations into their mode of action specifically focused on determining which protein was their target. Results from those investigations pointed to a plethora of proteins and signaling pathways, leading to a rather confusing scenario. Despite initial excitement based on their effectiveness in preclinical work, lack of success in clinical trials has resulted in a very limited use of these drugs as anticancer agents. Lack of understanding of their mode of action and the narrow expectation that these drugs must have a protein or specific signaling pathway as cellular targets have interfered with better outcomes. Our knowledge regarding the bioactivity of lipids has increased dramatically in the last 20 years, changing our view of the role and impact that lipids and lipid composition have on cellular membranes. As a result, the research community is currently better positioned to look at the mechanism of action of these drugs from a renewed lipid- and membrane-centered perspective. A more accurate understanding of the effect of these drugs on cells should improve their effective use as anticancer agents. In this chapter, we critically revise the body of work related to ATLs, trying to reconcile decades of disparate results with the current vision of how these lipids interact with other lipids and proteins in cellular membranes.

2 Mimicking Lysophosphatidylcholine: The Emergence of Antitumor Lipids

Immunomodulatory effects of lysophosphatidylcholine (lysolecithin, LysoPC) were first described in the early 1960s, when it was determined that LysoPC produced in a reaction catalyzed by phospholipase A2 stimulated the immune response by increasing macrophage activity (Munder et al. 1969; Munder and Modolell 1973). Since then, LysoPC has been recognized as a monocyte chemoattractant (Hoffman et al. 1982) been proposed as a bivalent factor that attracts phagocytes as a soluble "find me" signal, and that it is also involved in opsonization of apoptotic cells as a membrane-bound "eat me" signal (Lauber et al. 2003; Mueller et al. 2007). LysoPC, however, is not particularly stable, as it can be converted by acyltransferases or lysophospholipases to phosphatidylcholine (PC) or glycerophosphocholine, respectively (Arnold et al. 1978). To overcome the poor clinical efficacy of LysoPC, metabolically stable analogs were synthesized in a collaborative effort between Paul Gerhard Munder, Otto Westphal, Hans Ulrich Weltzien, and Herbert Fisher of the Max-Planck-Institut für Immunbiologie in Freiburg (Arnold et al. 1967). One of the strategies involved replacement of the ester linkages in the *sn-1* and *sn-2* positions of the glycerol backbone by ether bonds (Berdel 1982). Although some of these ether lipids indeed mimicked LysoPC immunomodulatory effects as intended (Munder et al. 1979), other compounds surprisingly displayed potent antitumor activity both in vivo and in vitro (Tarnowski et al. 1978), for which they received the collective name of antitumor lipids (ATLs). The wide-ranging antitumor properties of ATLs have been impressive. They include selective inhibition of tumor cell proliferation, induction of apoptosis in tumor cells, inhibition of tumor metastases, inhibition of angiogenesis, differentiation of tumor cells, and increase of host defenses against tumors (reviewed by Arthur and Bittman 1998; Berdel et al. 1981a; Gajate and Mollinedo 2002; Jaffrès et al. 2016; Vink et al. 2007a). Evidence from preclinical investigations has been well documented for both tumor cell lines and primary cells prepared from freshly explanted tumors including human and murine leukemias (Berdel et al. 1983a; Hoffman et al. 1984; Salari et al. 1992; Tidwell et al. 1981; Unger et al. 1987); rat (Berdel et al. 1983b) and human brain tumors (Ashagbley et al. 1996; Houlihan et al. 1987; Unger et al. 1987); human lung cancers (Ashagbley et al. 1996; Scheidt et al. 2003; Scholar 1986); ovarian carcinoma (Fujiwara et al. 1989; Herrmann and Neumann 1987); prostate carcinoma; urothelial carcinoma of the bladder; hypernephroid carcinoma and teratocarcinomas (Berdel et al. 1981b, 1983a; Herrmann and Neumann 1987); colon (Herrmann and Neumann 1987; Lu and Arthur 1992), breast (Ashagbley et al. 1996; Herrmann and Neumann 1987; Kosano and Takatani 1988), gallbladder, cervix, uterine, and corpus uteri tumors (Herrmann and Neumann 1987); and fibrosarcomas (Houlihan et al. 1987; Modolell et al. 1979; Tarnowski et al. 1978).

Edelfosine (1-*O*-octadecyl-2-*O*-methyl-rac-glycero-3-phosphocholine, ET-18-OCH3) is considered the architype of the first generation of ATLs featuring ether linkages on the glycerol backbone (Fig. 1). Interestingly, almost a decade after the chemical synthesis of edelfosine, a structurally related naturally occurring ether

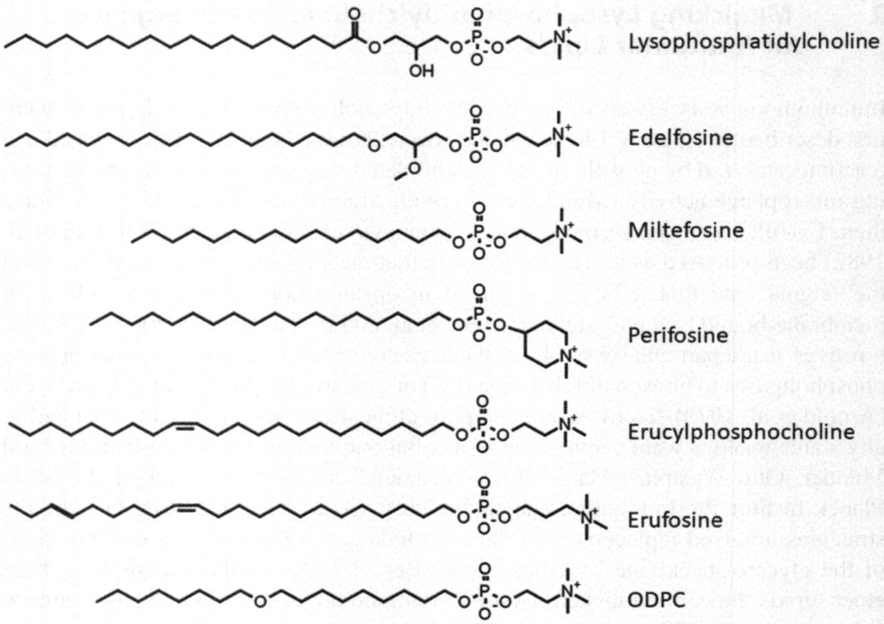

Fig. 1 Chemical structures of antitumor lipids compared to that of lysophosphatidylcholine (see text for details)

lipid, 1-*O*-alkyl-2-acetyl-*sn*-glycerol-3-phosphocholine (platelet-activating factor, PAF), was discovered (Chignard et al. 1979; Prescott et al. 1990; Snyder 1995). PAF differs from edelfosine in that it has an acetyl group attached via an ester linkage to the *sn*-2 position of the glycerol backbone. Despite this minor structural difference, PAF showed no antitumor activity in vivo or in vitro (Gajate and Mollinedo 2002). Moreover, PAF is recognized by a specific cell surface receptor, and edelfosine does not compete with PAF for binding to these receptors (Gajate and Mollinedo 2002).

Further studies demonstrated that the glycerol backbone was not essential for eliciting antitumor activity. The removal of this glycerol moiety gave rise to second-generation ATLs with hexadecylphosphocholine (HPC, *miltefosine*) (Fig. 1) being the prototypic drug of the alkylphosphocholine (APC) family (Hilgard et al. 1993) (Fig. 1). In an attempt to increase the therapeutic range of alkylphosphocholines, a few structural changes were made to miltefosine. Since miltefosine can be metabolized into choline and phosphocholine by phospholipases, it was proposed that elimination of this headgroup might increase its stability. Of the newly synthesized derivatives, *perifosine* (octadecyl-(1,1-dimethyl-4-piperidylio) phosphate, D-21266) (Fig. 1), with a piperidine moiety in place of the phosphocholine headgroup, showed the most promising clinical applications (Table 1; *ClinicalTrials.gov, U.S. National Library of Medicine, National Institutes of Health*). Among novel APCs structurally similar to miltefosine are *erucylphosphocholine* and *erufosine*, differing in the hydrocarbon chain length (22C) and the

Table 1 Summary of relevant clinical trials involving antitumor lipids

Drug	Phase	Treatment	Key findings
Edelfosine	I	Different forms of malignancies (intravenous and oral) (Berdel et al. 1987)	Partial remission in non-small cell lung cancers, reduction in leukemic blast in acute myelomonocytic leukemic with high gastrointestinal toxicity
		Acute leukemia (autologous) (Vogler et al. 1992)	Dose finding for successful purging of leukemic cells and safe dose was determined. Mucositis identified as a major side effect
	II	Non-small cell carcinoma (oral) (Drings et al. 1992)	Unfavorable outcome due to very low remission rate
		Acute leukemia (autologous) (Koenigsmann et al. 1996)	Effective for purging of bone barrow and better remission rate than phase I clinical trial
Miltefosine	I	Cutaneous lymphoma (topical) (Dummer et al. 1993), skin metastases in breast cancer (topical) (Unger et al. 1990)	Effective for treatment of these tumors with minimal side effects
		Variety of advanced solid tumors (oral) (Verweij et al. 1992; Crul et al. 2002)	Highly hemolytic, clinical trials were halted due to severe gastrointestinal toxicity
		Visceral leishmaniasis (oral) (Sundar et al. 1999)	Effective with minimal side effects such as diarrhea, vomiting, and gastrointestinal toxicity. Safe dose was determined
	II	Skin metastases in breast cancer (topical) (Smorenburg et al. 2000)	Very effective with minimal skin reactions and approved as Miltex for treatment
		Visceral leishmaniasis (oral) (Sundar et al. 2000; Jha et al. 1999)	90% cure rate with minimal toxicity and the schedule and dose were decided for effective treatment regime
	III	Visceral leishmaniasis (oral) (Sundar and Olliaro 2007)	94% cure rate with minimal toxicity and improved safety of drug due to reduced dose. The drug was approved in India

(continued)

Table 1 (continued)

Drug	Phase	Treatment	Key findings
	IV	Visceral leishmaniasis (oral) (Rahman et al. 2011; Bhattacharya et al. 2007)	Study was done in outpatient settings and found similar findings as phase III studies
		New clinical trials (see *ClinicalTrials.gov, U.S. National Library of Medicine, National Institutes of Health*)	
Perifosine	I	Variety of solid and leukemic tumors (Becher et al. 2017; Figg et al. 2014; Gills and Dennis 2009)	Promising only for sarcoma and Waldenström's macroglobulinemia
	II	Relapsed/refractory Waldenstrom's macroglobulinemia (Ghobrial et al. 2010)	Minimal response and gastrointestinal toxicity as side effect
		Recurrent prostate cancer, breast cancer, and squamous cell carcinoma of the head and neck (Gills and Dennis 2009)	Ineffective as a single agent
		Pancreatic adenocarcinoma (Marsh et al. 2007)	Study was suspended due to adverse effect
	III	Multiple myeloma (Nagler et al. 2013)	Combinatorial trial with two other antitumor drugs failed
		New clinical trials (see *ClinicalTrials.gov, U.S. National Library of Medicine, National Institutes of Health*)	
Erufosine[a]	I	Acute myeloid leukemia (Fiegl et al. 2008)	High leukemic activity observed in samples from patients
Erucylphosphocholine[a]	I	Malignant brain tumors (Erdlenbruch et al. 1998)	Preclinical study with positive result

[a]Mostly preclinical studies

presence of a monounsaturation (Fig. 1) (van Blitterswijk and Verheij 2008). Additionally, erufosine contains an extra carbon between the phosphate and the trimethylammonium headgroup. Another drug that has recently received attention is 10-(octyloxy)decyl-2-(trimethylammonium) ethyl phosphate (*ODPC*) (dos Santos et al. 2010; Gomide et al. 2013; Thome et al. 2012) (Fig. 1). Less investigated APC variants with different functional groups have been developed over the years including lipids containing halogens (Brachwitz et al. 1982), dioxanyl analogs (Duclos and Makriyannis 1992), and cyclopentane-containing derivatives (Alam et al. 2012).

3 Antitumor Lipid Drugs in Clinical Trials

A summary of relevant clinical trials involving the most promising ATLs is presented in Table 1 (*ClinicalTrials.gov, U.S. National Library of Medicine, National Institutes of Health*).

3.1 Edelfosine

A phase I clinical trial of edelfosine given as intravenous or oral treatment was initiated in 1987 with 16 patients suffering from different forms of malignancies (Berdel et al. 1987). This study had some promising results wherein partial remissions were observed in two patients with non-small cell lung cancers and a reduction in leukemic blasts was observed in patients with acute myelomonocytic leukemia (Berdel et al. 1987). Among the side effects observed in this study were altered liver function, pulmonary edema, and gastrointestinal toxicity (Berdel et al. 1987). In another clinical study, it was found that edelfosine was effective for purging leukemic cells from bone marrow obtained from patients during remissions (Vogler and Berdel 1993; Vogler et al. 1987). A phase II clinical trial with edelfosine was conducted in patients with non-small cell carcinoma, and despite very low tumor remission levels, the tumor progression rate was also very low (Drings et al. 1992). Similar side effects were observed in this study; hence the use of this drug intravenously or orally became undesirable (Drings et al. 1992). Later on, many clinical studies used edelfosine for bone marrow purging, and it was found to be effective and beneficial for leukemic patients requiring autologous bone marrow transplantation (Koenigsmann et al. 1996; Vogler and Berdel 1993). Currently, edelfosine is widely used for this purpose for acute leukemia patients (Andreesen et al. 1978; Vogler et al. 1992).

3.2 Miltefosine

Clinical trials using miltefosine were initiated for topical, intravenous, and oral treatment of cutaneous lymphoma and solid tumors (Dummer et al. 1993; Verweij et al. 1992). Among some of the side effects following oral treatment of miltefosine were gastrointestinal activity, diarrhea, nausea, and vomiting, but these were found to be dose-dependent (Verweij et al. 1992). Following this, a topical formulation of miltefosine was tested against skin metastases in breast cancer patients, which yielded highly promising results (Smorenburg et al. 2000; Terwogt et al. 1999; Unger et al. 1990). Miltefosine (Miltex) is currently being used as a topical agent to provide relief in breast cancer patients with skin metastases. The development of miltefosine as an oral agent for treatment of visceral leishmaniasis began in the late 1990s with many promising results during phase I and II of clinical trials (Croft et al. 1987; Kuhlencord et al. 1992). Miltefosine is presently the only oral treatment available for visceral leishmaniasis (Dorlo et al. 2012; Sundar and Olliaro 2007).

According to the *ClinicalTrials.gov* database from the US NIH National Library of Medicine, several phase II and III clinical trials involving miltefosine alone or in combination with other drugs for the treatment of parasitic related diseases have been initiated in the last 3 years and are currently either active or in the recruiting stages (*ClinicalTrials.gov, U.S. National Library of Medicine, National Institutes of Health*).

3.3 Perifosine

Perifosine has entered many phase I clinical trials to treat a variety of advanced solid and leukemic tumors (Becher et al. 2017; Figg et al. 2014; Gills and Dennis 2009). Perifosine treatment was promising in sarcoma and Waldenström's macroglobulinemia but unsatisfactory in breast, pancreatic, melanoma, and many other cancers during phase II clinical trials (Gills and Dennis 2009). Gastrointestinal toxicity and fatigue were common side effects associated with perifosine administration (Bailey et al. 2006). A phase III clinical trial of perifosine in combination with two other antitumor drugs, Velcade and Dexamethasone, was discontinued as no significant differences were observed with or without perifosine for the treatment of multiple myeloma (Nagler et al. 2013). According to the ClinicalTrials.gov database, close to 40 phase I, II, and III clinical trials involving perifosine in combination with other drugs for the treatment of a wide range of cancers have been completed since 2006, with the last one occurring as recently as February 2018 (*ClinicalTrials.gov, U.S. National Library of Medicine, National Institutes of Health*).

3.4 Erufosine and Erucylphosphocholine

Many preclinical studies were carried out with erufosine and erucylphosphocholine to target malignant brain tumors and acute myeloid leukemia (Erdlenbruch et al. 1998; Fiegl et al. 2008; Jendrossek et al. 2002). Chemical modifications of these drugs reduced gastrointestinal toxicity and increased solubility, especially for erufosine (Henke et al. 2009; Jendrossek et al. 2002). The ability of these drugs to cross the blood-brain barrier is promising, and clinical trials are required to evaluate the potential of these drugs to be used for human brain tumor treatment (Jendrossek et al. 2002).

4 Phase Behavior and Nanoparticle Formulations Involving Antitumor Lipids

In understanding the modes of entry and action for these drugs, an important consideration is the phase and aggregation behavior of the formulation. This aspect has been largely overlooked for ATL drugs. The thermotropic phase behavior of edelfosine has been characterized (Maurer et al. 1994) using dynamic light scattering, X-ray scattering, ultrasonic speed measurements, and differential scanning calorimetry, which demonstrated that edelfosine undergoes a micellar-to-lamellar phase transition upon cooling. Based on the small angle X-ray scattering data, large aggregates observed at low temperatures were determined to be interdigitated bilayers, and the micellar-to-lamellar transition was observed to take weeks to reach completion. This complex phase behavior has been reported for similar molecules such as stearoyllysophosphatidylcholine (Hui and Huang 1986; Wu et al. 1982), 1-stearoyl-2-acetyl-sn-glycerol-3-phosphorylcholine (Huang et al. 1984), and *n*-octadecylphosphocholine (Jain et al. 1985). PAF was shown to exist in three separate phases using infrared spectroscopy (Mushayakarara and Mantsch 1985), with the lowest-temperature state being an interdigitated gel phase, which transitions first into a lamellar gel phase, followed by micelles at higher temperatures. This behavior was later verified using ^{31}P-NMR and Raman spectroscopy (Huang et al. 1986). Other authors have proposed that edelfosine and related drugs act as surfactants with a defined critical micellar concentration (CMC). CMC determinations have been reported for edelfosine (Busto et al. 2007) and for ODPC (dos Santos et al. 2010). For edelfosine, the CMC was determined using surface pressure measurements as well as fluorescent dyes (Busto et al. 2007), which showed edelfosine had two CMCs, one at 3.5 μM and another at 19 μM in water corresponding to the formation of small micelles and large micelles, respectively. This however is unlikely, based on the phase behavior reported previously (Maurer et al. 1994). An alternative explanation (Busto et al. 2007) is that it corresponds to the formation of one aggregate and then transition to the other, as neither of the methods used provided direct structural information on the phase of the aggregate formed. The phase in which these drugs exist, whether it be micelles or interdigitated bilayers, would impact the properties of the drug and affect both the mode of cellular entry and the mode of action. Recently, edelfosine nanoparticles have been shown to elicit cytotoxicity for the previously-resistant K-562 leukemic cell line (Aznar et al. 2014) and to alleviate the in vivo toxicity of free edelfosine in mice (Lasa-Saracíbar et al. 2014), illustrating the relevance of considering phase and aggregation behavior in the development of effective formulations with minimal side effects. It is worth noting that according to the PubChem database (NCBI), more than 2,000 patents using edelfosine (PubChem CID: 1392) in different formulations have been deposited, with the most recent one being submitted in July 2017 for Cancer Stem Cell-Targeted Cancer Therapy (Patent ID: US2017274058).

5 Antitumor Lipid Selectivity Toward Cancerous Cells

In great contrast with many conventional chemotherapeutic drugs, ATLs are considered *non*-mutagenic (van der Luit et al. 2007) and to act selectively (Andreesen et al. 1978, 1979; Modolell et al. 1979). These properties reduce both the amount and severity of side effects associated with classical chemotherapeutics. The molecular basis for ATLs selectivity is not yet fully understood but has been linked to their preferred cellular uptake by tumoral cells (Mollinedo et al. 1997). It was shown that normal human fibroblasts are resistant to ATLs due to reduced uptake of the drugs. However, microinjection of edelfosine into them induces cell death (Gajate et al. 2000a; Mollinedo et al. 1997).

It is worth noting that cancer cells preferentially scavenge LysoPC species among all the lipids available in the serum (Kamphorst et al. 2013). Once inside the cell, these lysolipids serve as source of fatty acids or can be converted to membrane lipids, therefore supporting proliferation. Similarly, it has been recently discovered that serum LysoPC is a major building block of parasite phospholipid metabolism (Brancucci et al. 2017). Interestingly, ATLs are effective drugs for the treatment of both cancer and parasitic infections.

It was suggested that lack of the 1-*O*-alkyl-cleavage metabolizing enzyme in tumoral cells allows accumulation of these drugs, thus causing increased sensitivity of tumoral cells to ATLs compared to normal cells (Soodsma et al. 1970), but this remains speculative.

Other possible explanations allude to unique features associated with the lipid and protein compositions of the plasma membrane of tumor cells, which would favor interactions with and uptake of these drugs. Advances in lipid profiling and lipidomic approaches point to levels of cholesterol being increased in cancer cells (Clayman et al. 1983; Krycer and Brown 2013; Li et al. 2006). Interestingly, drugs that target and reduce cholesterol biosynthesis such as simvastatin have shown to reduce the risk of cancer malignancy. Simvastatin treatment reduced cholesterol content in detergent-resistant membranes (DRMs) isolated from pancreatic tumor cells and decreased Akt/PKB phosphorylation, which is generally hyperactive in tumor cells (Zhuang et al. 2005). As ATLs like edelfosine have been described to preferentially partition into DRMs rich in sterols (Gajate and Mollinedo 2001; Gajate et al. 2009), the high cholesterol accumulation in tumor cells could possibly enhance incorporation of ATLs into their membranes compared to those of normal cells. This hypothesis is supported by biophysical studies, which have demonstrated very strong interactions between ATLs and sterols. In fact, the strength of the interactions between edelfosine and different sterols was characterized as a way of screening for clinical efficacy (Busto et al. 2008). Whereas edelfosine alone (above 20 μM) caused hemolysis, formulations of edelfosine with cholesterol, campesterol, or β-sitosterol showed significant decrease of this side effect without reduction of the apoptotic effects of the drug. While injection of edelfosine alone was surface active, injections of edelfosine in combination with the abovementioned sterols were not. The authors surmised this decrease in surface activity to be responsible for the observed decrease in hemolytic activity.

Like edelfosine, miltefosine also forms strong interactions with sterols, and mixed monolayers of cholesterol and miltefosine are more stable than either component alone (Rey Gomez-Serranillos et al. 2004). All mixtures of cholesterol and miltefosine packed better than expected from ideal mixing, with the most stable mixture formed being 2:1 miltefosine: cholesterol (whereby each cholesterol is flanked by two miltefosine molecules via hydrophobic interactions). Monolayer experiments have also been performed with miltefosine injected under mixtures of POPC and either cholesterol or ergosterol (Rakotomanga et al. 2004). When the monolayer was held at constant pressure, miltefosine was observed to partition into both pure PC and pure sterol monolayers, whereas during compression, miltefosine caused greater expansion of the PC films over the sterol systems, suggesting that miltefosine is less perturbing due to the strong affinity of the drug for sterol molecules. Additionally, interactions between ATLs and either phospholipids or sphingolipids have been documented. One biophysical study using DSC, ^{31}P-NMR and X-ray scattering looked at the effect of edelfosine on the phase behavior of DMPC and DEPE (Torrecillas et al. 2006). Here, it was demonstrated that edelfosine added to DMPC below its phase transition induced interdigitation. Above the phase transition of DMPC, however, the presence of edelfosine resulted in the formation of small aggregates (micelles or small vesicles). As well, in the same study, DEPE, which has two transitions (the first corresponding to $L\beta$–$L\alpha$ transition and the second corresponding to a transition from $L\alpha$ to hexagonal phase), was shown to have an inhibition of the second transition by edelfosine. As some membrane-bound enzymes are stabilized by the hexagonal phase of PE (Epand 1990), this inhibition of hexagonal phase formation can disrupt enzymatic activity.

Mixed monolayers of PE with edelfosine, PAF, or lyso-PAF have also been characterized (Hąc-Wydro et al. 2012). Edelfosine was found to be immiscible with DSPE, causing pronounced phase separation, which was confirmed by Brewster angle microscopy. The authors suggested this is likely because edelfosine would break apart the hydrogen bond network of DSPE.

Monolayer studies have also been conducted on mixtures of sphingolipids with edelfosine (Hąc-Wydro and Dynarowicz-Łątka 2010a, b). Interactions between sphingomyelin (SM) and edelfosine were found to be unfavorable, as the inclusion of edelfosine was suggested to disrupt van der Waals interactions between the tails. In contrast, mixtures of gangliosides with edelfosine were proposed to decrease electrostatic repulsion, increasing the thermodynamic favorability of the interaction (Valentino et al. 1990).

6 Antitumor Lipids as Agents Targeting Membrane Organization

Membranes lipids have long been regarded as a passive, fluid solvent for proteins, which were considered the key components that provided membrane functionality. Cancer research and drug discovery have also been dominated by this idea, so is not surprising that investigations on the mode of action of ATLs have focused on finding the "protein target" of this class of drugs, with poor outcomes and a complex picture of several protein candidates depending on the cancer cell type (Fig. 2). In the last two decades, the lipid research field has exploded with compelling evidence that recognizes lipids as key players in signaling pathways and as regulatory molecules. Innovative ideas on membrane-organizing principles have challenged our view of how lipid-lipid and lipid-protein interactions affect membrane function, introducing a novel perspective also to the cancer research field. We believe that the important body of research investigating the effects of ATLs in cancer needs to be reinterpreted and further examined in light of recent advances in the lipid research field and the

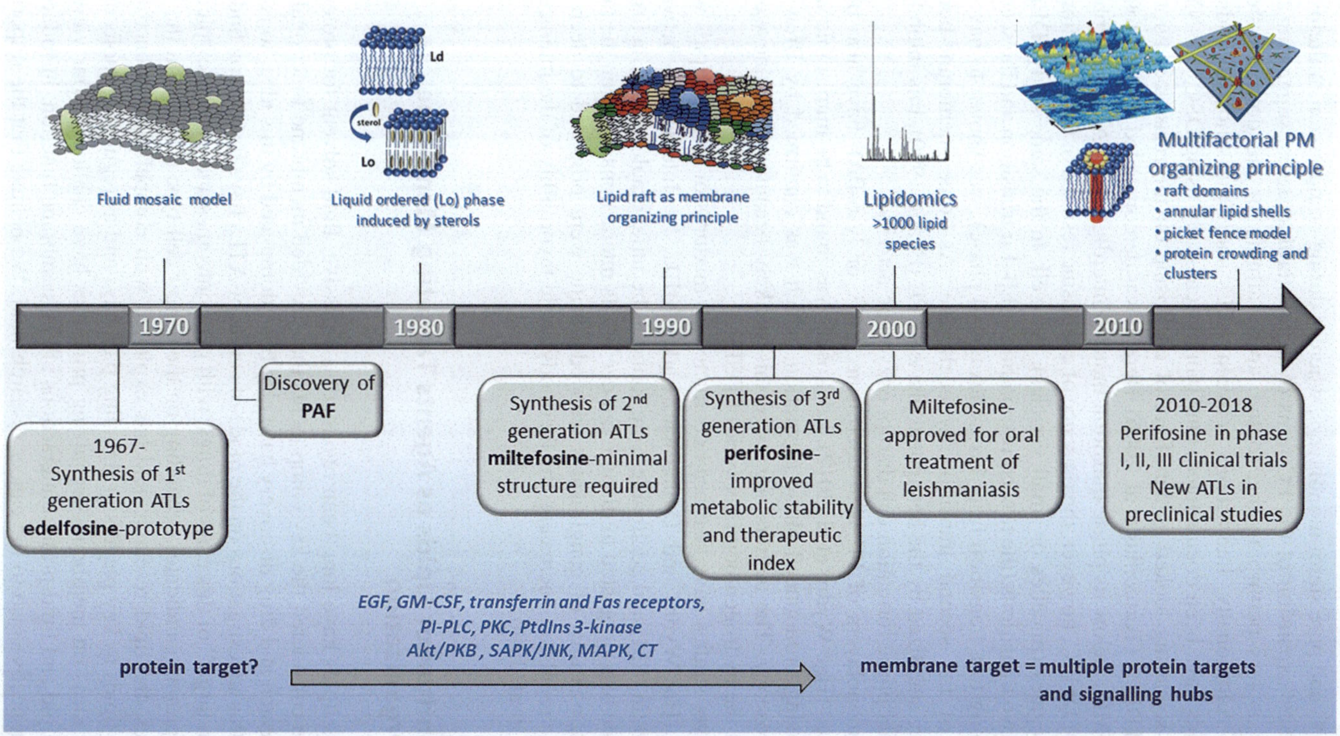

Fig. 2 Timeline of critical developments in antitumor lipid drugs and advances in understanding organizing membrane principles. *ATLs* antitumor lipids, *Ld* liquid disordered, *Lo* liquid ordered, *PAF* platelet-activating factor. See text for discussion of ATL protein targets

radical change of vision on the role of lipids in cellular processes (Fig. 2). At present, ATLs are considered agents that target membranes and disrupt their organization. Therefore, before discussing their mode of action, we will briefly highlight the key concepts that have shaped our current vision of how membranes are organized.

7 Evolving Concepts in Membrane-Organizing Principles: Membrane Domains

The cell membrane was first proposed to exist as a bilayer of phospholipids by Gorter and Grendel in 1925 (Gorter and Grendel 1925). Since then, the model for the cell membrane has evolved along with technological advances to reflect our understanding of its complexity. The "fluid mosaic model" proposed by Singer and Nicolson in 1972 (Singer and Nicolson 1972) included the presence of both integral and peripheral membrane proteins residing in a homogenous "sea of lipids." The phospholipid component of the membrane was devoid of any organization in either the lateral directions or between leaflets. Lateral organization was first proposed in 1977, resulting in a model that included changes in membrane thickness due to the presence of lipids with longer and more saturated tails (Israelachvili 1977). This was based on observations of temperature-dependent clustering in mixtures of saturated and unsaturated phosphatidylcholines (Lee et al. 1974) leading to the idea of two separate phases coexisting in the biologically relevant liquid crystalline (L_α) phase (Wunderlich et al. 1975). X-ray diffraction studies provided further evidence to the presence of discrete lipid domains existing within biomembranes (Wunderlich et al. 1978). Cholesterol was shown to be a crucial determinant of domain formation (Karnovsky et al. 1982). Early studies also demonstrated the formation of immiscible domains in mixtures of sphingolipids and glycerophospholipids (Thompson and Tillack 1985). Sphingolipids in these mixtures were found to segregate and cluster together (partly due to hydrogen bonding within the backbone), forming very rigid structures that were detergent-insoluble (Schroeder et al. 1994).

In addition to inducing separation of immiscible phases in phospholipids, cholesterol also formed very strong interactions with sphingolipids, due to hydrogen bonding between the hydroxyl group of the sterol with the backbone regions of sphingolipids. The thermodynamically favorable association of sterols and sphingolipids was also thought to occur based on the "umbrella model" (Huang and Feigenson 1999), wherein the larger headgroup of the sphingolipid better shields the sterol from exposure to water.

The formation of lateral domains within a single leaflet results from hydrophobic mismatch of membrane components. More rigid lipid domains, due to the elongated acyl tails, tend to form thicker segments of the membrane, whereas more fluid regions where the tails aren't extended tend to be thinner. Mismatch of the hydrophobic regions of the lipids at the boundary of the two immiscible phases is energetically unfavorable, generating line tension along the boundary (Benvegnu and McConnell 1992). This has been demonstrated in mixtures of unsaturated PC that form a fluid liquid-disordered (L_d) phase, with SM and cholesterol forming a rigid, liquid-ordered (L_o) phase. As the length of the PC acyl tails were shortened, the line tension increased due to greater mismatch (Garcia-Saez et al. 2007). The mixtures with greater line tension were also shown to form larger domains, thus decreasing the overall perimeter of the domains and the energetically unfavorable boundary surface. In addition to line tension, electrostatic and molecular dipoles were also shown to modulate domain size and shape (McConnell and De Koker 1996). Stronger molecular dipoles tend to result in the molecules orienting themselves in a more branched and elongated shape, rather than a circular one. Branched domains arise when the molecules pack into different orientations. In a study on mixed PC and SM monolayers, branched domains were observed, with six main branches each exhibiting an interesting internal anisotropy (Prenner et al. 2007). This suggests that each branch had a unique long-range ordering of the hydrocarbon chains resulting in the different molecular orientations. Domain shape is also influenced by the chirality of the lipids involved (Nandi et al. 2004).

The compelling evidence from biophysical studies supporting lateral domain segregation in mimetic systems paved the way to the emergence of the lipid raft hypothesis in 1988 as a means of explaining the principles behind the organization, localization, and trafficking of membrane components in the cellular context. Lipid rafts were first proposed during investigations aimed at understanding sorting of glycolipids by the trans-Golgi network and their delivery to the apical membrane of polarized mammalian epithelial cells (Simons and Van Meer 1988). This concept was further supported by the fact that glycosphingolipids were enriched in DRMs (Schroeder et al. 1994). Currently, lipid rafts are defined as dynamic nanoscale ordered membrane assemblies of specific proteins that are enriched in sterols and sphingolipids with long saturated acyl chains and hydroxylated ceramide backbones. The functional corollary of the hypothesis is that the resting state of these assemblies can be activated to coalesce by specific lipid-lipid, lipid-protein, and protein-protein interactions (Simons and Sampaio 2011). Lipid rafts were therefore proposed as platforms for integral and peripheral membrane proteins, providing a spatial and temporal organization that facilitates processes such as signal transduction and membrane trafficking. Cholesterol trafficking (Schroeder et al. 2001), signal transduction (Simons and Toomre 2000), apoptosis (George and Wu 2012), neurotransmitter signaling (Allen et al. 2007), and cytoskeletal interactions (Head et al. 2014) are among some of the cellular processes proposed to be regulated by lipid rafts. Since its inception, the theory has been passionately discussed by both proponents (Brown and London 1998a, b; Lingwood and Simons 2010; Pike 2003, 2009; Quinn 2010; Rietveld and Simons 1998; Simons and Ikonen 1997; Simons and Sampaio 2011) and critics (Edidin 2003; Munro 2003) of it. The main approaches used to study lipid rafts have involved manipulations of the levels of cholesterol in membranes and preparation of DRMs, but the main challenge has been (and still remains) their in vivo visualization. Furthermore, recent advances involving nanoscale imaging mass spectrometry allowed for the detection of sphingolipid microdomains in fibroblasts, though they were not enriched in cholesterol nor did they changed when cholesterol was removed from membranes (Frisz et al. 2013). In addition to the technical challenges of capturing lipid rafts in vivo is the fact that cholesterol alone has been found to be tightly associated with proteins forming annular shells or acting as a ligand. Many of the proteins identified as binding cholesterol participate in signaling hubs, including G-protein-coupled receptors, ion channels, caveolin, and peripheral scaffold proteins associated with synapsis (reviewed in Lu and Fairn 2018). Therefore, it has been argued that many of the processes proposed to be regulated by lipid rafts could be just ascribed to the cholesterol present in the Ld phase of the cellular membrane. A multifactorial view of the organizing principles of the plasma membrane has been recently proposed, resulting from the cooperative action of different mesoscale (2–300 nm) domains in the plasma membrane involving lipid domains, the cytoskeleton, and protein clusters (Kusumi et al. 2012; Lu and Fairn 2018).

It has been hypothesized that ATLs like edelfosine insert in the membranes of malignant cells and induce biophysical alterations in their organization, affecting growth regulatory signals that require a particular lipid domain used as scaffold for assembly and/or function. Different experimental lines of evidence have converged to support this mode of action for ATLs. Results obtained independently using a wide range of sensitive cancer cell lines (Gajate et al. 2000b, 2009; Gajate and Mollinedo 2001; Mollinedo et al. 2004) and cells that became resistant to ATLs (van der Luit et al. 2002, 2007) pointed to lipid rafts as target of ATLs in membranes. This was further supported by unbiased genetic screens using the model organism *Saccharomyces cerevisiae* (Zaremberg et al. 2005; Cuesta-Marbán et al. 2013; Czyz et al. 2013). In the next section, we will highlight the main signaling pathways altered by the interaction of ATLs with cellular membranes.

8 Inhibition of Survival Signaling Pathways by Antitumor Lipids

ATLs have been linked to the inhibition of several survival pathways known to associate with the plasma membrane, including the Ras-Raf-Mitogen Activating Protein Kinase (MAPK) (Samadder et al. 2003; Zhou et al. 1996) and the phosphatidylinositol 3-kinase/protein kinase B/Akt (PI3K/Akt) pathways (Kondapaka et al. 2003; Ruiter et al. 2003). Edelfosine, miltefosine, and perifosine inhibit the MAPK pathway by interfering with the ability of Raf to translocate to the plasma membrane (Samadder et al. 2003; Zhou et al. 1996). Additionally, edelfosine and miltefosine cause clustering and internalization of epidermal growth factor receptors (EGFR) (Kosano and Takatani 1988) localized upstream of MAPK. Phosphorylation of p38 MAPK and ERK1/ERK2 MAPK, which leads to their activation and binding of nuclear factor-kappa B to DNA, is prevented by edelfosine in a dose-dependent manner (Na and Surh 2008).

These ATLs have also inhibited the PI3K-Akt/PKB survival pathway, upstream of PI3K (Kondapaka et al. 2003; Ruiter et al. 2003). The exact mechanism by which ATLs inhibit this pathway is still unknown, but studies with perifosine suggest that the drug causes a conformational change in the Akt/PKB pleckstrin homology domain that makes it unable to bind to phosphatidylinositol-3,4,5-trisphosphate, therefore impairing its plasma membrane recruitment and activation. Furthermore, inhibition of PKB/Akt by ATLs also induces activation of pro-apoptotic pathways such as the SAPK/JNK (Ruiter et al. 2003). Interestingly, transcriptional profiling conducted using cells expressing constitutively active PKB/Akt (mimicking cancerous cells) showed increased expression of genes that are involved in cholesterol biosynthesis in a SREBP-dependent manner (Porstmann et al. 2005). The oncogenic form of Akt, which is myristoylated, has been shown to preferentially accumulate in cholesterol-enriched microdomains/lipid rafts at the plasma membrane (Adam et al. 2007), and the lipid raft-altering effect of ATLs may very well explain why PKB/Akt activation is impaired in cells treated with these drugs.

Protein kinase C (PKC) has also been implicated as a target of ATLs, as it is inhibited in a dose-dependent manner by edelfosine (Helfman et al. 1983). Edelfosine and miltefosine affect PKC-autophosphorylation and PKC-dependent phosphorylation of histones in cell-free systems and in NIH3T3 murine cells in a competitive manner (Gil et al. 1996; Salari et al. 1992; Uberall et al. 1991). It was speculated that edelfosine may possibly interfere with binding of PKC to phosphatidylserine/diacylglycerol (DAG) or phorbol esters, although no evidence has been presented to support this hypothesis.

Another signaling enzyme affected by treatment of cells with ATLs is phosphatidylinositol-phospholipase C (PI-PLC), which hydrolyzes PIP2 to produce DAG (Uberall et al. 1991; Powis et al. 1992). Thus, the inhibition of PKC by ATLs could also be a secondary effect downstream of PI-PLC. In fact, edelfosine has been widely marketed as a "specific" PI-PLC inhibitor to be used as a pharmacological tool to study the role of PI-PLC in membranes and cellular physiology (Horowitz et al. 2005; Wong et al. 2007). However, caution is required in the interpretation of results from such studies, as edelfosine and related ATLs affect many other membrane-associated proteins.

Edelfosine inhibits CTP/phosphocholine cytidylyltransferase (CCT) (Boggs et al. 1995; Baburina and Jackowski 1998), which catalyzes the rate-limiting step in the CDP-choline (Kennedy) pathway for de novo PC biosynthesis. CCT is a soluble enzyme that is recruited to the nuclear membrane where it becomes active (Wang et al. 1993; Watkins and Kent 1991). PC is the most abundant phospholipid found in eukaryotic membranes, and the CDP-choline pathway is the only way to generate PC, except in hepatocytes where PC can be also made from phosphatidylethanolamine through the methylation pathway. Therefore, inhibition of the Kennedy pathway will impair cell growth and eventually result in cell death. Moreover, PC is an important source for other lipids, as it can be broken down to lipid secondary messengers such as phosphatidic acid and DAG via phospholipase D and C activity, respectively. In addition, the phosphocholine headgroup of PC is transferred to ceramide to produce SM by SM synthase. As such, decreases in PC would result in decreased levels of SM and mitogenic signaling lipids such as DAG, with increased levels of pro-apoptotic signaling lipids such as ceramide (Wright et al. 2004; Baburina and Jackowski 1998). Interestingly, it has been reported that edelfosine inhibits PC biosynthesis in both HeLa and A549 cells, but not in Jurkat or Peer leukemic cells, before the triggering of apoptosis (Nieto-Miguel et al. 2006). Unfortunately, edelfosine is still used today as a "specific" inhibitor of CCT in high-profile studies aimed at targeting de novo PC synthesis, deliberately ignoring all other pleiotropic effects associated with this ATL.

In addition to inhibiting survival pathways, ATLs also stimulate pro-apoptotic pathways, such as those controlled by the ceramide-activated stress-activated protein kinase/c-Jun-N-terminal kinase (SAPK/JNK) and the Fas/CD95 death receptor (Ruiter et al. 2003; Gajate and Mollinedo 2001). The SAPK/JNK pathway is activated in response to stimuli such as radiation and ATLs and through sequential phosphorylation activates pro-apoptotic mechanisms. Although the exact mechanism of activation of the SAPK/JNK pathway by ATLs remains unknown, it has been proposed that the SAPK/JNK and MAPK pathways are inversely related and as such may function to regulate each other through cross talk involving secondary messenger lipids such as ceramide (Ruiter et al. 2003). Physiological activation of the Fas/CD95 receptor requires the presence of a Fas ligand to recruit the Fas-associated protein with death domain (FADD) and procaspase-8 to form the death-inducing signaling complex (DISC). Treatment with edelfosine has been shown to mimic the role of the Fas ligand, as it increased Fas/CD95-translocation and capping of the proteins into lipid rafts, leading to increased DISC formation and subsequent triggering of apoptosis. Furthermore, disruption of lipid rafts by extraction of sterols, using either filipin or methyl-ß-cyclodextrin, inhibited the effect of edelfosine on Fas/CD95 activation (Gajate and Mollinedo 2001, 2007; Chakrabandhu et al. 2007). It was shown that edelfosine partitioned into DRMs within 10–15 min following its addition into the cells, whereas clustering of Fas/CD95 was detected 6 h after treatment with edelfosine was initiated (Gajate et al. 2004).

9 Cellular Uptake of Antitumor Lipids

How cells uptake ATLs is not fully understood. Several mechanisms have been proposed including raft-mediated endocytosis and flippase-mediated uptake, although they may not be mutually exclusive. The main tools used to monitor uptake of ATLs are radioactive and fluorescent derivatives. Conclusive evidence against uptake of ATLs via classic clathrin-mediated endocytosis included the following: (1) treatment of cells with general endocytosis inhibitors, such as chloroquine, monensin, and cytochalasin B, does not alter uptake of radiolabeled ATLs (Kelley et al. 1993); (2) uptake of radiolabeled edelfosine and perifosine is unaffected at low temperature (4°C), whereas endocytosis is inhibited (van der Luit et al. 2007); and (3) uptake of Lucifer yellow and transferrin (which depend on endocytosis) is unaffected in macrophage-like cell lines that are resistant to ATLs due to lack of uptake (Zoeller et al. 1995).

As our understanding of membrane organization evolved, investigations focused on exploring new portals of entry for ATLs into eukaryotic cells were pursued. It has been proposed that uptake of ATLs in leukemic cells requires partitioning of these drugs into domains enriched in cholesterol and sphingolipids followed by their internalization via raft-mediated (caveolae-mediated) endocytosis (van der Luit et al. 2002, 2007). Pre-treatment of cells with the cholesterol-extracting agent methyl-β-cyclodextrin (MβCD) or with bacterial sphingomyelinase significantly reduced cellular uptake of radiolabeled ATLs, leading to the idea that intact lipid rafts are required for uptake of these drugs (van der Luit et al. 2007). In another study, uptake of radiolabeled perifosine and edelfosine was investigated using ATL-resistant KBr epidermal carcinoma and S49^{AR} mouse lymphoma cells (Vink et al. 2007b). KBr cells were obtained by chemical mutagenesis following by continuous culturing in the presence of perifosine, while S49^{AR} cells were obtained by continuous culturing in the presence of edelfosine (Smets et al. 1999; Vink et al. 2007b). It was discovered that S49^{AR} mouse lymphoma cells had reduced SM synthase activity, suggesting that abrogating lipid raft formation due to lack of SM prevented uptake of ATLs by these cells (Vink et al. 2007b). In contrast, KBr epidermal carcinoma cells showed no defect in SM synthesis, and it was suggested that uptake of ATLs in KBr cells is probably independent of raft-mediated endocytosis but could be dependent on a translocase present at the plasma membrane (Vink et al. 2007b; Muñoz-Martínez et al. 2010).

Much of what is known on edelfosine internalization comes from studies in budding yeast. The uptake of aminophospholipids in yeast is mediated by members of the P-type ATPase family of translocases (flippases). The results from a yeast genetic screen indicated that *lem3* mutants are resistant to edelfosine. Further research showed that edelfosine uptake is dependent on Lem3, a protein from the Cdc50 family that is a subunit of an aminophospholipid flippase (Hanson et al. 2003). Uptake assays using radiolabeled edelfosine further supported this finding (Zaremberg et al. 2005).

The human homologue, CDC50A was found to be responsible for uptake of ATLs in KB human epidermal carcinoma cells (Muñoz-Martínez et al. 2010). It is speculated that CDC50A formation of a functional translocase in combination with a P-type ATPase at the plasma membrane enables ATL uptake (Muñoz-Martínez et al. 2008, 2010). In addition, overexpression of human protein TMEM30a, an orthologue of the yeast Lem3 flippase subunit, increases import of radiolabeled platelet-activating factor into Chinese hamster ovary cells. Furthermore, expression of human TMEM30a in yeast lacking Lem3 restores NBC-PC uptake and sensitizes yeast cells to the presence of edelfosine in a concentration-dependent manner (Chen et al. 2011). Interestingly it has been shown that human CDC50A partitions into DRMs in both hepatocytes and liver sinusoidal endothelial cells (Folmer et al. 2012). We are accordingly tempted to speculate that the effects seen in uptake upon disruption of sterol and sphingolipid homeostasis could in fact alter proper flippase localization and/or activity. On another note, it is worth highlighting that supplementing cells with exogenous PC or LysoPC would compete with edelfosine for flippase-mediated uptake, protecting cells from the ATL (unpublished results). Indeed, this approach has been used to support the claim that CCT is the target of ATLs like edelfosine (Baburina and Jackowski 1998; van der Luit et al. 2002, 2003).

10 Concluding Remarks

The current mode of action of ATLs as agents targeting lipid platforms in tumor cell membranes has enormous significance with regard to:

1. *Targeting broad range of cancer types*: regulation of proliferative signals by membrane domains occurs in all cancer cells. In this regard it is well documented that ATLs affect a wide range of cancer cell types and current models of action reconcile the disparate effects reported for ATLs on a plethora of signaling pathways in different cell types. Therefore, upon cellular uptake, ATLs affect membrane organization in cancer cells altering signal cascades, regardless of which signaling pathway/s may govern their uncontrolled proliferation.
2. *Suppression of metastasis*: many mechanisms leading to metastasis are associated with functional coordination of signaling pathways by lipid domains. Thus, being lipid domain-disturbing agents, ATLs would promote dual suppression of tumor progression (1) and metastasis.
3. *Overcoming drug resistance*: since multidrug resistance pumps may require association with lipid domains to be active, ATLs have the potential to increase effectiveness of chemotherapeutic agents when added in combination (in addition to having a different mode of action).
4. *Advancing knowledge of unique traits in cancer cells*: an ideal chemotherapeutic drug should selectively kill tumor cells while sparing normal cells. That characterizes antitumor lipid drugs, but the molecular alterations that provide selective tumor toxicity are still unknown. Further investigation involving lipidomic and proteomic characterizations of cancer membranes should provide new insights into the molecular basis behind ATL selectivity for tumors and aid in the design of novel strategies to increase ATL efficacy.

References

Adam RM, Mukhopadhyay NK, Kim J, Di Vizio D, Cinar B, Boucher K et al (2007) Cholesterol sensitivity of endogenous and myristoylated Akt. Cancer Res 67(13):6238–6246

Alam MM, Joh EH, Kim Y, Oh YI, Hong J, Kim B et al (2012) Synthesis and biological evaluation of cyclopentane-linked alkyl phosphocholines as potential anticancer agents that act by inhibiting Akt phosphorylation. Eur J Med Chem 47:485–492

Allen JA, Halverson-Tamboli RA, Rasenick MM (2007) Lipid raft microdomains and neurotransmitter signalling. Nat Rev Neurosci 8:128–140

Andreesen R, Modolell M, Weltzien HU, Eibl H, Common HH, Löhr GW, Munder PG (1978) Selective destruction of human leukemic cells by alkyl-lysophospholipids. Cancer Res 38(11 Pt 1):3894–3899

Andreesen R, Modolell M, Munder PG (1979) Selective sensitivity of chronic myelogenous leukemia cell populations to alkyl-lysophospholipids. Blood 54:519–523

Arnold D, Weltzien HU, Westphal O (1967) Concerning the synthesis of lysolecithin and its ether analogs. Justus Liebigs Ann Chem 709:234–239

Arnold B, Reuther R, Weltzien HU (1978) Distribution and metabolism of synthetic alkyl analogs of lysophosphatidylcholine in mice. Biochim Biophys Acta 530:47–55

Arthur G, Bittman R (1998) The inhibition of cell signaling pathways by antitumor ether lipids. Biochim Biophys Acta 1390(1):85–102

Ashagbley A, Samadder P, Bittman R, Erukulla RK, Byun HS, Arthur G (1996) Synthesis of ether-linked analogues of lysophosphatidate and their effect on the proliferation of human epithelial cancer cells in vitro. Anticancer Res 16(4A):1813–1818

Aznar MÁ, Lasa-Saracíbar B, Blanco-Prieto MJ (2014) Edelfosine lipid nanoparticles overcome multidrug resistance in K-562 leukemia cells by a caspase-independent mechanism. Mol Pharm 11:2650–2658

Baburina I, Jackowski S (1998) Apoptosis triggered by 1-O-octadecyl-2-O-methyl-rac-glycero-3-phosphocholine is prevented by increased expression of CTP:phosphocholine cytidylyltransferase. J Biol Chem 273(4):2169–2173

Bailey HH, Mahoney MR, Ettinger DS, Maples WJ, Fracasso PM, Traynor AM et al (2006) Phase II study of daily oral perifosine in patients with advanced soft tissue sarcoma. Cancer 107(10):2462–2467

Becher OJ, Millard NE, Modak S, Kushner BH, Haque S, Spasojevic I et al (2017) A phase I study of single-agent perifosine for recurrent or refractory pediatric CNS and solid tumors. PLoS One 12(6):e0178593

Benvegnu DJ, McConnell HM (1992) Line tension between liquid domains in lipid monolayers. J Phys Chem 96:6820–6824

Berdel WE (1982) Antineoplastic activity of synthetic lysophospholipid analogs. Blut 44:71–78

Berdel WE, Bausert WR, Fink U, Rastetter J, Munder PG (1981a) Anti-tumor action of alkyl-lysophospholipids (review). Anticancer Res 1(6):345–352

Berdel WE, Fink U, Egger B, Reichert A, Munder PG, Rastetter J (1981b) Inhibition by alkyl-lysophospholipids of tritiated thymidine uptake in cells of human malignant urologic tumors. J Natl Cancer Inst 66(5):813–817

Berdel WE, Fromm M, Fink U, Pahlke W, Bicker U, Reichert A, Rastetter J (1983a) Cytotoxicity of thioether-lysophospholipids in leukemias and tumors of human origin. Cancer Res 43(11): 5538–5543

Berdel WE, Greiner E, Fink U, Stavrou D, Reichert A, Rastetter J et al (1983b) Cytotoxicity of alkyl-lysophospholipid derivatives and low-alkyl-cleavage enzyme activities in rat brain tumor cells. Cancer Res 43(2):541–545

Berdel WE, Fink U, Rastetter J (1987) Clinical phase I pilot study of the alkyl lysophospholipid derivative ET-18-OCH3 1. Lipids 22(11):967–969

Bhattacharya SK et al (2007) Phase 4 trial of miltefosine for the treatment of Indian visceral leishmaniasis. J Infect Dis 196:591–598

Boggs KP, Rock CO, Jackowski S (1995) Lysophosphatidylcholine and 1-O-octadecyl-2-O-methyl-rac-glycero-3-phosphocholine inhibit the CDP-choline pathway of phosphatidylcholine synthesis at the CTP:phosphocholine cytidylyltransferase step. J Biol Chem 270(13):7757–7764

Brachwitz H, Langen P, Hintsche R, Schildt J (1982) Halo lipids. V. Synthesis, nuclear magnetic resonance spectra and cytostatic properties of halo analogues of alkyllysophospholipids. Chem Phys Lipids 31:33–52

Brancucci NMB, Gerdt JP, Wang C, De Niz M, Philip N, Adapa SR et al (2017) Lysophosphatidylcholine regulates sexual stage differentiation in the human malaria parasite *Plasmodium falciparum*. Cell 171(7):1532–1544.e15

Brown DA, London E (1998a) Functions of lipid rafts in biological membranes. Annu Rev Cell Dev Biol 14:111–136

Brown DA, London E (1998b) Structure and origin of ordered lipid domains in biological membranes. J Membr Biol 164:103–114

Busto JV, Sot J, Goni FM, Mollinedo F, Alonso A (2007) Surface-active properties of the antitumour ether lipid 1-O-octadecyl-2-O-methyl-rac-glycero-3-phosphocholine (edelfosine). Biochim Biophys Acta 1768:1855–1860

Busto JV, del Canto-Jañez E, Goñi F, Mollinedo F, Alonso A (2008) Combination of the antitumour cell ether lipid edelfosine with sterols abolishes haemolytic side effects of the drug. J Chem Biol 1:89–94

Chakrabandhu K, Hérincs Z, Huault S, Dost B, Peng L, Conchonaud F et al (2007) Palmitoylation is required for efficient Fas cell death signaling. EMBO J 26(1):209–220

Chen R, Brady E, McIntyre TM (2011) Human TMEM30a promotes uptake of antitumor and bioactive choline phospholipids into mammalian cells. J Immunol 186(5):3215–3225

Chignard M, Le Couedic JP, Tence M, Vargaftig BB, Benveniste J (1979) The role of platelet-activating factor in platelet aggregation. Nature 279(5716):799–800

Clayman RV, Gonzalez R, Elliott AY, Gleason DE, Dempsey ME (1983) Cholesterol accumulation in heterotransplanted renal cell cancer. J Urol 129(3):621–624

Croft SL, Neal RA, Pendergast W, Chan JH (1987) The activity of alkyl phosphorylcholines and related derivatives against Leishmania donovani. Biochem Pharmacol 36(16):2633–2636

Crul M et al (2002) Phase I and pharmacological study of daily oral administration of perifosine (D-21266) in patients with advanced solid tumours. Eur J Cancer 38:1615–1621

Cuesta-Marbán Á, Botet J, Czyz O, Cacharro LM, Gajate C, Hornillos V et al (2013) Drug uptake, lipid rafts, and vesicle trafficking modulate resistance to an anticancer lysophosphatidylcholine analogue in yeast. J Biol Chem 288(12):8405–8418

Czyz O, Bitew T, Cuesta-Marbán A, McMaster CR, Mollinedo F, Zaremberg V (2013) Alteration of plasma membrane organization by an anticancer lysophosphatidylcholine analogue induces intracellular acidification and internalization of plasma membrane transporters in yeast. J Biol Chem 288(12):8419–8432

Dorlo TPC, Balasegaram M, Beijnen JH, de Vries PJ (2012) Miltefosine: a review of its pharmacology and therapeutic efficacy in the treatment of leishmaniasis. J Antimicrob Chemother 67(11): 2576–2597

dos Santos GA, Thome CH, Ferreira GA, Yoneda JS, Nobre TM, Daghastanli KR et al (2010) Interaction of 10-(octyloxy) decyl-2-(trimethylammonium) ethyl phosphate with mimetic membranes and cytotoxic effect on leukemic cells. Biochim Biophys Acta 1798:1714–1723

Drings P, Günther I, Gatzemeier U, Ulbrich F, Khanavkar B, Schreml W et al (1992) Final evaluation of a phase II study on the effect of edelfosine (an ether lipid) in advanced non-small-cell bronchogenic carcinoma. Oncol Res Treat 15(5):375–382

Duclos RI Jr, Makriyannis A (1992) Syntheses of all four stereoisomers which are conformationally constrained 1, 4-dioxanyl analogs of the antineoplastic ether lipid ET-18-OCH3. J Org Chem 57:6156–6163

Dummer R, Krasovec M, Röger J, Sindermann H, Burg G (1993) Topical administration of hexadecylphosphocholine in patients with cutaneous lymphomas: results of a phase I/II study. J Am Acad Dermatol 29(6):963–970

Edidin M (2003) The state of lipid rafts: from model membranes to cells. Annu Rev Biophys Biomol Struct 32:257–283

Epand RM (1990) Relationship of phospholipid hexagonal phases to biological phenomena. Biochem Cell Biol 68:17–23

Erdlenbruch B, Jendrossek V, Marx M, Hunold A, Eibl H, Lakomek M (1998) Antitumor effects of erucylphosphocholine on brain tumor cells in vitro and in vivo. Anticancer Res 18(4A): 2551–2557

Fiegl M, Lindner LH, Juergens M, Eibl H, Hiddemann W, Braess J (2008) Erufosine, a novel alkylphosphocholine, in acute myeloid leukemia: single activity and combination with other antileukemic drugs. Cancer Chemother Pharmacol 62(2):321–329

Figg WD, Monga M, Headlee D, Shah A, Chau CH, Peer C et al (2014) A phase I and pharmacokinetic study of oral perifosine with different loading schedules in patients with refractory neoplasms. Cancer Chemother Pharmacol 74(5):955–967

Folmer DE, Mok KS, de Wee SW, Duijst S, Hiralall JK, Seppen J et al (2012) Cellular localization and biochemical analysis of mammalian CDC50A, a glycosylated β-subunit for P4 ATPases. J Histochem Cytochem 60(3):205–218

Frisz JF, Lou K, Klitzing HA, Hanafin WP, Lizunov V, Wilson RL, Carpenter KJ, Kim R, Hutcheon ID, Zimmerberg J et al (2013) Direct chemical evidence for sphingolipid domains in the plasma membranes of fibroblasts. Proc Natl Acad Sci U S A 110:E613–E622

Fujiwara K, Modest EJ, Welander CE, Wallen CA (1989) Cytotoxic interactions of heat and an ether lipid analogue in human ovarian carcinoma cells. Cancer Res 49(22):6285–6289

Gajate C, Mollinedo F (2001) The antitumor ether lipid ET-18-OCH(3) induces apoptosis through translocation and capping of Fas/CD95 into membrane rafts in human leukemic cells. Blood 98(13):3860–3863

Gajate C, Mollinedo F (2002) Biological activities, mechanisms of action and biomedical prospect of the antitumor ether phospholipid ET-18-OCH(3) (edelfosine), a proapoptotic agent in tumor cells. Curr Drug Metab 3(5):491–525

Gajate C, Mollinedo F (2007) Edelfosine and perifosine induce selective apoptosis in multiple myeloma by recruitment of death receptors and downstream signaling molecules into lipid rafts. Blood 109(2):711–719

Gajate C, Fonteriz RI, Cabaner C, Alvarez-Noves G, Alvarez-Rodriguez Y, Modolell M, Mollinedo F (2000a) Intracellular triggering of Fas, independently of FasL, as a new mechanism of antitumor ether lipid-induced apoptosis. Int J Cancer 85(5):674–682

Gajate C, Santos-Beneit AM, Macho A, Lazaro M d C, Hernandez-De Rojas A, Modolell M et al (2000b) Involvement of mitochondria and caspase-3 in ET-18-OCH3-induced apoptosis of human leukemic cells. Int J Cancer 86(2):208–218

Gajate C, del Canto-Jañez E, Acuña AU, Amat-Guerri F, Geijo E, Santos-Beneit AM et al (2004) Intracellular triggering of fas aggregation and recruitment of apoptotic molecules into fas-enriched rafts in selective tumor cell apoptosis. J Exp Med 200(3):353–365

Gajate C, Gonzalez-Camacho F, Mollinedo F (2009) Involvement of raft aggregates enriched in Fas/CD95 death-inducing signaling complex in the antileukemic action of edelfosine in Jurkat cells. PLoS One 4(4):e5044

Garcia-Saez AJ, Chiantia S, Schwille P (2007) Effect of line tension on the lateral organization of lipid membranes. J Biol Chem 282:33537–33544

George KS, Wu S (2012) Lipid raft: a floating island of death or survival. Toxicol Appl Pharmacol 259:311–319

Ghobrial IM et al (2010) Clinical and translational studies of a phase II trial of the novel oral Akt inhibitor perifosine in relapsed or relapsed/refractory Waldenstrom's macroglobulinemia. Clin Cancer Res 16:1033–1041

Gil C, Molina E, Plana M, Carabaza A, Cabré F, Mauleón D et al (1996) Differential effect of alkyl chain-modified ether lipids on protein kinase C autophosphorylation and histone phosphorylation. Biochem Pharmacol 52(12):1843–1847

Gills JJ, Dennis PA (2009) Perifosine: update on a novel Akt inhibitor. Curr Oncol Rep 11(2): 102–110

Gomide AB, Thome CH, dos Santos GA, Ferreira GA, Faca VM, Rego EM et al (2013) Disrupting membrane raft domains by alkylphospholipids. Biochim Biophys Acta 1828:1384–1389

Gorter E, Grendel F (1925) On bimolecular layers of lipoids on the chromocytes of the blood. J Exp Med 41:439–443

Hąc-Wydro K, Dynarowicz-Łątka P (2010a) Searching for the role of membrane sphingolipids in selectivity of antitumor ether lipid–edelfosine. Colloids Surf B: Biointerfaces 81:492–497

Hąc-Wydro K, Dynarowicz-Łątka P (2010b) The relationship between the concentration of ganglioside GM1 and antitumor activity of edelfosine—the Langmuir monolayer study. Colloids Surf B: Biointerfaces 81:385–388

Hąc-Wydro K, Flasiński M, Wydro P, Dynarowicz-Łątka P (2012) Towards the understanding of the behavior of single-chained ether phospholipids in model biomembranes: interactions with phosphatidylethanolamines in Langmuir monolayers. Colloids Surf B: Biointerfaces 97: 162–170

Hanson PK, Malone L, Birchmore JL, Nichols JW (2003) Lem3p is essential for the uptake and potency of alkylphosphocholine drugs, edelfosine and miltefosine. J Biol Chem 278(38):36041–36050

Head BP, Patel HH, Insel PA (2014) Interaction of membrane/lipid rafts with the cytoskeleton: impact on signaling and function: membrane/lipid rafts, mediators of cytoskeletal arrangement and cell signaling. Biochim Biophys Acta 1838:532–545

Helfman DM, Barnes KC, Kinkade JM, Vogler WR, Shoji M, Kuo JF (1983) Phospholipid-sensitive Ca2+-dependent protein phosphorylation system in various types of leukemic cells from human patients and in human leukemic cell lines HL60 and K562, and its inhibition by alkyl-lysophospholipid. Cancer Res 43(6):2955–2961

Henke G, Lindner LH, Vogeser M, Eibl H-J, Wörner J, Müller AC et al (2009) Pharmacokinetics and biodistribution of erufosine in nude mice--implications for combination with radiotherapy. Radiat Oncol 4:46

Herrmann DB, Neumann HA (1987) Cytotoxic activity of the thioether phospholipid analogue BM 41.440 in primary human tumor cultures. Lipids 22(11):955–957

Hilgard P, Klenner T, Stekar J, Unger C (1993) Alkylphosphocholines: a new class of membrane-active anticancer agents. Cancer Chemother Pharmacol 32(2):90–95

Hoffman RD, Kligerman M, Sundt TM, Anderson ND, Shin HS (1982) Stereospecific chemo-attraction of lymphoblastic cells by gradients of lysophosphatidylcholine. Proc Natl Acad Sci 79(10):3285–3289

Hoffman DR, Hajdu J, Snyder F (1984) Cytotoxicity of platelet activating factor and related alkyl-phospholipid analogs in human leukemia cells, polymorphonuclear neutrophils, and skin fibro-blasts. Blood 63(3):545–552

Horowitz LF, Hirdes W, Suh B-C, Hilgemann DW, Mackie K, Hille B (2005) Phospholipase C in living cells. J Gen Physiol 126(3):243–262

Houlihan WJ, Lee ML, Munder PG, Nemecek GM, Handley DA, Winslow CM et al (1987) Antitumor activity of SRI 62-834, a cyclic ether analog of ET-18-OCH3. Lipids 22(11): 884–890

Huang J, Feigenson GW (1999) A microscopic interaction model of maximum solubility of chole-sterol in lipid bilayers. Biophys J 76:2142–2157

Huang C, Mason JT, Stephenson FA, Levin IW (1984) Raman and phosphorus-31 NMR spectro-scopic identification of a highly ordered lamellar phase in aqueous dispersions of 1-stearoyl-2-acetyl-sn-glycero-3-phosphorylcholine. J Phys Chem 88:6454–6458

Huang C, Mason JT, Stephenson FA, Levin IW (1986) Polymorphic phase behavior of platelet-activating factor. Biophys J 49:587–595

Hui SW, Huang CH (1986) X-ray diffraction evidence for fully interdigitated bilayers of 1-stearoyllysophosphatidylcholine. Biochemistry 25:1330–1335

Israelachvili JN (1977) Refinement of the fluid-mosaic model of membrane structure. Bio-chim Biophys Acta 469:221–225

Jaffrès P-A, Gajate C, Bouchet AM, Couthon-Gourvès H, Chantôme A, Potier-Cartereau M et al (2016) Alkyl ether lipids, ion channels and lipid raft reorganization in cancer therapy. Pharmacol Ther 165:114–131

Jain MK, Crecely RW, Hille JDR, de Haas GH, Gruner SM (1985) Phase properties of the aqueous dispersions of n-octadecylphosphocholine. Biochim Biophys Acta 813:68–76

Jendrossek V, Hammersen K, Erdlenbruch B, Kugler W, Krügener R, Eibl H, Lakomek M (2002) Structure-activity relationships of alkylphosphocholine derivatives: antineoplastic action on brain tumor cell lines in vitro. Cancer Chemother Pharmacol 50(1):71–79

Jha TK et al (1999) Miltefosine, an oral agent, for the treatment of Indian visceral leishmaniasis. N Engl J Med 341:1795–1800

Kamphorst JJ, Cross JR, Fan J, de Stanchina E, Mathew R, White EP et al (2013) Hypoxic and Ras-transformed cells support growth by scavenging unsaturated fatty acids from lysophospho-lipids. Proc Natl Acad Sci 110(22):8882–8887

Karnovsky MJ, Kleinfeld AM, Hoover RL, Klausner RD (1982) The concept of lipid domains in membranes. J Cell Biol 94:1–6

Kelley EE, Modest EJ, Burns CP (1993) Unidirectional membrane uptake of the ether lipid antineoplastic agent edelfosine by L1210 cells. Biochem Pharmacol 45(12):2435–2439

Koenigsmann MP, Notter M, Knauf WU, Papadimitriou CA, Oberberg D, Reufi B et al (1996) Chemopurging of peripheral blood-derived progenitor cells by alkyl-lysophospholipid and its effect on haematopoietic rescue after high-dose therapy. Bone Marrow Transplant 18(3): 549–557

Kondapaka SB, Singh SS, Dasmahapatra GP, Sausville EA, Roy KK (2003) Perifosine, a novel alkylphospholipid, inhibits protein kinase B activation. Mol Cancer Ther 2(11):1093–1103

Kosano H, Takatani O (1988) Reduction of epidermal growth factor binding in human breast cancer cell lines by an alkyl-lysophospholipid. Cancer Res 48(21):6033–6036

Krycer JR, Brown AJ (2013) Cholesterol accumulation in prostate cancer: a classic observation from a modern perspective. Biochim Biophys Acta 1835(2):219–229

Kuhlencord A, Maniera T, Eibl H, Unger C (1992) Hexadecylphosphocholine: oral treatment of visceral leishmaniasis in mice. Antimicrob Agents Chemother 36(8):1630–1634

Kusumi A, Fujiwara TK, Morone N, Yoshida KJ, Chadda R, Xie M et al (2012) Membrane mechanisms for signal transduction: the coupling of the meso-scale raft domains to membrane-skeleton-induced compartments and dynamic protein complexes. Semin Cell Dev Biol 23(2): 126–144

Lasa-Saracíbar B, Aznar MÁ, Lana H, Aizpún I, Gil AG, Blanco-Prieto MJ (2014) Lipid nanoparticles protect from edelfosine toxicity in vivo. Int J Pharm 474:1–5

Lauber K, Bohn E, Kröber SM, Xiao Y, Blumenthal SG, Lindemann RK et al (2003) Apoptotic cells induce migration of phagocytes via caspase-3-mediated release of a lipid attraction signal. Cell 113(6):717–730

Lee AG, Birdsall NJM, Metcalfe JC, Toon PA, Warren GB (1974) Clusters in lipid bilayers and the interpretation of thermal effects in biological membranes. Biochemistry 13:3699–3705

Li YC, Park MJ, Ye S-K, Kim C-W, Kim Y-N (2006) Elevated levels of cholesterol-rich lipid rafts in cancer cells are correlated with apoptosis sensitivity induced by cholesterol-depleting agents. Am J Pathol 168(4):1107–1118

Lingwood D, Simons K (2010) Lipid rafts as a membrane-organizing principle. Science 327:46–50

Lu X, Arthur G (1992) Perturbations of cellular acylation processes by the synthetic alkyl-lysophospholipid 1-O-octadecyl-2-O-methylglycero-3-phosphocholine do not correlate with inhibition of proliferation of MCF7 and T84 cell lines. Cancer Res 52(10):2806–2812

Lu SM, Fairn GD (2018) Mesoscale organization of domains in the plasma membrane – beyond the lipid raft. Crit Rev Biochem Mol Biol 53(2):192–207

Marsh R d W et al (2007) A phase II trial of perifosine in locally advanced, unresectable, or metastatic pancreatic adenocarcinoma. Am J Clin Oncol 30:26–31

Maurer N, Prenner E, Paltauf F, Glatter O (1994) Phase behavior of the antineoplastic ether lipid 1-O-octadecyl-2-O-methyl-glycero-3-phosphocholine. Biochim Biophys Acta 1192:167–176

McConnell HM, De Koker R (1996) Equilibrium thermodynamics of lipid monolayer domains. Langmuir 12:4897–4904

Modolell M, Andreesen R, Pahlke W, Brugger U, Munder PG (1979) Disturbance of phospholipid metabolism during the selective destruction of tumor cells induced by alkyl-lysophospholipids. Cancer Res 39:4681–4686

Mollinedo F, Fernández-Luna JL, Gajate C, Martín-Martín B, Benito A, Martínez-Dalmau R, Modolell M (1997) Selective induction of apoptosis in cancer cells by the ether lipid ET-18-OCH3 (edelfosine): molecular structure requirements, cellular uptake, and protection by Bcl-2 and Bcl-X(L). Cancer Res 57(7):1320–1328

Mollinedo F, Gajate C, Martín-Santamaría S, Gago F (2004) ET-18-OCH3 (edelfosine): a selective antitumour lipid targeting apoptosis through intracellular activation of Fas/CD95 death receptor. Curr Med Chem 11(24):3163–3184

Mueller RB, Sheriff A, Gaipl US, Wesselborg S, Lauber K (2007) Attraction of phagocytes by apoptotic cells is mediated by lysophosphatidylcholine. Autoimmunity 40(4):342–344

Munder PG, Modolell M (1973) Adjuvant induced formation of lysophosphatides and their role in the immune response. Int Arch Allergy Appl Immunol 45(1):133–135

Munder PG, Ferber E, Modolell M, Fischer H (1969) The influence of various adjuvants on the metabolism of phospholipids in macrophages. Int Arch Allergy Appl Immunol 36(1):117–128

Munder PG, Modolell M, Andreesen R, Weltzien HU, Westphal O (1979) Lysophosphatidylcholine (lysolecithin) and its synthetic analogues. Immunemodulating and other biologic effects. Springer Semin Immunopathol 2(2):187–203

Muñoz-Martínez F, Torres C, Castanys S, Gamarro F (2008) The anti-tumor alkylphospholipid perifosine is internalized by an ATP-dependent translocase activity across the plasma membrane of human KB carcinoma cells. Biochim Biophys Acta 1778(2):530–540

Muñoz-Martínez F, Torres C, Castanys S, Gamarro F (2010) CDC50A plays a key role in the uptake of the anticancer drug perifosine in human carcinoma cells. Biochem Pharmacol 80(6): 793–800

Munro S (2003) Lipid rafts: elusive or illusive? Cell 115:377–388

Mushayakarara EC, Mantsch HH (1985) Thermotropic phase behavior of the platelet-activating factor: an infrared spectroscopic study. Can J Biochem Cell Biol 63:1071–1076

Na H-K, Surh Y-J (2008) The antitumor ether lipid edelfosine (ET-18-O-CH3) induces apoptosis in H-ras transformed human breast epithelial cells: by blocking ERK1/2 and p38 mitogen-activated protein kinases as potential targets. Asia Pac J Clin Nutr 17(Suppl 1):204–207

Nagler A, Ben-Yehuda D, Badros A, Hari P, Hajek R, Spicka I et al (2013) Randomized placebo-controlled phase III study of perifosine combined with bortezomib and dexamethasone in relapsed, refractory multiple myeloma patients previously treated with bortezomib. Blood 122(21):3189

Nandi N, Vollhardt D, Brezesinski G (2004) Chiral discrimination effects in Langmuir monolayers of 1-O-hexadecyl glycerol. J Phys Chem B 108:327–335

Nieto-Miguel T, Gajate C, Mollinedo F (2006) Differential targets and subcellular localization of antitumor alkyl-lysophospholipid in leukemic *Versus* solid tumor cells. J Biol Chem 281(21): 14833–14840

Pike LJ (2003) Lipid rafts: bringing order to chaos. J Lipid Res 44(4):655–667

Pike LJ (2009) The challenge of lipid rafts. J Lipid Res 50:S323–S328

Porstmann T, Griffiths B, Chung Y-L, Delpuech O, Griffiths JR, Downward J, Schulze A (2005) PKB/Akt induces transcription of enzymes involved in cholesterol and fatty acid biosynthesis via activation of SREBP. Oncogene 24(43):6465–6481

Powis G, Seewald MJ, Gratas C, Melder D, Riebow J, Modest EJ (1992) Selective inhibition of phosphatidylinositol phospholipase C by cytotoxic ether lipid analogues. Cancer Res 52(10): 2835–2840

Prenner E, Honsek G, Hönig D, Möbius D, Lohner K (2007) Imaging of the domain organization in sphingomyelin and phosphatidylcholine monolayers. Chem Phys Lipids 145:106–118

Prescott SM, Zimmerman GA, McIntyre TM (1990) Platelet-activating factor. J Biol Chem 265(29):17381–17384

Quinn PJ (2010) A lipid matrix model of membrane raft structure. Prog Lipid Res 49:390–406

Rahman M et al (2011) Phase IV trial of miltefosine in adults and children for treatment of visceral leishmaniasis (kala-azar) in Bangladesh. Am J Trop Med Hyg 85:66–69

Rakotomanga M, Loiseau PM, Saint-Pierre-Chazalet M (2004) Hexadecylphosphocholine interaction with lipid monolayers. Biochim Biophys Acta 1661:212–218

Rey Gomez-Serranillos I, Minones J, Dynarowicz-Latka P, Minones J, Iribarnegaray E (2004) Miltefosine-cholesterol interactions: a monolayer study. Langmuir 20:928–933

Rietveld A, Simons K (1998) The differential miscibility of lipids as the basis for the formation of functional membrane rafts. Biochim Biophys Acta 1376:467–479

Ruiter GA, Zerp SF, Bartelink H, van Blitterswijk WJ, Verheij M (2003) Anti-cancer alkyl-lysophospholipids inhibit the phosphatidylinositol 3-kinase-Akt/PKB survival pathway. Anti-Cancer Drugs 14(2):167–173

Salari H, Dryden P, Davenport R, Howard S, Jones K, Bittman R (1992) Inhibition of protein kinase C by ether-linked lipids is not correlated with their antineoplastic activity on WEHI-3B and R6X-B15 cells. Biochim Biophys Acta 1134(1):81–88

Samadder P, Richards C, Bittman R, Bhullar RP, Arthur G (2003) The antitumor ether lipid 1-Q-octadecyl-2-O-methyl-rac-glycerophosphocholine (ET-18-OCH3) inhibits the association between Ras and Raf-1. Anticancer Res 23(3B):2291–2295

Scheidt HA, Muller P, Herrmann A, Huster D (2003) The potential of fluorescent and spin-labeled steroid analogs to mimic natural cholesterol. J Biol Chem 278(46):45563–45569

Scholar EM (1986) Inhibition of the growth of human lung cancer cells by alkyl-lysophospholipid analogs. Cancer Lett 33(2):199–204

Schroeder R, London E, Brown D (1994) Interactions between saturated acyl chains confer detergent resistance on lipids and glycosylphosphatidylinositol (GPI)-anchored proteins: GPI-anchored proteins in liposomes and cells show similar behavior. Proc Natl Acad Sci 91: 12130–12134

Schroeder F, Gallegos AM, Atshaves BP, Storey SM, McIntosh AL, Petrescu AD et al (2001) Recent advances in membrane microdomains: rafts, caveolae, and intracellular cholesterol trafficking. Exp Biol Med 226:873–890

Simons K, Ikonen E (1997) Functional rafts in cell membranes. Nature 387:569–572

Simons K, Sampaio JL (2011) Membrane organization and lipid rafts. Cold Spring Harb Perspect Biol 3(10):a004697

Simons K, Toomre D (2000) Lipid rafts and signal transduction. Nat Rev Mol Cell Biol 1:31–39

Simons K, Van Meer G (1988) Lipid sorting in epithelial cells. Biochemistry 27:6197–6202

Singer SJ, Nicolson GL (1972) The fluid mosaic model of the structure of cell membranes. Science 175:720–731

Smets LA, Van Rooij H, Salomons GS (1999) Signalling steps in apoptosis by ether lipids. Apoptosis 4(6):419–427

Smorenburg CH, Seynaeve C, Bontenbal M, Planting AS, Sindermann H, Verweij J (2000) Phase II study of miltefosine 6% solution as topical treatment of skin metastases in breast cancer patients. Anti-Cancer Drugs 11(10):825–828

Snyder F (1995) Platelet-activating factor: the biosynthetic and catabolic enzymes. Biochem J 305(Pt 3):689–705

Soodsma JF, Piantadosi C, Snyder F (1970) The biocleavage of alkyl glyceryl ethers in Morris hepatomas and other transplantable neoplasms. Cancer Res 30(2):309–311

Sundar S, Olliaro PL (2007) Miltefosine in the treatment of leishmaniasis: clinical evidence for informed clinical risk management. Ther Clin Risk Manag 3(5):733–740

Sundar S et al (1999) Oral treatment of visceral leishmaniasis with miltefosine. Ann Trop Med Parasitol 93:589–597

Sundar S et al (2000) Short-course of oral miltefosine for treatment of visceral leishmaniasis. Clin Infect Dis 31:1110–1113

Tarnowski GS, Mountain IM, Stock CC, Munder PG, Weltzien HU, Westphal O (1978) Effect of lysolecithin and analogs on mouse ascites tumors. Cancer Res 38(2):339–344

Terwogt JMM, Mandjes IAM, Sindermann H, Beijnen JH, ten Bokkel Huinink WW (1999) Phase II trial of topically applied miltefosine solution in patients with skin-metastasized breast cancer. Br J Cancer 79(7–8):1158–1161

Thome CH, dos Santos GA, Ferreira GA, Scheucher PS, Izumi C, Leopoldino AM et al (2012) Linker for activation of T-cell family member2 (LAT2) a lipid raft adaptor protein for AKT signaling, is an early mediator of alkylphospholipid anti-leukemic activity. Mol Cell Proteomics 11:1898–1912

Thompson TE, Tillack TW (1985) Organization of glycosphingolipids in bilayers and plasma membranes of mammalian cells. Annu Rev Biophys Biophys Chem 14:361–386

Tidwell T, Guzman G, Vogler WR (1981) The effects of alkyl-lysophospholipids on leukemic cell lines. I. Differential action on two human leukemic cell lines, HL60 and K562. Blood 57(4): 794–797

Torrecillas A, Aroca-Aguilar JD, Aranda FJ, Gajate C, Mollinedo F, Corbalán-García S et al (2006) Effects of the anti-neoplastic agent ET-18-OCH3 and some analogs on the biophysical properties of model membranes. Int J Pharm 318:28–40

Uberall F, Oberhuber H, Maly K, Zaknun J, Demuth L, Grunicke HH (1991) Hexadecylphosphocholine inhibits inositol phosphate formation and protein kinase C activity. Cancer Res 51(3):807–812

Unger C, Eibl H, Kim DJ, Fleer EA, Kötting J, Bartsch HH et al (1987) Sensitivity of leukemia cell lines to cytotoxic alkyl-lysophospholipids in relation to O-alkyl cleavage enzyme activities. J Natl Cancer Inst 78(2):219–222

Unger C, Peukert M, Sindermann H, Hilgard P, Nagel G, Eibl H (1990) Hexadecylphosphocholine in the topical treatment of skin metastases in breast cancer patients. Cancer Treat Rev 17(2–3): 243–246

Valentino L, Moss T, Olson E, Wang H-J, Elashoff R, Ladisch S (1990) Shed tumor gangliosides and progression of human neuroblastoma. Blood 75:1564–1567

van Blitterswijk WJ, Verheij M (2008) Anticancer alkylphospholipids: mechanisms of action, cellular sensitivity and resistance, and clinical prospects. Curr Pharm Des 14:2061–2074

van der Luit AH, Budde M, Ruurs P, Verheij M, van Blitterswijk WJ (2002) Alkyl-lysophospholipid accumulates in lipid rafts and induces apoptosis via raft-dependent endocytosis and inhibition of phosphatidylcholine synthesis. J Biol Chem 277(42):39541–39547

Van Der Luit AH, Budde M, Verheij M, Van Blitterswijk WJ (2003) Different modes of internalization of apoptotic alkyl-lysophospholipid and cell-rescuing lysophosphatidylcholine. Biochem J 374(Pt 3):747–753

van der Luit AH, Vink SR, Klarenbeek JB, Perrissoud D, Solary E, Verheij M, van Blitterswijk WJ (2007) A new class of anticancer alkylphospholipids uses lipid rafts as membrane gateways to induce apoptosis in lymphoma cells. Mol Cancer Ther 6(8):2337–2345

Verweij J, Planting A, van der Burg M, Stoter G (1992) A dose-finding study of miltefosine (hexadecylphosphocholine) in patients with metastatic solid tumours. J Cancer Res Clin Oncol 118(8):606–608

Vink SR, van Blitterswijk WJ, Schellens JHM, Verheij M (2007a) Rationale and clinical application of alkylphospholipid analogues in combination with radiotherapy. Cancer Treat Rev 33(2):191–202

Vink SR, van der Luit AH, Klarenbeek JB, Verheij M, van Blitterswijk WJ (2007b) Lipid rafts and metabolic energy differentially determine uptake of anti-cancer alkylphospholipids in lymphoma versus carcinoma cells. Biochem Pharmacol 74(10):1456–1465

Vogler WR, Berdel WE (1993) Autologous bone marrow transplantation with alkyl-lysophospholipid-purged marrow. J Hematother 2(1):93–102

Vogler WR, Olson AC, Okamoto S, Somberg LB, Glasser L (1987) Experimental studies on the role of alkyl lysophospholipids in autologous bone marrow transplantation. Lipids 22(11): 919–924

Vogler W, Berdel W, Olson A, Winton E, Heffner L, Gordon D (1992) Autologous bone marrow transplantation in acute leukemia with marrow purged with alkyl-lysophospholipid. Blood 80(6):1423

Wang Y, Sweitzer TD, Weinhold PA, Kent C (1993) Nuclear localization of soluble CTP:phosphocholine cytidylyltransferase. J Biol Chem 268(8):5899–5904

Watkins JD, Kent C (1991) Regulation of CTP:phosphocholine cytidylyltransferase activity and subcellular location by phosphorylation in Chinese hamster ovary cells. The effect of phospholipase C treatment. J Biol Chem 266(31):21113–21117

Wong R, Fabian L, Forer A, Brill JA (2007) Phospholipase C and myosin light chain kinase inhibition define a common step in actin regulation during cytokinesis. BMC Cell Biol 8(1):15

Wright MM, Howe AG, Zaremberg V (2004) Cell membranes and apoptosis: role of cardiolipin, phosphatidylcholine, and anticancer lipid analogues. Biochem Cell Biol 82:18–26

Wu WG, Huang CH, Conley TG, Martin RB, Levin IW (1982) Lamellar-micellar transition of 1-stearoyllysophosphatidylcholine assemblies in excess water. Biochemistry 21:5957–5961

Wunderlich F, Ronai A, Speth V, Seelig J, Blume A (1975) Thermotropic lipid clustering in tetrahymena membranes. Biochemistry 14:3730–3735

Wunderlich F, Kreutz W, Mahler P, Ronai A, Heppeler G (1978) Thermotropic fluid→ordered "discontinuous" phase separation in microsomal lipids of tetrahymena. An X-ray diffraction study. Biochemistry 17:2005–2010

Zaremberg V, Gajate C, Cacharro LM, Mollinedo F, McMaster CR (2005) Cytotoxicity of an anticancer lysophospholipid through selective modification of lipid raft composition. J Biol Chem 280(45):38047–38058

Zhou X, Lu X, Richard C, Xiong W, Litchfield DW, Bittman R, Arthur G (1996) 1-O-octadecyl-2-O-methyl-glycerophosphocholine inhibits the transduction of growth signals via the MAPK cascade in cultured MCF-7 cells. J Clin Investig 98(4):937–944

Zhuang L, Kim J, Adam RM, Solomon KR, Freeman MR (2005) Cholesterol targeting alters lipid raft composition and cell survival in prostate cancer cells and xenografts. J Clin Investig 115(4):959–968

Zoeller RA, Layne MD, Modest EJ (1995) Animal cell mutants unable to take up biologically active glycerophospholipids. J Lipid Res 36(9):1866–1875

Part VI

Nuclear Trafficking of Lipids

Inositide-Dependent Nuclear Signalling in Health and Disease

Matilde Y. Follo, Stefano Ratti, Lucia Manzoli, Giulia Ramazzotti, Irene Faenza, Roberta Fiume, Sara Mongiorgi, Pann Ghill Suh, James A. McCubrey, and Lucio Cocco

Contents

Matilde Y. Follo, Stefano Ratti, and Lucia Manzoli contributed equally to this work.

M. Y. Follo · S. Ratti · L. Manzoli · G. Ramazzotti · I. Faenza · R. Fiume · S. Mongiorgi · L. Cocco (✉)
Cellular Signalling Laboratory, Department of Biomedical and Neuromotor Sciences, University of Bologna, Bologna, Italy
e-mail: lucio.cocco@unibo.it

P. G. Suh
Korea Brain Research Institute, Daegu, Republic of Korea

School of Life Sciences, UNIST, Ulsan, Republic of Korea

J. A. McCubrey
Department of Microbiology and Immunology, Brody School of Medicine, East Carolina University, Greenville, NC, USA

J. Gomez-Cambronero, M. A. Frohman (eds.), *Lipid Signaling in Human Diseases*, Handbook of Experimental Pharmacology 259, https://doi.org/10.1007/164_2019_321

Abstract
Nuclear inositides have a specific subcellular distribution that is linked to specific functions; thus their regulation is fundamental both in health and disease. Emerging evidence shows that alterations in multiple inositide signalling pathways are involved in pathophysiology, not only in cancer but also in other diseases. Here, we give an overview of the main features of inositides in the cell, and we discuss their potential as new molecular therapeutic targets.

Keywords
Cancer · Disease · Nuclear inositides

1 Eukaryotic Cell Nuclear Structure and Function: The Big Picture

1.1 General Characteristics

The eukaryotic cell nucleus is bounded by a double membrane of phospholipid bilayers, the nuclear envelope. With the exception of mitochondrial DNA, the rest of the genome is conserved inside the nucleus where long, linear DNA molecules complexed with histones forming the chromosomes that host the genes have different fundamental cell functions. The nucleus maintains the integrity of the genes, regulates gene expression, and mediates DNA replication during the cell cycle. It is responsible for cell compartmentalization and nuclear transport that can be either through the nuclear membrane itself or through the nuclear pores with carrier proteins that differ according to the size and characteristics of the molecules (e.g., proteins, ions, and RNA).

Inside the nucleus there are several structures and nuclear bodies that can be identified and that play different roles (Fig. 1). Among these structures, the nucleolus is mainly responsible for ribosome assembly before the ribosomes are exported to the cytoplasm to engage in mRNA translation, while the speckles are the sites on which phosphoinositides and their metabolizing enzymes (Cocco et al. 1994; Manzoli et al. 1997; Martelli et al. 2000) are localized along with splicing factors, transcription factors, diacylglycerol kinases (DGKs), and phosphatidylinositol (PI) (Jacobsen et al. 2019; Poli et al. 2016, 2017, 2018; Ramazzotti et al. 2019a; Ratti et al. 2017, 2018, 2019; Sztacho et al. 2019; Trubiani et al. 2016). The nucleus is approximately 6 μm, but its size and shape can change in different cells. The number of nuclei can also be different in some eukaryotic cell types, from zero in red blood cells to many nuclei in osteoclasts, reflecting the different function and requirements of these different cell types.

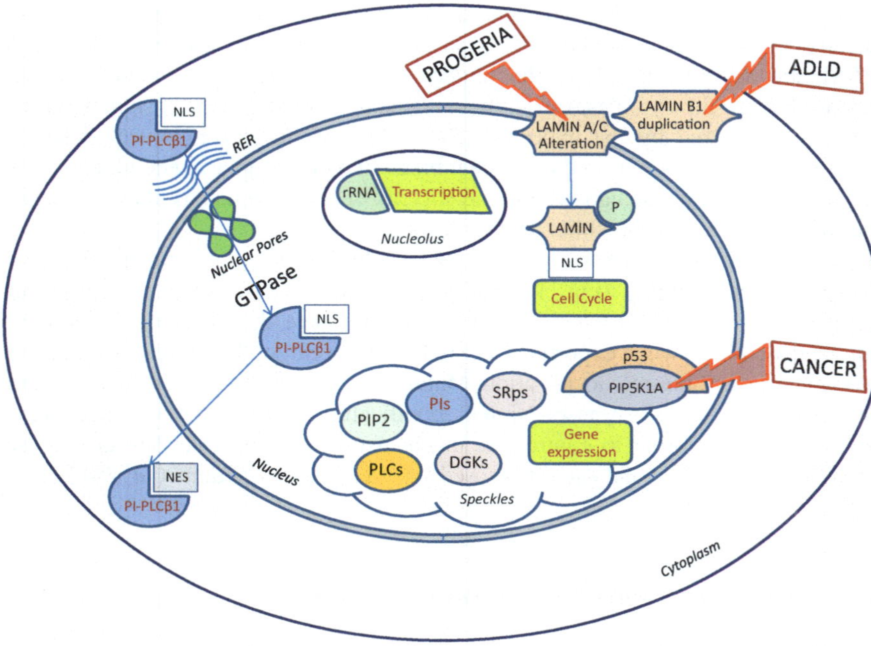

Fig. 1 The figure depicts the localization of the main players of inositide signalling molecules and, namely, the relationship between plasma membrane, cytoplasm, and nucleus, including the nuclear domains (i.e., nucleolus and speckles) in physiological conditions. Red arrows highlight the disease targets

1.2 Nuclear Membrane and Transport

The nuclear membrane is made of an inner and outer lipid bilayer membrane, divided by a perinuclear space. The outer membrane is continuous with the rough endoplasmic reticulum (RER). The nuclear pores, about 3,000–4,000 in mammalian cells, are fully extended through the nuclear envelope to enable the transport of specific molecules (Glass and Wente 2019). The complex of the nuclear pore and its related proteins, whose number vary in different animal species, is called nucleoporin. The pore molecular weight is about 125 million Da and the diameter is about 100 nm, resulting in a limitation of the molecular free diffusion to proteins no more than 9 nm wide. The passage of small water-soluble molecules is therefore passive, whereas larger molecules, such as nucleic acids and proteins, have to be actively transported. The pores have an eightfold-symmetric ring-shaped structure that attaches to the nuclear basket on the nucleoplasm side and to filaments that extend into the cytoplasm to enable protein nuclear transport.

Karyopherins are transport factors that are divided into importins and exportins according to the direction of the transport of the many proteins, ribosomal subunits, and some DNAs that they facilitate the movement of. They are assisted in this function by adaptor proteins. The "cargo" proteins that have to be translocated into the nucleus have short amino acid sequences called nuclear localization signals (NLS) that are recognized by the importins. Conversely, the proteins that are transported into the cytoplasm from the nucleus have nuclear export signals (NES) that are recognized by the exportins. Small lipid molecules involved in signal transduction can diffuse from the cell membrane into the cytoplasm and bind nuclear receptor proteins that are carried into the nucleus. Inside the nucleus, they can act as transcription factors if they bind to their ligand.

Active transport is driven by GTPases that hydrolyze guanosine triphosphate (GTP) to release energy (Fig. 1). Ran is the main GTPase involved in nuclear transport and binds GTP when importins have to leave their cargo or guanosine diphosphate (GDP) when exportins have to bind their cargo; therefore it is related to the nuclear or cytoplasmic localization. Mature mRNA and tRNA translocation into the cytoplasm after posttranscriptional modification is mediated by specialized export proteins in order to control the mechanism and to degrade RNAs that are incompletely modified and cannot be used for translation (Cautain et al. 2015).

1.3 Nuclear Lamina and Its Modifications

The nuclear lamina is formed by lamins and nuclear lamin-associated membrane proteins and is essential to support the nuclear envelope structure and assist with the assembly and disassembly of the nuclear membrane. Lamins are type V intermediate filament proteins with NLSs. They are divided into A type (lamin A, C) and B type (lamin B1, B2) (de Leeuw et al. 2018). Lamin phosphorylation by CDC2 protein kinases at the beginning of mitosis creates structural changes that trigger disassembly of the nuclear lamina. The nuclear lamina is reassembled by dephosphorylating the lamins. During apoptosis, caspases cleave the lamins and degrade the integrity of the nucleus, underlying the central role of lamins in nuclear processes such as cell cycle or apoptosis (Fig. 1). Indeed, the nuclear lamina is essential in chromatin organization during the different phases of cell cycle. The major nuclear lamin-associated membrane proteins are lamina-associated polypeptides 1 and 2 (LAP1, LAP2), emerin, lamin B receptor, MAN 1, otefin, and nesprin. They help to mediate the attachment of the nuclear lamina to the nuclear envelope and/or the cytoskeleton for structural support. The nuclear lamina network is synthetized in the cytoplasm, transported inside the nucleus, and assembled and incorporated into the nuclear envelope (Naetar et al. 2017). Mutations of lamin genes (Lamin A/C) can lead to defects in filament assembly resulting in laminopathies such as progeria (Ullrich and Gordon 2015). Conversely, duplication of lamin genes (lamin B1), as depicted in Fig. 1, can result in diseases such as the adult-onset autosomal dominant leukodystrophy (ADLD) (Padiath et al. 2006). The exact mechanisms of these pathologies are still under investigation (Dobrzynska et al. 2016).

1.4 Chromatin and Nucleosome

DNA is organized into a DNA-protein complex, the chromatin, that during cell division is organized into chromosomes (Cutter and Hayes 2015). Considering the function of chromatin in relation to DNA replication, repair, and recombination, its structure needs to be very dynamic in relation to the different stages of the cell cycle and the varying needs of the cell (Lai and Pugh 2017). The fundamental unit of chromatin is the nucleosome, which is composed of DNA and histone proteins. Nucleosomes can have different levels of DNA compaction, with the most highly condensed state being visible in metaphase chromosome. In contrast, chromatin is called euchromatin where the DNA is less compact and contains genes that are frequently expressed, and it is called heterochromatin where the DNA is more compact and contains genes that are infrequently transcribed (Venkatesh and Workman 2015). Moreover, epigenetic modifications via methylation and acetylation have different effects on chromatin structure and therefore gene expression.

1.5 Nucleolus and Other Nuclear Bodies

The nucleolus, the largest structure inside the nucleus, is the site of ribosomal RNA (rRNA) transcription, pre-rRNA processing, and ribosome subunit assembly (Pederson 2011). It assembles around rRNA gene repeat clusters in a dynamic manner related to the cell cycle. These regions are also named nuclear organizer regions (NOR). RNA polymerase I transcribes rDNA that forms a pre-rRNA precursor that is cleaved into 5.8S, 18S, and 28S rRNAs. Subsequently, inside the nucleolus, the transcription, posttranscriptional processing, and rRNA and ribosomal proteins assembly are performed (Fig. 1). Inside a nucleolus there are between 1 and 10 coiled bodies (CB) or Cajal bodies (Meier 2017). CB are involved in RNA processing, especially small nucleolar RNA (snoRNA) and small nuclear RNA (snRNA) maturation, but also in histone mRNA modification. In addition, polymorphic interphase karyosomal associations, or PIKA domains, are nuclear bodies that appear to be associated with the transcription of snRNA. Usually associated with CB are the promyelocytic leukemia bodies (PML bodies). These small nuclear bodies associated with the nuclear matrix are involved in many nuclear functions, from DNA replication to transcription, and epigenetic modifications (Chang et al. 2018). Among nuclear bodies, it is interesting to highlight the speckles, that are full of pre-messenger RNA splicing factors (Galganski et al. 2017). They localize in the interchromatin regions of the nucleoplasm in mammalian cells. As well as other nuclear bodies, speckles are very dynamic structures with a continuous protein cycle between different speckles and active transcriptional sites. The changes in the speckles are related to mRNA transcription and regulation. As Fig. 1 shows, nuclear inositides often co-localize with nuclear speckles, where they can directly regulate gene expression (Fiume et al. 2019; Martelli et al. 2005). In addition, there are also paraspeckles that are nuclear bodies involved in nuclear mechanisms in response to changes in cellular metabolic activity. They are considered to be "parallel," in being very close to the speckles (Fox and Lamond 2010). Another nuclear body is represented by the clastosomes that are present in the nucleus in high proteolytic conditions, but not in normal cells. Indeed, osmotic stress can induce clastosome activity that is related to catalytic activity in response to stress events (Lafarga et al. 2002).

2 Discovery and Hints to a Peculiar Function of Nuclear Inositide Signalling

Even though the presence of phospholipids in the nucleus has been reported since the 1970s (Manzoli et al. 1977), it was difficult to assign a role to these molecules at that time. Early in the 1980s, Smith and Wells (Smith and Wells 1983) reported the presence of phosphatidylinositol kinase and phosphatidylinositol phosphate kinase in rat liver nuclei, whose level of purity, i.e., contamination by membranes, did rise some doubts, but in 1987 a *Biochemical Journal* article by Cocco and Irvine (Cocco et al. 1987) clearly showed that highly purified nuclei from Friend cells, freed from nuclear membrane by Triton, can incorporate radiolabelled [gamma-32P]ATP into phosphatidic acid, phosphatidylinositol phosphate, and phosphatidylinositol 4,5-bisphosphate. The degree of radiolabelling of phosphatidylinositol bisphosphate was highly dependent on the state of differentiation of the cells, being barely detectable in growing cells and much greater after dimethyl sulfoxide-induced differentiation; this difference was mostly due to different amounts of phosphatidylinositol phosphate in the isolated nuclei. Interestingly, these changes were present only in the nuclear compartment.

This was the beginning of the story that has been furthered by the evidence of specific PIP kinase and diacylglycerol kinase (DGK) isoforms (Clarke et al. 2007; Raben and Tu-Sekine 2008; Goto et al. 2014). A new twist came from evidence of an inositide-dependent phospholipase C (PI-PLC) activity ascribed to the isoform β1 in the nuclei of several cell types, and more interestingly, this PLC is regulated in a different way than the cytoplasmatic one and acts in a separate manner (Divecha et al. 1991; Martelli et al. 1992; Xu et al. 2001).

A hint for the possible involvement of PI-PLCβ1 in the control of cell growth and differentiation came from its specific localization inside the nucleus. PI-PLCβ1 was found to be located in speckles (Fig. 1), which contain PIP2, DGK, transcription factors, and splicing factors as well (Bavelloni et al. 2006).

Very recently, it has been shown that a nuclear phosphoinositide kinase complex regulates p53 that protects the genome against cellular stress and is frequently mutated in cancer (Fig. 1), which provides a new hint for the importance of inositide signalling in health and disease (Choi et al. 2019).

3 Involvement of Nuclear Inositide-Dependent Signalling in Disease

3.1 General Characteristics

Nuclear inositides are finely regulated in stem cell metabolism (Manzoli et al. 1995), and their modifications can lead to disease or cancer (Mongiorgi et al. 2016a; Cocco et al. 2015; Blalock et al. 2011). That is why the role and localization of several kinases, phosphatases, and phospholipases are essential for the normal cell function (Follo et al. 2014; Ramazzotti et al. 2011; Follo et al. 2010; Cocco et al. 2010), as depicted in Fig. 2. This is true for a number of systems and organs, including brain, blood, breast, and muscle.

3.2 PI-PLCβ1/PI-PLCγ1: Brain and Nervous System

PI-PLCβ1 can be found in several parts of the brain, such as the cerebral cortex, hippocampus, amygdala, lateral septum, and olfactory bulb (Ross et al. 1989).

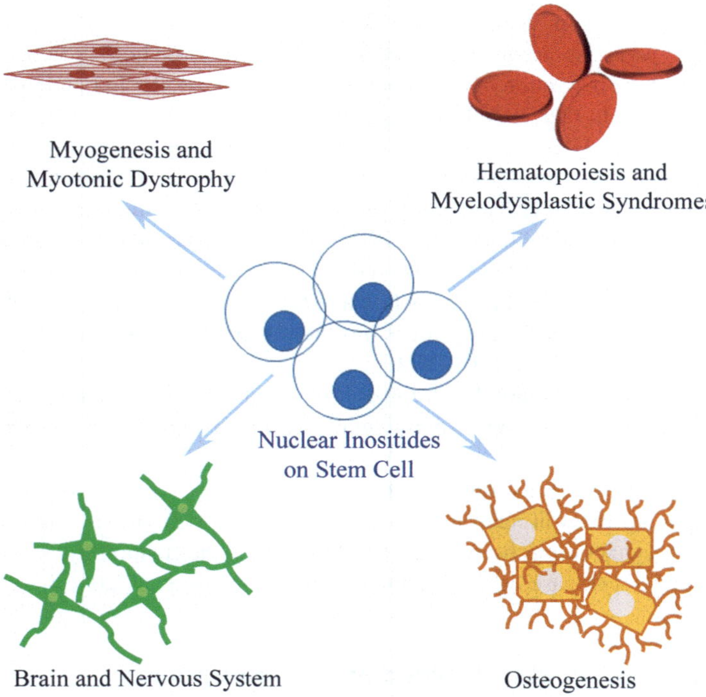

Fig. 2 The figure depicts the involvement of inositide signalling in stem cell differentiation, whose alteration is involved in diseases such as myelodysplastic syndromes, myotonic dystrophy, brain disorders, cancer, and osteogenesis

PI-PLCβ1 is particularly involved in both synaptic plasticity and cortical development, thanks to the regulation of gene expression in brain cortical neurons (Garcia del Cano et al. 2014) and the activation of hippocampal muscarinic acetylcholine receptor signal transduction pathways (Hannan et al. 1998).

Therefore, several brain disorders could stem from an impairment of PI-PLCβ1-dependent signal transduction pathways. In fact, PI-PLCβ1 deficiency can lead to epilepsy, abnormal neurogenesis, and aberrant migration of adult-born neurons (Choi et al. 1989; Kim et al. 1997).

PI-PLCβ1 has also been genetically associated with brain diseases, as human epileptic encephalopathies have been linked to specific PI-PLCβ1 gene mutations (Kurian et al. 2010). Moreover, a homozygous deletion of the PI-PLCβ1 gene was associated with the onset of malignant migrating partial seizures in infancy (Poduri et al. 2012), and PI-PLCβ1 gene deletions were detected also in orbitofrontal cortex samples from patients diagnosed with schizophrenia and bipolar disorders (Lo Vasco et al. 2012, 2013). As for the latter, PI-PLCβ1 and phosphoinositide-specific pathways represented good targets for therapies. This is the case for lithium, which is used for its ability to reduce the oxidative stress that occurs with multiple episodes of mania and depression. At a molecular level, lithium dampens excessive excitatory neurotransmission through PKC modulation, increases the expression of brain-derived neurotrophic factor, and inhibits glycogen synthase kinase 3, thus reducing neuronal apoptotic processes and showing protective effects (Malhi et al. 2013).

PI-PLCβ1 was also indirectly associated also with psychological stress and cancer, through the activation of α-adrenergic receptor (α-ADR) signalling pathways (Shin et al. 2016). In fact, α-ADRs can activate MAPKs or the PI3K/Akt pathway, thus enhancing cellular survival, blocking apoptosis, and finally promoting tumorigenesis (Follo et al. 2010; Cocco et al. 2010; Ross et al. 1989). Moreover, activation of α-ADR/PI-PLC signalling can also increase the amount of arachidonic acid, which is associated with the cAMP/PKA signal cascade and phosphorylation of CREB. In turn, phosphorylated CREB binds to the cyclin D promoter, and elevated cyclin D controls the G1/S phase transition and induces cell proliferation (Shin et al. 2016). Remarkably, α-ADR antagonists or other agents that inhibit the α-ADR/PI-PLC signalling but are not direct ADR blockers could be candidate anticancer drugs: this is the case for propranolol, norepinephrine, and the β2-adrenergic antagonist ICI118,551, which are being experimentally tested as novel anticancer agents (Zhang et al. 2011).

PI-PLCγ1 is additionally highly expressed in a broad range of brain regions, playing important roles in neuronal function, like neurite outgrowth, neuronal cell migration and synaptic plasticity (Park and Poo 2013), and pathology, i.e., depression, Huntington's disease, and Alzheimer's disease (Yang et al. 2016).

3.3 PI-PLCβ1/PI-PLCγ1: Blood and Hematopoiesis

Nuclear PI-PLCβ1 is essential for the regulation of hematopoiesis, particularly for myeloid and erythroid lineages, for which it has opposing behaviors: during erythroid differentiation it decreases, whereas its expression is induced during myeloid differentiation (Manzoli et al. 2014; Mongiorgi et al. 2016b).

More specifically, both in murine erythroleukemia cells and in normal CD34+ cells subjected to erythropoietin stimulation, PI-PLCβ1 expression decreases (Follo et al. 2012a). Furthermore, PI-PLCβ1 and nuclear inositide signalling pathways show the same trend also in myelodysplastic syndrome (MDS) cells responding to erythropoiesis-stimulating agents, i.e., erythropoietin or lenalidomide (Poli et al. 2018; Follo et al. 2012b, 2013). These data suggest that PI-PLCβ1 plays an inhibiting role in erythroid differentiation that, however, is countered by PI-PLCγ1, another PI-PLC isozyme whose nuclear-specific subcellular localization is associated with erythropoiesis in mouse models (Liao et al. 2002).

Remarkably, PI-PLCγ1, but also PI-PLCγ2, play important roles also in myeloid differentiation, being involved in the monocytic differentiation (Alimandi et al. 1997; Barbosa et al. 2014). Again, PI-PLCβ1 also participates in these processes, showing a specific increase in MDS cells (Follo et al. 2011, 2012c). In fact, MDS patients that respond to azacitidine, an epigenetic drug that induces myeloid differentiation, show a specific early increase of nuclear PI-PLCβ1 expression, decreased expression of phosphorylated Akt, an induction of normal myeloid differentiation (through MZF-1 recruitment), and a longer favorable clinical response (Cocco et al. 2015; Finelli et al. 2016). Surprisingly, PI-PLCβ1 is a dynamic marker of response, as its reduction is associated with a loss of response even in patients that initially had a positive response to azacitidine (Follo et al. 2012c; Fili et al. 2013).

A recent study analyzed the molecular effect of the current azacitidine and lenalidomide combination therapy on the mutation profile of cancer-specific genes associated with myeloid neoplasms, as well as a selection of inositide genes (Follo et al. 2019). The study reported a correlation between patients showing decreasing variant allele frequency during therapy and a favorable response to therapy (Follo et al. 2019). In particular, the analyses showed that the most frequently mutated cancer-related myeloid genes were ASXL1 (47%), TET2 (37%), RUNX1 (27%), and SRSF2 (17%), with an association between mutated SRSF2 and AML evolution. As for the inositide-specific genes, a cluster of eight genes never showed mutations, neither at baseline nor during therapy. Among them were inositide genes directly involved in cell cycle regulation (PKCα) or genes associated with myeloid differentiation that were linked to inositide metabolism (MZF-1, which is associated with PI-PLCβ1). On the other hand, 21/31 genes showed mutations at baseline and during the treatment, and 19/31 genes acquired specific variants. A deeper analysis of the inositide-specific mutation profile revealed a small cluster of six genes commonly mutated only in non-responder patients or in patients losing response. More interestingly, three of these genes (PIK3CD, AKT3, and PLCG2) acquired the same three point mutations: D133E in the PIK3CD gene, D280G in the AKT3 gene, and Q548R in the PLCG2 gene. Remarkably, the presence of this inositide-mutated three-gene cluster was significantly associated with shortened overall survival, leukemia-free survival, and shorter duration of response. This is important, as the detection of these three point mutations could provide an early prediction of an unfavorable response to azacitidine and lenalidomide combination therapy in MDS patients.

3.4 PI-PLCβ1/PI-PLCγ1: Myogenic/Osteogenic Differentiation

PI-PLCβ1, but not PI-PLCγ1, is directly involved in myogenesis and osteogenic differentiation, primarily in connection to vascular smooth cells (Mackenzie et al. 2013), where it is activated downstream of the PI3K/Akt signalling pathway, possibly through PIP5K1α intervention and the subsequent modulation of Ca2+ levels (Chen et al. 2018).

PI-PLCβ1 role in this setting is related to its nuclear localization (Faenza et al. 2005), as overexpression of a PI-PLCβ1 mutant lacking the nuclear localization sequence, and therefore entirely located in the cytoplasm, conversely blocks myogenic differentiation (Faenza et al. 2007; O'Carroll et al. 2009). PI-PLCβ1 catalytic activity is necessary to initiate the differentiation program, especially in human disease (Ramazzotti et al. 2017). In fact, myogenic cells obtained from patients with myotonic dystrophy showed a marked decrease in PI-PLCβ1/cyclin D3 expression and elongated myotube formation, which was reversed by PI-PLCβ1-forced overexpression (Faenza et al. 2012).

Nuclear PI-PLCβ1 also promotes osteogenic differentiation, as first observed in C2C12 cells responding to BMP-2 administration that upregulated osteogenic markers such as ALP and OSX when PI-PLCβ1 was overexpressed (Ramazzotti et al. 2016a). This phenomenon was also seen in proliferating adipose-derived stem cells (ADSCs) during early stages of osteogenic differentiation, accompanied by decreased PI-PLCβ1 levels (Ramazzotti et al. 2019b). Interestingly, cyclin D3 levels did not increase during osteogenesis, with or without PI-PLCβ1 overexpression. Therefore, cyclin D3 seems to play an important role in promoting myogenic but not osteogenic differentiation (Ramazzotti et al. 2016b).

3.5 PI-PLCβ1/PI-PLCγ1 and Other Phospholipases in Disease: Breast Cancer

PI-PLCβ1 plays a relatively small role in breast cancer, but it can promote metastatic breast cancer cell migration through a PIP_2-dependent actin remodelling. Moreover, PI-PLCβ1 is upregulated in highly metastatic breast cancer cells, and its increased expression is associated with metastatic relapse (Sengelaub et al. 2016). Within the PI-PLCβ family, PI-PLCβ2 is thought to be the most relevant isoform, being implicated in breast cancer and potentially representing a new target for therapy. The PI-PLCβ2 role in breast cancer was recently uncovered through analysis of moderate hypoxia in ductal carcinoma in situ (DCIS)-derived cells, showing motility, epithelial-to-mesenchymal transition (EMT), and expression of the stem cell marker CD133, indicative of their increased malignant potential (Al-Qassab et al. 2018). In these cells, cultured in vitro under hypoxia, administration of ATRA supported the epithelial-like phenotype and suppressed the number of CD133 positive cells, abrogating almost completely the effects of poor oxygenation. Interestingly, these effects were mediated by PI-PLCβ2, which was responsible for countering the effects of low oxygen availability on CD133 levels (Al-Qassab et al. 2018).

PI-PLCγ1 is associated with breast cancer in connection to cancer cell migration and metastasis (Mongiorgi et al. 2016a; Sala et al. 2008), while its inhibition is linked to a reduction of tumor cell motility in vitro and of tumor metastasis in vivo (Lattanzio et al. 2013; Yang et al. 2014). PI-PLCγ1 regulates integrin-mediated cell migration, as well as the cell motility induced by growth factors such as epidermal growth factor and hepatocyte growth factor (Choi et al. 2007; Xie et al. 2010; Davies et al. 2008). Recent studies showed a novel signalling pathway required for PI-PLCγ1 activation, involving the formation of a protein complex with 3-phosphoinositide-dependent protein kinase 1 (PDK1). This signalling pathway can be targeted by novel therapeutic approaches, such as the one mediated by 2-*O*-Bn-$InsP_5$, that binds to the PH domain of PDK1 with high affinity, thus preventing the formation of the PDK1/PI-PLCγ1 complex and resulting in inhibition of cell migration in vitro and metastasis in vivo (Raimondi et al. 2016).

As for other phospholipases, phospholipase D (PLD) is involved in promoting breast cancer cell growth, proliferation, and metastasis (Chen et al. 2012; Gomez-Cambronero et al. 2018). In particular, PLD gene and protein expression are upregulated in breast carcinoma human samples, where PLD-dependent posttranscriptional processes are activated, enabling PLD accumulation and ultimately breast cancer cell growth. First, PA, a mitogen, functions as a protein and mRNA stabilizer that counteracts natural decay and degradation. Second, there is a repertoire of microRNAs (miRs) that keep PLD mRNA translation at low levels in normal cells, but their effects change with starvation and during endothelial-to-mesenchymal transition (EMT) in breast cancer cells. Third, there is a novel way of posttranscriptional regulation of PLD involving 3′-exonucleases, specifically the deadenylase, poly(A)-specific ribonuclease (PARN), which tags mRNA for mRNA for degradation (Gomez-Cambronero et al. 2018).

In breast cancer, inositide signalling is particularly important, above all for novel therapies based on nutraceuticals that target PI3K/PTEN/Akt/mTOR and Ras/Raf/MEK/ERK pathways (Steelman et al. 2016). Indeed, sulforaphane is a natural compound derived from broccoli/broccoli sprouts that is able to suppress mammosphere formation of breast cancer stem cells (CSCs) in vitro as well as tumor formation in mice studies (Li et al. 2010). The natural phenol isoliquiritigenin (ISL), a licorice chalconoid, is also effective on breast CSCs (Khan et al. 2011). Indeed, nutraceuticals and drugs used in the treatment of other diseases are being investigated as potential supplemental approaches to treat or to prevent the development of breast cancer. Some of these potential treatments include drugs which are currently clinically used in the therapies of other diseases (e.g., diabetes, alcoholism, and others), and they are approved for those treatments. In some cases the effectiveness of some of these potential treatments may be obtained by analysis of the effects of their usage in the long-term treatment of other diseases and determination if the patients developed breast cancer, especially if the patient belonged to a family with a history of breast cancer (Steelman et al. 2016). To come back to a traditional pharmaceutical approach, Akt is one of the main targets in breast cancer, as it affects the maintenance of breast CSCs. Moreover, Akt localization is also important, as introduction of a modified Akt gene tagged with the nuclear localization signal into breast cancer cell lines resulted in an increased number of cells with the CD44+/CD24- and ALDH+ phenotypes, i.e., highly tumorigenic breast cancer cells (Li et al. 2017). Interestingly, these effects could be reversed upon treatment with the Akt inhibitor triciribine (Jain et al. 2015).

3.6 Other Phospholipases in Disease: Fertility

A specific PI-PLC isozyme is responsible for the mammalian oocyte activation: PI-PLCζ (Saunders et al. 2002). At first, PI-PLCζ was identified in sperm from numerous mammalian species. Generally, it appears to be localized within the sperm head and in particular in cytoplasmic vesicles, where it co-localizes with PIP2 (Amdani et al. 2016). More interestingly, an abnormal PI-PLCζ localization pattern was detected in the sperm of infertile men, which lacked or showed reduced PI-PLCζ levels due to gene mutations and a peculiar PI-PLCζ localization within the nucleus (Amdani et al. 2016). Nuclear PI-PLCζ has been specifically connected with molecular oocyte activation, but the PI-PLC nuclear translocation mechanism still remains unknown (Amdani et al. 2016).

Mammalian oocytes are extremely sensitive to the precise Ca2+ oscillation profile elicited at fertilization and contain multiple PI-PLC isoforms, including β, γ, and δ, whose role in Ca2+ metabolism can be relevant for oocyte activation (Igarashi et al. 2007). Indeed, reducing PI-PLCβ1 altered, but did not prevent, Ca2+ oscillation profiles, thus oocyte activation. Conversely, overexpression of PI-PLCβ1 elicited spontaneous Ca2+ oscillations, altering (but not preventing) the Ca2+ oscillation profiles observed at fertilization (Igarashi et al. 2007). On the other hand, a novel PI-PLCδ isoform with an increasing activity at fertilization has also been identified in sea urchin gametes. Interestingly, recombinant protein or cRNA corresponding to the sea urchin PI-PLCδ failed to elicit Ca2+ release when injected into mouse oocytes and sea urchin eggs (Coward et al. 2007). Furthermore, recombinant PI-PLCβ1, PI-PLCγ1, PI-PLCγ2, PI-PLCδ1, PI-PLCδ3, and PI-PLCδ4 protein and cRNA failed to elicit Ca2+ release upon injection into mouse oocytes. Collectively, such findings indicate that oocyte PLC isoforms are not directly involved in oocyte activation but may potentially exert an effect further downstream of fertilization (Igarashi et al. 2007; Runft et al. 2004; Yin and Eckberg 2009; Kashir et al. 2014).

Acknowledgments This work was supported by grants from Intesa San Paolo Foundation and the Italian Ministry of University and Research – Projects of National Interest 2015.

References

Alimandi M, Heidaran MA, Gutkind JS, Zhang J, Ellmore N, Valius M, Kazlauskas A, Pierce JH, Li W (1997) PLC-gamma activation is required for PDGF-betaR-mediated mitogenesis and monocytic differentiation of myeloid progenitor cells. Oncogene 15:585–593

Al-Qassab Y, Grassilli S, Brugnoli F, Vezzali F, Capitani S, Bertagnolo V (2018) Protective role of all-trans retinoic acid (ATRA) against hypoxia-induced malignant potential of non-invasive breast tumor derived cells. BMC Cancer 18:1194

Amdani SN, Yeste M, Jones C, Coward K (2016) Phospholipase C zeta (PLCzeta) and male infertility: clinical update and topical developments. Adv Biol Regul 61:58–67

Barbosa CM, Bincoletto C, Barros CC, Ferreira AT, Paredes-Gamero EJ (2014) PLCgamma2 and PKC are important to myeloid lineage commitment triggered by M-SCF and G-CSF. J Cell Biochem 115:42–51

Bavelloni A, Faenza I, Cioffi G, Piazzi M, Parisi D, Matic I, Maraldi NM, Cocco L (2006) Proteomic-based analysis of nuclear signaling: PLCbeta1 affects the expression of the splicing factor SRp20 in Friend erythroleukemia cells. Proteomics 6:5725–5734

Blalock WL, Bavelloni A, Piazzi M, Tagliavini F, Faenza I, Martelli AM, Follo MY, Cocco L (2011) Multiple forms of PKR present in the nuclei of acute leukemia cells represent an active kinase that is responsive to stress. Leukemia 25:236–245

Cautain B, Hill R, de Pedro N, Link W (2015) Components and regulation of nuclear transport processes. FEBS J 282:445–462

Chang HR, Munkhjargal A, Kim MJ, Park SY, Jung E, Ryu JH, Yang Y, Lim JS, Kim Y (2018) The functional roles of PML nuclear bodies in genome maintenance. Mutat Res 809:99–107

Chen Q, Hongu T, Sato T, Zhang Y, Ali W, Cavallo JA, van der Velden A, Tian H, Di Paolo G, Nieswandt B, Kanaho Y, Frohman MA (2012) Key roles for the lipid signaling enzyme phospholipase D1 in the tumor microenvironment during tumor angiogenesis and metastasis. Sci Signal 5:ra79

Chen X, Wan J, Yu B, Diao Y, Zhang W (2018) PIP5K1alpha promotes myogenic differentiation via AKT activation and calcium release. Stem Cell Res Ther 9:33

Choi WC, Gerfen CR, Suh PG, Rhee SG (1989) Immunohistochemical localization of a brain isozyme of phospholipase C (PLC III) in astroglia in rat brain. Brain Res 499:193–197

Choi JH, Yang YR, Lee SK, Kim IS, Ha SH, Kim EK, Bae YS, Ryu SH, Suh PG (2007) Phospholipase C-gamma1 potentiates integrin-dependent cell spreading and migration through Pyk2/paxillin activation. Cell Signal 19:1784–1796

Choi S, Chen M, Cryns VL, Anderson RA (2019) A nuclear phosphoinositide kinase complex regulates p53. Nat Cell Biol 21:462–475

Clarke JH, Richardson JP, Hinchliffe KA, Irvine RF (2007) Type II PtdInsP kinases: location, regulation and function. Biochem Soc Symp:149–159

Cocco L, Gilmour RS, Ognibene A, Letcher AJ, Manzoli FA, Irvine RF (1987) Synthesis of polyphosphoinositides in nuclei of friend cells. Evidence for polyphosphoinositide metabolism inside the nucleus which changes with cell differentiation. Biochem J 248:765–770

Cocco L, Martelli AM, Gilmour RS (1994) Inositol lipid cycle in the nucleus. Cell Signal 6:481–485

Cocco L, Follo MY, Faenza I, Billi AM, Ramazzotti G, Martelli AM, Manzoli L, Weber G (2010) Inositide signaling in the nucleus: from physiology to pathology. Adv Enzyme Regul 50:2–11

Cocco L, Finelli C, Mongiorgi S, Clissa C, Russo D, Bosi C, Quaranta M, Malagola M, Parisi S, Stanzani M, Ramazzotti G, Mariani GA, Billi AM, Manzoli L, Follo MY (2015) An increased expression of PI-PLCbeta1 is associated with myeloid differentiation and a longer response to azacitidine in myelodysplastic syndromes. J Leukoc Biol 98:769–780

Coward K, Owen H, Tunwell R, Swann K, Parrington J (2007) Phospholipid binding properties and functional characterization of a sea urchin phospholipase Cdelta in urchin and mouse eggs. Biochem Biophys Res Commun 357:964–970

Cutter AR, Hayes JJ (2015) A brief review of nucleosome structure. FEBS Lett 589:2914–2922

Davies G, Martin TA, Ye L, Lewis-Russell JM, Mason MD, Jiang WG (2008) Phospholipase-C gamma-1 (PLCgamma-1) is critical in hepatocyte growth factor induced in vitro invasion and migration without affecting the growth of prostate cancer cells. Urol Oncol 26:386–391

de Leeuw R, Gruenbaum Y, Medalia O (2018) Nuclear lamins: thin filaments with major functions. Trends Cell Biol 28:34–45

Divecha N, Banfic H, Irvine RF (1991) The polyphosphoinositide cycle exists in the nuclei of Swiss 3T3 cells under the control of a receptor (for IGF-I) in the plasma membrane, and stimulation of the cycle increases nuclear diacylglycerol and apparently induces translocation of protein kinase C to the nucleus. EMBO J 10:3207–3214

Dobrzynska A, Gonzalo S, Shanahan C, Askjaer P (2016) The nuclear lamina in health and disease. Nucleus 7:233–248

Faenza I, Billi AM, Follo MY, Fiume R, Martelli AM, Cocco L, Manzoli L (2005) Nuclear phospholipase C signaling through type 1 IGF receptor and its involvement in cell growth and differentiation. Anticancer Res 25:2039–2041

Faenza I, Ramazzotti G, Bavelloni A, Fiume R, Gaboardi GC, Follo MY, Gilmour RS, Martelli AM, Ravid K, Cocco L (2007) Inositide-dependent phospholipase C signaling mimics insulin in skeletal muscle differentiation by affecting specific regions of the cyclin D3 promoter. Endocrinology 148:1108–1117

Faenza I, Blalock W, Bavelloni A, Schoser B, Fiume R, Pacella S, Piazzi M, D'Angelo A, Cocco L (2012) A role for PLCbeta1 in myotonic dystrophies type 1 and 2. FASEB J 26:3042–3048

Fili C, Malagola M, Follo MY, Finelli C, Iacobucci I, Martinelli G, Cattina F, Clissa C, Candoni A, Fanin R, Gobbi M, Bocchia M, Defina M, Spedini P, Skert C, Manzoli L, Cocco L, Russo D (2013) Prospective phase II study on 5-days azacitidine for treatment of symptomatic and/or erythropoietin unresponsive patients with low/INT-1-risk myelodysplastic syndromes. Clin Cancer Res 19:3297–3308

Finelli C, Follo MY, Stanzani M, Parisi S, Clissa C, Mongiorgi S, Barraco M, Cocco L (2016) Clinical impact of hypomethylating agents in the treatment of myelodysplastic syndromes. Curr Pharm Des 22:2349–2357

Fiume R, Faenza I, Sheth B, Poli A, Vidalle MC, Mazzetti C, Abdul SH, Campagnoli F, Fabbrini M, Kimber ST, Mariani GA, Xian J, Marvi MV, Mongiorgi S, Shah Z, Divecha N (2019) Nuclear phosphoinositides: their regulation and roles in nuclear functions. Int J Mol Sci 20(12). pii: E2991. doi: https://doi.org/10.3390/ijms20122991

Follo MY, Mongiorgi S, Finelli C, Clissa C, Ramazzotti G, Fiume R, Faenza I, Manzoli L, Martelli AM, Cocco L (2010) Nuclear inositide signaling in myelodysplastic syndromes. J Cell Biochem 109:1065–1071

Follo MY, Finelli C, Mongiorgi S, Clissa C, Chiarini F, Ramazzotti G, Paolini S, Martinelli G, Martelli AM, Cocco L (2011) Synergistic induction of PI-PLCbeta1 signaling by azacitidine and valproic acid in high-risk myelodysplastic syndromes. Leukemia 25:271–280

Follo MY, Faenza I, Fiume R, Ramazzotti G, McCubrey JA, Martelli AM, Manzoli FA, Cocco L (2012a) Revisiting nuclear phospholipase C signalling in MDS. Adv Biol Regul 52:2–6

Follo MY, Mongiorgi S, Clissa C, Paolini S, Martinelli G, Martelli AM, Fioravanti G, Manzoli L, Finelli C, Cocco L (2012b) Activation of nuclear inositide signalling pathways during erythropoietin therapy in low-risk MDS patients. Leukemia 26:2474–2482

Follo MY, Russo D, Finelli C, Mongiorgi S, Clissa C, Fili C, Colombi C, Gobbi M, Manzoli L, Piazzi M, Martelli AM, Cocco L (2012c) Epigenetic regulation of nuclear PI-PLCbeta1 signaling pathway in low-risk MDS patients during azacitidine treatment. Leukemia 26:943–950

Follo MY, Marmiroli S, Faenza I, Fiume R, Ramazzotti G, Martelli AM, Gobbi P, McCubrey JA, Finelli C, Manzoli FA, Cocco L (2013) Nuclear phospholipase C beta1 signaling, epigenetics and treatments in MDS. Adv Biol Regul 53:2–7

Follo MY, Faenza I, Piazzi M, Blalock WL, Manzoli L, McCubrey JA, Cocco L (2014) Nuclear PI-PLCbeta1: an appraisal on targets and pathology. Adv Biol Regul 54:2–11

Follo MY, Pellagatti A, Armstrong RN, Ratti S, Mongiorgi S, De Fanti S, Bochicchio MT, Russo D, Gobbi M, Miglino M, Parisi S, Martinelli G, Cavo M, Luiselli D, McCubrey JA, Suh PG, Manzoli L, Boultwood J, Finelli C, Cocco L (2019) Response of high-risk MDS to azacitidine and lenalidomide is impacted by baseline and acquired mutations in a cluster of three inositide-specific genes. Leukemia 33(9):2276–2290

Fox AH, Lamond AI (2010) Paraspeckles. Cold Spring Harb Perspect Biol 2:a000687

Galganski L, Urbanek MO, Krzyzosiak WJ (2017) Nuclear speckles: molecular organization, biological function and role in disease. Nucleic Acids Res 45:10350–10368

Garcia del Cano G, Montana M, Aretxabala X, Gonzalez-Burguera I, Lopez de Jesus M, Barrondo S, Salles J (2014) Nuclear phospholipase C-beta1 and diacylglycerol LIPASE-alpha in brain cortical neurons. Adv Biol Regul 54:12–23

Glass L, Wente SR (2019) Gle1 mediates stress granule-dependent survival during chemotoxic stress. Adv Biol Regul 71:156–171

Gomez-Cambronero J, Fite K, Miller TE (2018) How miRs and mRNA deadenylases could post-transcriptionally regulate expression of tumor-promoting protein PLD. Adv Biol Regul 68:107–119

Goto K, Tanaka T, Nakano T, Okada M, Hozumi Y, Topham MK, Martelli AM (2014) DGKzeta under stress conditions: "to be nuclear or cytoplasmic, that is the question". Adv Biol Regul 54:242–253

Hannan AJ, Kind PC, Blakemore C (1998) Phospholipase C-beta1 expression correlates with neuronal differentiation and synaptic plasticity in rat somatosensory cortex. Neuropharmacology 37:593–605

Igarashi H, Knott JG, Schultz RM, Williams CJ (2007) Alterations of PLCbeta1 in mouse eggs change calcium oscillatory behavior following fertilization. Dev Biol 312:321–330

Jacobsen RG, Mazloumi Gavgani F, Edson AJ, Goris M, Altankhuyag A, Lewis AE (2019) Polyphosphoinositides in the nucleus: roadmap of their effectors and mechanisms of interaction. Adv Biol Regul 72:7–21

Jain MV, Jangamreddy JR, Grabarek J, Schweizer F, Klonisch T, Cieslar-Pobuda A, Los MJ (2015) Nuclear localized Akt enhances breast cancer stem-like cells through counter-regulation of p21 (Waf1/Cip1) and p27(kip1). Cell Cycle 14:2109–2120

Kashir J, Nomikos M, Lai FA, Swann K (2014) Sperm-induced Ca2+ release during egg activation in mammals. Biochem Biophys Res Commun 450:1204–1211

Khan SI, Zhao J, Khan IA, Walker LA, Dasmahapatra AK (2011) Potential utility of natural products as regulators of breast cancer-associated aromatase promoters. Reprod Biol Endocrinol 9:91

Kim D, Jun KS, Lee SB, Kang NG, Min DS, Kim YH, Ryu SH, Suh PG, Shin HS (1997) Phospholipase C isozymes selectively couple to specific neurotransmitter receptors. Nature 389:290–293

Kurian MA, Meyer E, Vassallo G, Morgan NV, Prakash N, Pasha S, Hai NA, Shuib S, Rahman F, Wassmer E, Cross JH, O'Callaghan FJ, Osborne JP, Scheffer IE, Gissen P, Maher ER (2010) Phospholipase C beta 1 deficiency is associated with early-onset epileptic encephalopathy. Brain 133:2964–2970

Lafarga M, Berciano MT, Pena E, Mayo I, Castano JG, Bohmann D, Rodrigues JP, Tavanez JP, Carmo-Fonseca M (2002) Clastosome: a subtype of nuclear body enriched in 19S and 20S proteasomes, ubiquitin, and protein substrates of proteasome. Mol Biol Cell 13:2771–2782

Lai WKM, Pugh BF (2017) Understanding nucleosome dynamics and their links to gene expression and DNA replication. Nat Rev Mol Cell Biol 18:548–562

Lattanzio R, Piantelli M, Falasca M (2013) Role of phospholipase C in cell invasion and metastasis. Adv Biol Regul 53:309–318

Li Y, Zhang T, Korkaya H, Liu S, Lee HF, Newman B, Yu Y, Clouthier SG, Schwartz SJ, Wicha MS, Sun D (2010) Sulforaphane, a dietary component of broccoli/broccoli sprouts, inhibits breast cancer stem cells. Clin Cancer Res 16:2580–2590

Li W, Ma H, Zhang J, Zhu L, Wang C, Yang Y (2017) Unraveling the roles of CD44/CD24 and ALDH1 as cancer stem cell markers in tumorigenesis and metastasis. Sci Rep 7:13856

Liao HJ, Kume T, McKay C, Xu MJ, Ihle JN, Carpenter G (2002) Absence of erythrogenesis and vasculogenesis in Plcg1-deficient mice. J Biol Chem 277:9335–9341

Lo Vasco VR, Cardinale G, Polonia P (2012) Deletion of PLCB1 gene in schizophrenia-affected patients. J Cell Mol Med 16:844–851

Lo Vasco VR, Longo L, Polonia P (2013) Phosphoinositide-specific phospholipase C beta1 gene deletion in bipolar disorder affected patient. J Cell Commun Signal 7:25–29

Mackenzie LS, Lymn JS, Hughes AD (2013) Linking phospholipase C isoforms with differentiation function in human vascular smooth muscle cells. Biochim Biophys Acta 1833:3006–3012

Malhi GS, Tanious M, Das P, Coulston CM, Berk M (2013) Potential mechanisms of action of lithium in bipolar disorder. Current understanding. CNS Drugs 27:135–153

Manzoli FA, Maraldi NM, Cocco L, Capitani S, Facchini A (1977) Chromatin phospholipids in normal and chronic lymphocytic leukemia lymphocytes. Cancer Res 37:843–849

Manzoli L, Billi AM, Gilmour RS, Martelli AM, Matteucci A, Rubbini S, Weber G, Cocco L (1995) Phosphoinositide signaling in nuclei of friend cells: tiazofurin down-regulates phospholipase C beta 1. Cancer Res 55:2978–2980

Manzoli L, Billi AM, Rubbini S, Bavelloni A, Faenza I, Gilmour RS, Rhee SG, Cocco L (1997) Essential role for nuclear phospholipase C beta1 in insulin-like growth factor I-induced mitogenesis. Cancer Res 57:2137–2139

Manzoli L, Mongiorgi S, Clissa C, Finelli C, Billi AM, Poli A, Quaranta M, Cocco L, Follo MY (2014) Strategic role of nuclear inositide signalling in myelodysplastic syndromes therapy. Mini Rev Med Chem 14:873–883

Martelli AM, Gilmour RS, Bertagnolo V, Neri LM, Manzoli L, Cocco L (1992) Nuclear localization and signalling activity of phosphoinositidase C beta in Swiss 3T3 cells. Nature 358:242–245

Martelli AM, Tabellini G, Bortul R, Manzoli L, Bareggi R, Baldini G, Grill V, Zweyer M, Narducci P, Cocco L (2000) Enhanced nuclear diacylglycerol kinase activity in response to a mitogenic stimulation of quiescent Swiss 3T3 cells with insulin-like growth factor I. Cancer Res 60:815–821

Martelli AM, Fiume R, Faenza I, Tabellini G, Evangelista C, Bortul R, Follo MY, Fala F, Cocco L (2005) Nuclear phosphoinositide specific phospholipase C (PI-PLC)-beta 1: a central intermediary in nuclear lipid-dependent signal transduction. Histol Histopathol 20:1251–1260

Meier UT (2017) RNA modification in Cajal bodies. RNA Biol 14:693–700

Mongiorgi S, Finelli C, Yang YR, Clissa C, McCubrey JA, Billi AM, Manzoli L, Suh PG, Cocco L, Follo MY (2016a) Inositide-dependent signaling pathways as new therapeutic targets in myelodysplastic syndromes. Expert Opin Ther Targets 20:677–687

Mongiorgi S, Follo MY, Yang YR, Ratti S, Manzoli L, McCubrey JA, Billi AM, Suh PG, Cocco L (2016b) Selective activation of nuclear PI-PLCbeta1 during normal and therapy-related differentiation. Curr Pharm Des 22:2345–2348

Naetar N, Ferraioli S, Foisner R (2017) Lamins in the nuclear interior – life outside the lamina. J Cell Sci 130:2087–2096

O'Carroll SJ, Mitchell MD, Faenza I, Cocco L, Gilmour RS (2009) Nuclear PLCbeta1 is required for 3T3-L1 adipocyte differentiation and regulates expression of the cyclin D3-cdk4 complex. Cell Signal 21:926–935

Padiath QS, Saigoh K, Schiffmann R, Asahara H, Yamada T, Koeppen A, Hogan K, Ptácek LJ, Fu YH (2006) Lamin B1 duplications cause autosomal dominant leukodystrophy. Nat Genet 38:1114–1123

Park H, Poo MM (2013) Neurotrophin regulation of neural circuit development and function. Nat Rev Neurosci 14:7–23

Pederson T (2011) The nucleolus. Cold Spring Harb Perspect Biol 3(3). pii: a000638. doi: https://doi.org/10.1101/cshperspect.a000638

Poduri A, Chopra SS, Neilan EG, Elhosary PC, Kurian MA, Meyer E, Barry BJ, Khwaja OS, Salih MA, Stodberg T, Scheffer IE, Maher ER, Sahin M, Wu BL, Berry GT, Walsh CA, Picker J, Kothare SV (2012) Homozygous PLCB1 deletion associated with malignant migrating partial seizures in infancy. Epilepsia 53:e146–e150

Poli A, Billi AM, Mongiorgi S, Ratti S, McCubrey JA, Suh PG, Cocco L, Ramazzotti G (2016) Nuclear phosphatidylinositol signaling: focus on phosphatidylinositol phosphate kinases and phospholipases C. J Cell Physiol 231:1645–1655

Poli A, Fiume R, Baldanzi G, Capello D, Ratti S, Gesi M, Manzoli L, Graziani A, Suh PG, Cocco L, Follo MY (2017) Nuclear localization of diacylglycerol kinase alpha in K562 cells is involved in cell cycle progression. J Cell Physiol 232:2550–2557

Poli A, Ratti S, Finelli C, Mongiorgi S, Clissa C, Lonetti A, Cappellini A, Catozzi A, Barraco M, Suh PG, Manzoli L, McCubrey JA, Cocco L, Follo MY (2018) Nuclear translocation of PKC-alpha is associated with cell cycle arrest and erythroid differentiation in myelodysplastic syndromes (MDSs). FASEB J 32:681–692

Raben DM, Tu-Sekine B (2008) Nuclear diacylglycerol kinases: regulation and roles. Front Biosci 13:590–597

Raimondi C, Calleja V, Ferro R, Fantin A, Riley AM, Potter BV, Brennan CH, Maffucci T, Larijani B, Falasca M (2016) A small molecule inhibitor of PDK1/PLCgamma1 interaction blocks breast and melanoma cancer cell invasion. Sci Rep 6:26142

Ramazzotti G, Faenza I, Fiume R, Matteucci A, Piazzi M, Follo MY, Cocco L (2011) The physiology and pathology of inositide signaling in the nucleus. J Cell Physiol 226:14–20

Ramazzotti G, Bavelloni A, Blalock W, Piazzi M, Cocco L, Faenza I (2016a) BMP-2 induced expression of PLCbeta1 that is a positive regulator of osteoblast differentiation. J Cell Physiol 231:623–629

Ramazzotti G, Billi AM, Manzoli L, Mazzetti C, Ruggeri A, Erneux C, Kim S, Suh PG, Cocco L, Faenza I (2016b) IPMK and beta-catenin mediate PLC-beta1-dependent signaling in myogenic differentiation. Oncotarget 7:84118–84127

Ramazzotti G, Faenza I, Fiume R, Billi AM, Manzoli L, Mongiorgi S, Ratti S, McCubrey JA, Suh PG, Cocco L, Follo MY (2017) PLC-beta1 and cell differentiation: an insight into myogenesis and osteogenesis. Adv Biol Regul 63:1–5

Ramazzotti G, Ratti S, Fiume R, Yung Follo M, Billi AM, Rusciano I, Owusu Obeng E, Manzoli L, Cocco L, Faenza I (2019a) Phosphoinositide 3 kinase signaling in human stem cells from reprogramming to differentiation: a tale in cytoplasmic and nuclear compartments. Int J Mol Sci 20(8). pii: E2026. doi: https://doi.org/10.3390/ijms20082026

Ramazzotti G, Fiume R, Chiarini F, Campana G, Ratti S, Billi AM, Manzoli L, Follo MY, Suh PG, McCubrey J, Cocco L, Faenza I (2019b) Phospholipase C-beta1 interacts with cyclin E in adipose-derived stem cells osteogenic differentiation. Adv Biol Regul 71:1–9

Ratti S, Mongiorgi S, Ramazzotti G, Follo MY, Mariani GA, Suh PG, McCubrey JA, Cocco L, Manzoli L (2017) Nuclear inositide signaling via phospholipase C. J Cell Biochem 118:1969–1978

Ratti S, Ramazzotti G, Faenza I, Fiume R, Mongiorgi S, Billi AM, McCubrey JA, Suh PG, Manzoli L, Cocco L, Follo MY (2018) Nuclear inositide signaling and cell cycle. Adv Biol Regul 67:1–6

Ratti S, Follo MY, Ramazzotti G, Faenza I, Fiume R, Suh PG, McCubrey JA, Manzoli L, Cocco L (2019) Nuclear phospholipase C isoenzyme imbalance leads to pathologies in brain, hematologic, neuromuscular, and fertility disorders. J Lipid Res 60:312–317

Ross CA, MacCumber MW, Glatt CE, Snyder SH (1989) Brain phospholipase C isozymes: differential mRNA localizations by in situ hybridization. Proc Natl Acad Sci U S A 86:2923–2927

Runft LL, Carroll DJ, Gillett J, Giusti AF, O'Neill FJ, Foltz KR (2004) Identification of a starfish egg PLC-gamma that regulates Ca2+ release at fertilization. Dev Biol 269:220–236

Sala G, Dituri F, Raimondi C, Previdi S, Maffucci T, Mazzoletti M, Rossi C, Iezzi M, Lattanzio R, Piantelli M, Iacobelli S, Broggini M, Falasca M (2008) Phospholipase Cgamma1 is required for metastasis development and progression. Cancer Res 68:10187–10196

Saunders CM, Larman MG, Parrington J, Cox LJ, Royse J, Blayney LM, Swann K, Lai FA (2002) PLC zeta: a sperm-specific trigger of Ca(2+) oscillations in eggs and embryo development. Development 129:3533–3544

Sengelaub CA, Navrazhina K, Ross JB, Halberg N, Tavazoie SF (2016) PTPRN2 and PLCbeta1 promote metastatic breast cancer cell migration through PI(4,5)P2-dependent actin remodeling. EMBO J 35:62–76

Shin KJ, Lee YJ, Yang YR, Park S, Suh PG, Follo MY, Cocco L, Ryu SH (2016) Molecular mechanisms underlying psychological stress and cancer. Curr Pharm Des 22:2389–2402

Smith CD, Wells WW (1983) Phosphorylation of rat liver nuclear envelopes. II. Characterization of in vitro lipid phosphorylation. J Biol Chem 258:9368–9373

Steelman LS, Fitzgerald T, Lertpiriyapong K, Cocco L, Follo MY, Martelli AM, Neri LM, Marmiroli S, Libra M, Candido S, Nicoletti F, Scalisi A, Fenga C, Drobot L, Rakus D, Gizak A, Laidler P, Dulinska-Litewka J, Basecke J, Mijatovic S, Maksimovic-Ivanic D, Montalto G, Cervello M, Milella M, Tafuri A, Demidenko Z, Abrams SL, McCubrey JA (2016) Critical roles of EGFR family members in breast cancer and breast cancer stem cells: targets for therapy. Curr Pharm Des 22:2358–2388

Sztacho M, Sobol M, Balaban C, Escudeiro Lopes SE, Hozak P (2019) Nuclear phosphoinositides and phase separation: important players in nuclear compartmentalization. Adv Biol Regul 71:111–117

Trubiani O, Guarnieri S, Diomede F, Mariggio MA, Merciaro I, Morabito C, Cavalcanti MF, Cocco L, Ramazzotti G (2016) Nuclear translocation of PKCalpha isoenzyme is involved in neurogenic commitment of human neural crest-derived periodontal ligament stem cells. Cell Signal 28:1631–1641

Ullrich NJ, Gordon LB (2015) Hutchinson-Gilford progeria syndrome. Handb Clin Neurol 132:249–264

Venkatesh S, Workman JL (2015) Histone exchange, chromatin structure and the regulation of transcription. Nat Rev Mol Cell Biol 16:178–189

Xie Z, Peng J, Pennypacker SD, Chen Y (2010) Critical role for the catalytic activity of phospholipase C-gamma1 in epidermal growth factor-induced cell migration. Biochem Biophys Res Commun 399:425–428

Xu A, Suh PG, Marmy-Conus N, Pearson RB, Seok OY, Cocco L, Gilmour RS (2001) Phosphorylation of nuclear phospholipase C beta1 by extracellular signal-regulated kinase mediates the mitogenic action of insulin-like growth factor I. Mol Cell Biol 21:2981–2990

Yang J, Song X, Chen Y, Lu XA, Fu Y, Luo Y (2014) PLCgamma1-PKCgamma signaling-mediated Hsp90alpha plasma membrane translocation facilitates tumor metastasis. Traffic 15:861–878

Yang YR, Kang DS, Lee C, Seok H, Follo MY, Cocco L, Suh PG (2016) Primary phospholipase C and brain disorders. Adv Biol Regul 61:80–85

Yin X, Eckberg WR (2009) Characterization of phospholipases C beta and gamma and their possible roles in Chaetopterus egg activation. Mol Reprod Dev 76:460–470

Zhang D, Ma Q, Wang Z, Zhang M, Guo K, Wang F, Wu E (2011) beta2-adrenoceptor blockage induces G1/S phase arrest and apoptosis in pancreatic cancer cells via Ras/Akt/NFkappaB pathway. Mol Cancer 10:146

Lipids in Exosome Biology

Antonio Luis Egea-Jimenez and Pascale Zimmermann

Contents

Abstract

Extracellular vesicles (EVs), and exosomes in particular, were initially considered as "garbage bags" for secretion of undesired cellular components. This view has changed considerably over the last two decades, and exosomes have now emerged as important organelles controlling cell-to-cell signaling. They are present in biological fluids and have important roles in the communication

A. L. Egea-Jimenez · P. Zimmermann (✉)
Centre de Recherche en Cancérologie de Marseille, Equipe labellisée Ligue 2018, Aix-Marseille Université, Inserm, CNRS, Institut Paoli Calmettes, Marseille, France

Department of Human Genetics, K. U. Leuven, Leuven, Belgium
e-mail: pascale.zimmermann@kuleuven.be

J. Gomez-Cambronero, M. A. Frohman (eds.), *Lipid Signaling in Human Diseases*, Handbook of Experimental Pharmacology 259, https://doi.org/10.1007/164_2019_220

between cells in physiological and pathological processes. They are envisioned for clinical use as carriers of biomarkers, therapeutic targets, and vehicles for drug delivery. Important efforts are being made to characterize the contents of these vesicles and to understand the mechanisms that govern their biogenesis and modes of action. This chapter aims to recapitulate the place given to lipids in our understanding of exosome biology. Besides their structural role and their function as carriers, certain lipids and lipid-modifying enzymes seem to exert privileged functions in this mode of cellular communication. By extension, the use of selective "lipid inhibitors" might turn out to be interesting modulators of exosomal-based cell signaling.

Keywords
Cell signaling · Ceramide · Exosomes · Neutral sphingomyelinase 2 · Phosphatidic acid · Phospholipase D2

1 Extracellular Vesicles as Signaling Organelles

1.1 Extracellular Vesicles: Definition and Types

Extracellular vesicles (EVs) are lipid bilayer-limited vesicles released by any type of cell. They have the same topology as the cells (inside-in and outside-out) and contain cytosolic and transmembrane proteins, lipids, and various types of nucleic acids. It has been known for decades that membrane-enclosed vesicles originating from cells are present in the extracellular environment (Anderson 1969; Trams et al. 1981; George et al. 1982). Their functional importance was disregarded, being dismissed as "garbage bags" (Harding et al. 1983; Pan and Johnstone 1983), until immunologists realized their role in antigen presentation (Raposo et al. 1996), and several papers revealed that EVs can transport messenger RNA (mRNA) and microRNA (miRNA) and influence gene expression in recipient cells (Baj-Krzyworzeka et al. 2006; Valadi et al. 2007; Hunter et al. 2008; Skog et al. 2008). There is still a lot of confusion regarding EV nomenclature, and the field suffers from a lack of established protocols and methods to purify and characterize these organelles in an accurate and reproducible manner. In an effort to clarify definitions and promote solid EV-related work, the International Society of Extracellular Vesicles (ISEV) was created in 2011 (www.isev.org). The first set of guidelines (MISEV for Minimal Information for Studies of Extracellular Vesicles) was proposed in 2014 (Lotvall et al. 2014) including rules for nomenclature, i.e., to refer solely to three types of EVs, namely, exosomes, microvesicles, and apoptotic bodies (Fig. 1).

Exosomes are now defined as EVs that originate from endosomal membranes, specifically intraluminal vesicles (ILVs) that accumulate inside late endosomes or multivesicular bodies (MVB). MVB fusion with the plasma membrane secretes ILVs into the extracellular environment, where these small vesicles are then designated as "exosomes." Their diameter can vary from 40 to 120 nm. Microvesicles, which originate from cell surface budding, have diameters that vary from 50 to 1,000 nm.

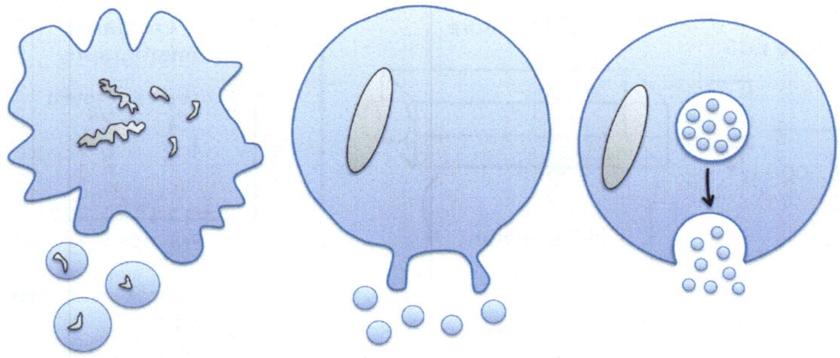
APOPTOTIC BODIES
1000-5000 nm
MICROVESICLES
50-1000 nm
EXOSOMES
40-120 nm

Fig. 1 Types of extracellular vesicles. A classification based on the cellular origin was proposed in 2011

Finally, apoptotic bodies result from cell fragmentation and can reach up to 5,000 nm in diameter. These populations can be enriched (but not fully separated) and concentrated by differential centrifugation (Fig. 2a–g). Exosomes can then be further purified/enriched by size exclusion chromatography, density gradients, or immunocapture (Fig. 2h–j). Complementary cell biology approaches (and in particular imaging approaches) are necessary to validate a specific EV subpopulation. It should be noted though that the new nomenclature is not yet uniformly used; the term "exosome" has been, and still is, sometimes abusively used to qualify any type of EV.

Because in some applications it is not realistic to clarify the nature of EVs according to their biogenesis, the MISEV recommendations have recently been revised. In the MISEV2018 update, authors are alternately given the option to refer to EV physical characteristics such as their size ("small EVs" (sEVs) and "medium/large EVs" (m/lEVs)), density (light, medium, or heavy), or their biochemical composition, such as CD81+/CD9− EVs. In fact, precise description of such pre-analytical parameters is very important because they have major impact on EV secretion and function.

Taking all of these issues into consideration, we will use the term "exosome" in referring to the studies cited here, even when it corresponds only to an exosome-enriched fraction derived from a high-speed (100,000 × *g*) pellet that had removed most of the apoptotic bodies and microvesicles through differential ultracentrifugation (Fig. 2a–g).

1.2 Extracellular Vesicles: Function

Work over the past few years has led to the view that EVs should now be considered organelles that mediate cell-cell communication over short and long distances. EVs have been shown to signal to target tissues in at least three different ways (Turturici et al. 2014) (Fig. 3): through transfer of their cargo into recipient cells

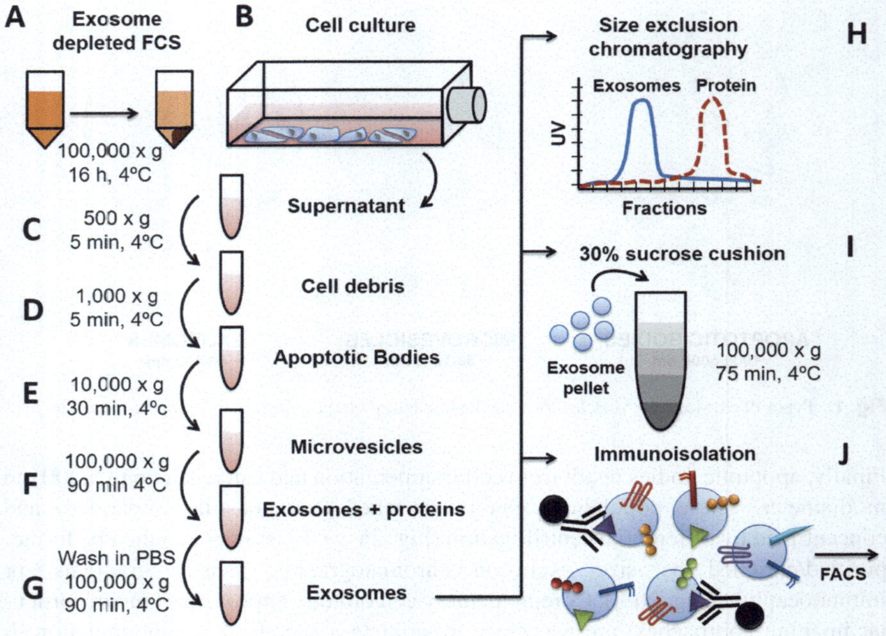

Fig. 2 Schematic representation of EV purification using differential centrifugation (**a–g**). (**a**) Fetal calf serum (FCS) must be exosome depleted if the cells cannot be cultured under serum-free conditions. (**b**) Conditioned medium is usually collected within 24–48 h from cells that have reached 70–80% confluency. (**c–g**) The purification of exosomes necessitates a series of differential ultracentrifugation steps. The first steps (**c–d**) are designed to remove large components such as cell debris and apoptotic bodies. Microvesicles are pelleted with 10,000 × *g* centrifugation (**e**). The exosome pellet is recovered after ultracentrifugation (**f**) and washed in PBS to remove contaminating proteins (**g**). Further procedures can be performed to increase exosome purity (**h–j**). (Théry et al. 2006). These procedures include size exclusion chromatography (**h**), density gradients (**i**), or immunoaffinity capture (**j**). Specific antibodies against tetraspanins, for example, can be used to isolate EVs in some settings. There is no universal immunocapture protocol, however, since tetraspanin distribution among EV subpopulations can vary depending on the cell type of origin

subsequent to (1) fusion with the plasma membrane (Fig. 3a) or (2) fusion with endosomal membranes after internalization (Fig. 3b) or (3) through direct interaction with cell surface receptors (Fig. 3c).

1.2.1 Physiological vs Pathological Roles of EVs

The prevalence of "disease EVs" has been validated in various pathological contexts including cancer and neurodegeneration (Rajendran et al. 2014; Costa-Silva et al. 2015). These "bad EVs" can transport pathological molecules including proteins, lipids, and nucleic acids and participate in disease progression.

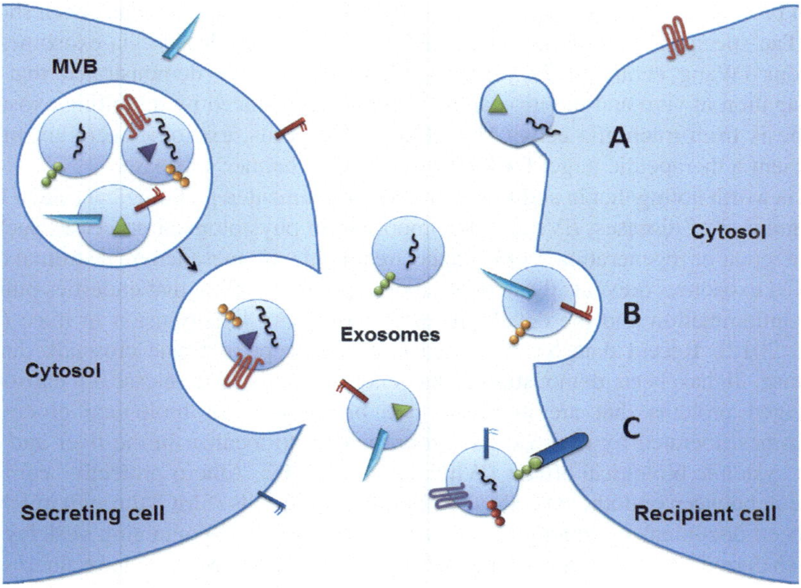

Fig. 3 Schematic representation illustrating how exosomes can convey signals to target cells: membrane fusion (**a**), endocytosis (**b**), or direct ligand-receptor interaction at the plasma membrane (**c**)

In cancer, for example, tumor cells establish an intricate network of communication with non-tumor cells that is supported by EV exchange. These exchanges promote a microenvironment favorable for support of the cancer progression (Ruivo et al. 2017). Tumor-derived exosomes are implicated in cancer onset, progression, and metastasis. In particular, EVs participate in sustaining hallmarks of cancer such as increased proliferation (1), resistance to cell death (2), tumor angiogenesis (3), immune escape (4), resistance to therapy (5), and metastasis (6) (Meehan and Vella 2016). For example, exosomes secreted by breast cancer can promote metastasis by adapting the metabolic environment of the premetastatic niche (Fong et al. 2015), and glioblastoma tumor cells release exosomes enriched in angiogenic proteins that induce the formation of new blood vessels (Skog et al. 2008). Exosomes from human prostate cancer cells can induce apoptosis of T cells (Abusamra et al. 2005), and exosomes from pancreatic adenocarcinoma cells impact on the extracellular matrix to support cell motility and invasiveness (Mu et al. 2013). Exosomes derived from pancreatic ductal adenocarcinomas are able to prepare the liver premetastatic niche (Costa-Silva et al. 2015). In neuropathological diseases, abnormally folded or partially unfolded proteins cause toxic protein aggregation spreading in the brain. These aggregates can trigger a group of diseases, called protein misfolding disorders (PMDs), such as Alzheimer's disease, Parkinson's disease, or prion disease. EVs have been shown to transport and to support the release of abnormally phosphorylated tau protein, alpha-synuclein (α-Syn), and prion protein (PrP^C) (Aguzzit and Lakkaraju 2016). For example, it has been shown that Tau species including oligomers and aggregates are released via exosomes by neurons (Wang et al. 2017a). Asai and coworkers have demonstrated that tau propagation in vivo and in vitro can be significantly reduced by inhibiting exosome synthesis from microglia cells (Asai et al. 2015). Thus, exosome secretion might represent a therapeutic target for PMDs such as Alzheimer's disease.

It is worth noting that in addition to the well-documented pathological role of EVs in a number of diseases, EVs are also important in physiological processes such as tissue repair or regeneration. For instance, treatment with mesenchymal stromal cell-derived exosomes prevents the activation of hypoxic signaling that underlies pulmonary inflammation and the development of pulmonary hypertension in mice (Lee et al. 2012). Recent data have pointed to the concept of tissue crosstalk during exercise. It has been demonstrated that exercise induces a release of exosome-packaged proteins that are involved in a broad array of biological processes. Exosomes liberated by exercise have a propensity to localize in the liver and can exert systemic biological effects (Whitham et al. 2018). Athero-protective communication between endothelial cells and smooth muscle cells (SMC) through miRNAs has been documented: endothelial-derived miRNA143/145-containing vesicles can be transferred to SMC to prevent SMC dedifferentiation and to reduce atherosclerotic lesion formation in vivo (Hergenreider et al. 2012).

1.3 EVs as Disease Biomarkers

EVs, and exosomes in particular, are attractive as a potential source of biomarkers for disease diagnosis and prognosis because of their ability to protect and transport pathological molecules in biofluids, creating an analysis opportunity using relatively noninvasive procedures. Noteworthy, several reports suggest that of exosomal protein concentration is higher in cancer patients than in tumor-free individuals (Peinado et al. 2012; Li et al. 2017). For example, RAS protein and activating transcription factor 1 (ATF1) have been proposed as biomarkers for the early diagnosis of cervical cancer; both proteins are detected in plasma exosomes in a mouse model of cervical cancer (Shi et al. 2017). The diagnostic value of exosomes could also be exploited in neurodegenerative diseases. One good example is the presence of tau protein in exosomes in the cerebrospinal fluid of patients with Alzheimer's disease (Saman et al. 2012).

Not just proteins but also noncoding RNAs, particularly miRNAs, circulate in EVs. The role of miRNAs in cancer pathways is well documented (Kai et al. 2017). For example, high levels of miRNA-122 in the blood circulation of breast cancer patients have been associated with metastatic progression (Fong et al. 2015). Exosomal miRNA-105 expressed by metastatic breast cancer cells can disrupt endothelial cell tight junctions and disrupt the blood-brain barrier, promoting brain metastases (Zhou et al. 2014).

Changes in exosome lipid profiles could provide information about pathological processes as well; however, this area is less well investigated. It has been shown that injured hepatocytes release exosomes enriched in C16:0 ceramide, which activates macrophage chemotaxis via formation of sphingosine-1-phosphate (S1P) from C16:0 ceramide in nonalcoholic steatohepatitis (NASH) (Kakazu et al. 2016). C16:0 ceramide has been proposed as a marker of lipotoxic stress due to its high levels in plasma exosomes in both mouse and human models of NASH (Kakazu et al. 2016) Hexosylceramide (HexCer) is another potential diagnostic marker in prostate cancer, and HexCer species have been reported to be more abundant in urinary exosomes from prostate cancer patients than from controls (Skotland et al. 2017).

1.4 Exosomes as Drug Delivery Vehicles

EVs are also attracting considerable attention as potential drug delivery vehicles. They offer biocompatibility and high physicochemical stability (Clayton et al. 2003) compared with other synthetic vectors such as liposomes or nanoparticles. While drug-loaded nanoparticles in the bloodstream are rapidly cleared by mononuclear phagocytosis (Peng et al. 2013), exosomes escape such phagocytosis (van den Boorn et al. 2011).

Interestingly, exosomes are able to cross the blood-brain barrier. Alvarez-Erviti and coworkers used exosomes to deliver short-interfering RNA (siRNA) to the brains of mice. The targeting to brain cells was achieved by engineering dendritic cells to express an exosomal membrane protein fused with rabies viral glycoprotein (RVG) peptide, which binds the acetylcholine receptor. siRNA against the protein BACE1 was exosome-loaded using electroporation. After intravenous injection, BACE1 knockdown in neurons, microglia, and oligodendrocytes was observed at both the mRNA and protein levels (Alvarez-Erviti et al. 2011). Using the same cell line, Yang and collaborators showed that exosomes can efficiently deliver miRNA-124 to the infarct site in a focal ischemia mouse model to promote cortical neurogenesis (Yang et al. 2017). EVs loaded with catalase, which is a promising drug in the treatment of Parkinson's disease, were able to reach target neurons and accumulate in them in a Parkinson's mouse model (Haney et al. 2015). Exosomes could also help achieve targeted delivery to minimize the side effects of drugs.

2 Lipids in Exosomes

2.1 Lipid Composition of Exosomes

The lipid composition of exosomes varies in a manner that correlates with the pre-analytical parameters described earlier (which is also true for other constituents of exosomes). Cell density (Kavaliauskiene et al. 2014) and the composition of the culture medium (Stoll and Spector 1984) impact on cellular lipid composition and intracellular trafficking of the cell and thereby will influence exosome composition as well (Skotland et al. 2017). After differential ultracentrifugation (Fig. 2), exosomes can still be contaminated with lipid droplets, lipoproteins, and other lipoparticles, and these contaminants can interfere with lipidomic analyses. For instance, cholesterol esters and triacylglycerides form part of the core of lipoproteins, and their presence might indicate contamination (van Meer et al. 2008). Taken together, different studies point to an enrichment of exosomes with cholesterol, sphingomyelin (SM), ceramide, and phosphatidylserine (PS) and suggest that exosome composition resembles that of plasma membrane rafts (Laulagnier et al. 2004b; Trajkovic et al. 2008; Llorente et al. 2013; Wubbolts et al. 2003). Interestingly, human immunodeficiency virus type 1 (HIV-1) particles resemble exosomes in terms of lipid content (Brugger et al. 2006), consistent with reports that HIV-1 can "hijack" the exosome biogenesis pathway (Grigorov et al. 2006). For more details about exosomal lipids, the reader is invited to consult an excellent recent review (Skotland et al. 2017).

2.2 Transport of Bioactive Lipids

Exosomes carry bioactive lipids that traffic between cells and can promote inflammatory disease (Esser et al. 2010) or immunosuppression (Xiang et al. 2009; Salimu et al. 2017). Exosomes from RBL-2H3 cells contain arachidonic acid and derivatives such as prostaglandin E2 (PGE2) and 15-deoxy-$\Delta^{12,14}$-prostaglandinJ2 (Subra et al. 2010). PGE2 has also been identified in exosomes from 4T-1 cells, a murine mammary adenocarcinoma cell line (Xiang et al. 2009), and in DU145, a prostate cancer cell line (Salimu et al. 2017). Xiang et al. observed induction of myeloid-derived suppressor cells, which promote tumor progression, after the intravenous injection of PGE2-enriched exosomes in mice (Xiang et al. 2009). These immunosuppressive effects were also observed when PGE2-enriched exosomes from prostatic cancer cell line were incubated with dendritic cells (Salimu et al. 2017). This treatment led to an impairment of cross-presentation function in dendritic cells. Taken together, these findings suggest that tumor exosomes containing PGE2 have a role in immune regulation. Noteworthy, exosomes can also contain enzymes responsible for the biosynthesis of bioactive lipids. For example, exosomes released from macrophages and dendritic cells transport enzymes for biosynthesis of leukotrienes, which are potent proinflammatory lipid mediators (Esser et al. 2010). γ-glutamyl transpeptidase (GGT) is an enzyme involved in leukotriene metabolism and is present in A549 cells, a human lung carcinoma cell line (Lukic et al. 2016). GGT converts leukotriene C4 (LTC4) to leukotriene D4 (LTD4), which has a 10- to 50-fold higher potency than LTC4 for activation of cysteinyl LTs, which contributes to symptoms in several chronic inflammatory diseases including asthma (Lukic et al. 2016).

3 Role of Lipids in the Biogenesis of Exosomes

The endosomal sorting complex required for transport (ESCRT) is the best-described mechanism for the formation of ILV and MVB (Henne et al. 2011; Hanson and Cashikar 2012). It consists of four multimeric complexes (ESCRT-0, ESCRT-I, ESCRT-II, and ESCRT-III) and associated proteins (e.g., VPS4 and ALIX) that are assembled in an orderly manner at the endosome, recognizing and sequestering ubiquitinated membrane proteins for ultimate budding and incorporation into ILVs (Raiborg and Stenmark 2009; Hurley et al. 2010).

Besides ESCRTs, syndecans, syntenin (Baietti et al. 2012), heparanase (Roucourt et al. 2015), SRC (Imjeti et al. 2017), and ARF6 (Ghossoub et al. 2014) have been shown to participate in the budding of ILVs that contribute significantly to the pool of exosomal vesicles, at least in a cell type like MCF-7. Noteworthy, specific lipids and lipid-modifying enzymes such as neutral sphingomyelinase 2 (Trajkovic et al. 2008) and phospholipase D2 (Ghossoub et al. 2014) have been shown to participate in the budding of ILVs and to impact on exosome production.

3.1 Neutral Sphingomyelinase 2 and Its Reaction Product Ceramide

Sphingolipids represent one of the major classes of eukaryotic lipids. This large family, which includes bioactive sphingolipids such as sphingosine, ceramide, or S1P, not only is an important structural component of membranes but also has important roles in a wide range of signaling pathways (Hannun and Obeid 2017). Among the bioactive species of sphingolipids, ceramide has been identified as an important molecule in exosome biology (Trajkovic et al. 2008). Ceramide can be synthesized by multiple pathways including the ceramide salvage pathway (Kitatani et al. 2008), the de novo synthetic pathway in the endoplasmic reticulum (Perry 2002), and the hydrolysis of complex sphingolipids such as SM in the cytosol or endosomal compartments (Stoffel 1999) (Fig. 4). Consistent with the role of the SM pathway in exosome formation (Trajkovic et al. 2008), lipidomic studies show that exosomes are enriched for SM and ceramide in comparison to whole cells (Trajkovic et al. 2008; Llorente et al. 2013).

Sphingomyelinases (SMases) catalyze the hydrolysis of the phosphocholine headgroup from SM to generate ceramide and phosphorylcholine (Fig. 4). SMases are classified based on their pH optimum into acid, neutral, and alkaline subtypes, respectively. The neutral SMases (nSMases) family is composed of four members: nSMase1, nSMase2, nSMase3, and the recently identified nSMase that associates to mitochondria (MA-nSMase) (Wu et al. 2010a). The biological function of the latter is still unknown (Rajagopalan et al. 2015). These enzymes catalyze the hydrolysis of SM, at least in vitro. NSMase2 (Marchesini et al. 2003) and nSMase3 (Corcoran et al. 2008) have been reported to possess both in vitro and in vivo activities, whereas nSMase1 was found to function as a lysophospholipase C and not as a nSMase in vivo (Sawai et al. 1999). All nSMases identified so far have an absolute

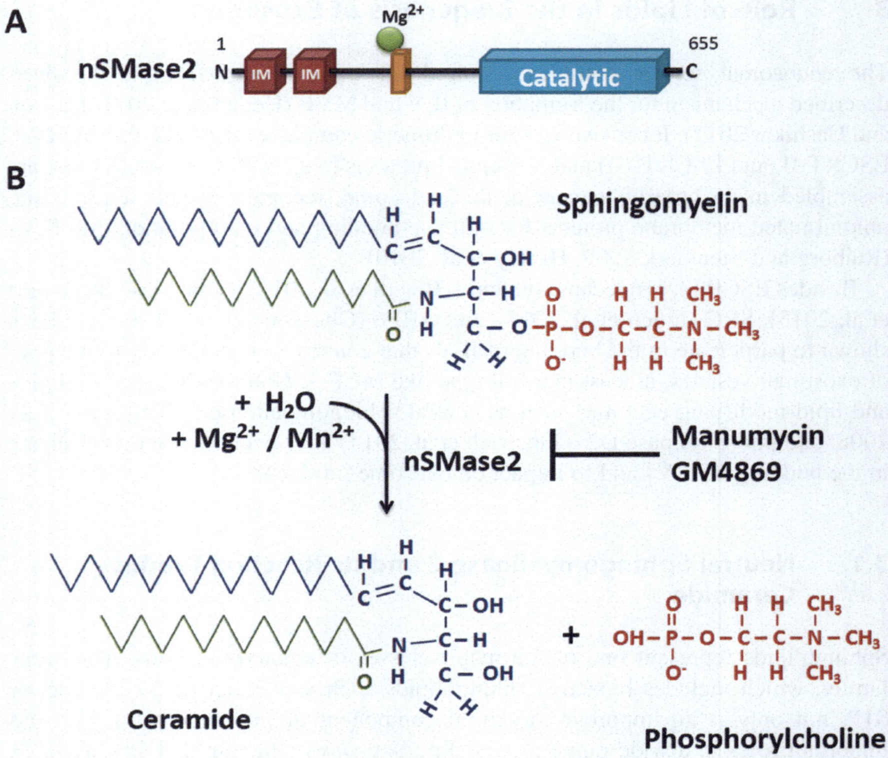

Fig. 4 (**a**) Domain structure of mammalian nSMase2. The amino (N) and carboxyl (C) terminal amino acids are indicated. In red, intramembrane hydrophobic domains (IM); in orange, cation-binding domain; and in blue, catalytic domain. UniProt code: nSMase2 Q9NY59. (**b**) Sphingomyelin consists of a phosphocholine headgroup (red), a sphingosine (blue), and a fatty acid chain (green). Sphingomyelin can be hydrolyzed by nSMase2 to form ceramide and phosphorylcholine in the presence of one molecule of water and divalent cations such as Mg^{2+} or Mn^{2+}. Manumycin and GM4869 are competitive and noncompetitive inhibitors, respectively, that block nSMase2 activity

requirement for cations such as $Mg^{(2+)}$ and $Mn^{(2+)}$ for their catalytic activity. Furthermore, nSMase2 (Marchesini et al. 2003), nSMase3 (Krut et al. 2006), and MA-nSMase (Wu et al. 2010b) can be activated by anionic phospholipids, especially PS and the mitochondrial cardiolipin. NSMases are known to display different steady-state localizations in the cell. NSMase1 is ubiquitously expressed in various tissues and concentrates in the endoplasmic reticulum (ER) and the Golgi (Tomiuk et al. 2000); nSMase2 is found in the Golgi and at the plasma membrane (Milhas et al. 2010); nSMase3 is localized in the ER where it is anchored via a C-terminal transmembrane domain (Krut et al. 2006); and finally, MA-nSMase associates with the outer mitochondrial membrane (Rajagopalan et al. 2015).

Only nSMase2 has been implicated in the biogenesis of EVs/exosomes (Trajkovic et al. 2008; Kowal et al. 2014). Moreover, its importance might be cell type-dependent. Studies performed with HEK293 cells (Kosaka et al. 2010), mouse neuroblastoma N2a cells (Yuyama et al. 2012), and oligodendroglial Oli-neu cells (Trajkovic et al. 2008) indicate that inhibition or depletion of nSMase2 affects ILV budding. Yet, ceramide seems not to be involved in the formation of ILVs for MNT-1 melanoma cells (van Niel et al. 2011) or the human prostatic cancer cell line PC-3 (Phuyal et al. 2014).

3.1.1 Ceramide Production in Exosome Biology and Composition

Ceramide has the unique biophysical property of inducing coalescence of small microdomains to form large, ceramide-enriched macrodomains (Holopainen et al. 1998). This can lead to the oligomerization of selected cell surface receptors and promote domain-induced budding. For example, ceramide-enriched domains are important for the internalization or budding of viruses (Gulbins and Kolesnick 2003; Tani et al. 2010). The cone-shaped structure of ceramide can induce spontaneous negative curvature that supports spontaneous endosomal intraluminal budding. Furthermore, ceramide induces spontaneous fusion of lipid vesicles even at very low concentrations (Abdul-Hammed et al. 2010). Ceramide also excludes cholesterol from membranes. Cholesterol is known to stabilize membranes and enables the liquid-ordered phase of lipid bilayers (Vance and Van den Bosch 2000) that is disrupted by ceramide. It has widely been reported that depletion of cholesterol by methyl-β-cyclodextrin treatment in human prostate cancer cell line PC-3 enhances exosome release (Llorente et al. 2007).

Selection of RNAs for incorporation into ILVs depends on their affinity for ceramide-enriched regions at the outer layer of the MVB membrane (Janas et al. 2015). Kosaka and coworkers have proposed that a ceramide-dependent secretory pathway is involved in miRNA secretion, observing that inhibiting nSMase2 with the chemical inhibitor GW4869 or siRNA reduces miRNA secretion, whereas the expression of protein exosomal markers such as CD63 did not change (Kosaka et al. 2010). Conversely, nSMase2 overexpression increases extracellular amounts of miRNA (Kosaka et al. 2010). For example, nSMase2 and/or ceramide promotes exosome-mediated miRNA-10b secretion, whereas ceramide inhibitor suppresses it (Singh et al. 2014). miRNA-10b is highly expressed in metastatic breast cancer and is actively secreted into medium via exosomes (Singh et al. 2014). Noteworthy, RNA motifs can also selectively interact with raft-like regions that are sorted into exosomes, for example, the heterogeneous nuclear ribonucleoprotein A2B1 (hnRNPA2B1) controls RNA loading into exosomes and co-localizes with ceramide markers (Villarroya-Beltri et al. 2013). hnRNPA2B1 could thus contribute to the packaging of RNAs into exosomes in a ceramide-dependent manner.

The nSMase pathway, nSMase2 activity, and ceramide production in particular have also been proposed to help pack infectious prions into exosomes (Guo et al. 2015) and to promote aggregation of neurotoxic amyloid-β peptides, consequently exacerbating Alzheimer's disease-related pathologies (Dinkins et al. 2016).

3.1.2 Neutral Sphingomyelinase 2 Inhibitors

Manumycin-A is a natural product that was first isolated from *Streptomyces parvulus* and has been reported to act as an irreversible inhibitor of nSMase (Arenz et al. 2001b). Other manumycin-A analogues, such as scyphostatin, have been reported to inhibit acidic SMase (aSMase) in a competitive manner (Arenz et al. 2001a). Manumycin-A and the nSMase substrate SM have been proposed to compete for binding at the nSMase active site (Arenz et al. 2001b). However, the use of manumycin-A as a nSMase2 inhibitor is controversial and should be avoided (Hofmann et al. 2000; Jung et al. 2000; Mittelbrunn et al. 2011; Datta et al. 2017; Shi et al. 2017).

GW4869, another nSMase inhibitor, functions as a noncompetitive inhibitor at low concentrations (IC50 of 1 μM) and at high concentrations (>150 μM) also inhibits aSMase (Luberto et al. 2002). For manumycin-A, activity measurements were obtained using rat brain and bacterial nSMases, and thus it is unclear whether their activity is specific for nSMase2 (Luberto et al. 2002). The treatment of cells with GW4869 decreases exosome release (Trajkovic et al. 2008; Kosaka et al. 2010) and exosomal miRNAs, but not cellular miRNAs (Kosaka et al. 2010). However, the field would benefit from better pharmacological characterization of these nSMase2 inhibitors.

3.2 Phospholipase D2 and Its Reaction Product Phosphatidic Acid

Phospholipase D (PLD) catalyzes the hydrolysis of phosphatidylcholine (PC), the most abundant membrane phospholipid, to yield phosphatidic acid (PA) and choline (Fig. 5). There are six mammalian isoforms, designated PLD1–6 (Frohman 2015).

Thus far, only PLD2 (Colley et al. 1997) has been implicated in the biogenesis of extracellular vesicles/exosomes (Laulagnier et al. 2004a; Ghossoub et al. 2014). In a cell line model of human mammary carcinoma (MCF-7), ARF6 depletion decreased exosomal proteins such as syntenin, ALIX, CD63, and syndecan and reduced ILV budding (Ghossoub et al. 2014). Similar observations were obtained upon depletion of the ARF nucleotide-binding site opener (ARNO), which is an ARF6-specific guanine nucleotide exchange factor (GEF). Investigation of the ARF6 effectors mediating these effects pointed to a role for PLD2, which ARF6 stimulates (Honda et al. 1999). In contrast, roles for other ARF6 effectors including PLD1 and phosphatidylinositol 4-phosphate 5-kinase-α or -γ (PIP5K-α and -γ), which produces phosphatidylinositol 4,5-bisphosphate (PI(4,5)P2) (Ghossoub et al. 2014), were ruled out. PI(4,5)P2 is an important cofactor/activator of PLD2, leading to increased PA formation that further stimulates PIP5K activity (Honda et al. 1999; Divecha et al. 2000). However, this does not seem to be a rate-limiting factor for MVB formation, since PIP5K knockdown doesn't affect syntenin intra-endosomal budding (Ghossoub et al. 2014). Interestingly, on endosomal membranes, ARF6-PIP5K supports the recycling of syntenin and associated transmembrane protein cargo through direct syntenin-PI(4,5)P2 interaction (Zimmermann et al. 2005; Egea-Jimenez et al. 2016). In contrast, ARF6-PLD2 appears to drive formation of MVBs

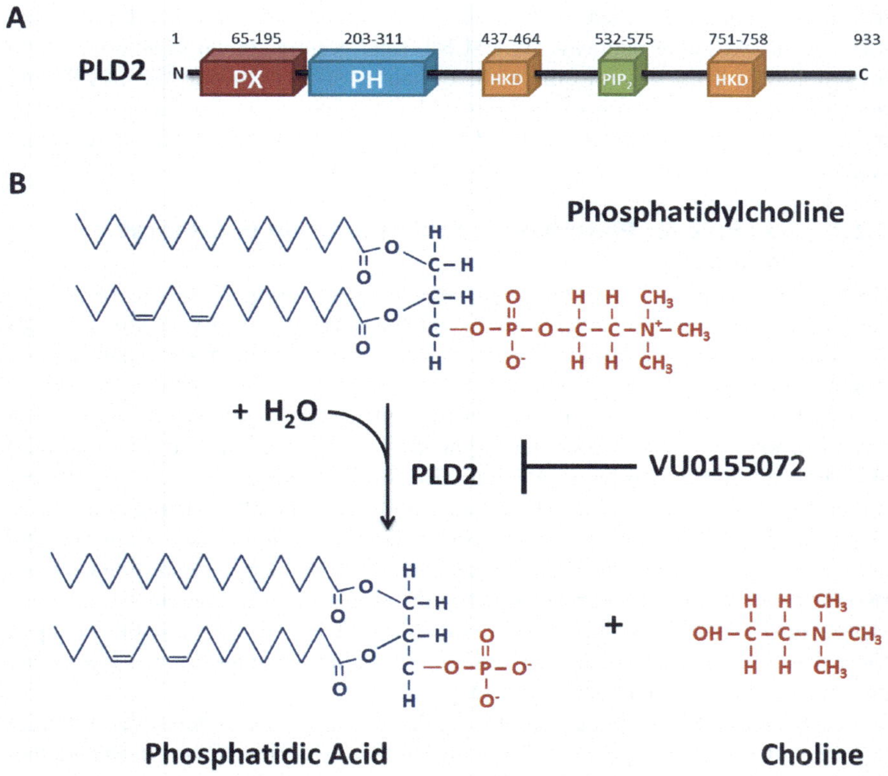

Fig. 5 (**a**) Domain structure of mammalian PLD2. The amino (N) and carboxyl (C) terminals are shown. Domains: in red, the *phox* domain (PX); in blue, the pleckstrin homology (PH) domain; in orange, the catalytic sequence HxxxxxxxKxD/E (HKD domain); and in green, the PIP2 binding site. UniProt code: PLD2 O14393. (**b**) Phosphatidylcholine is a glycerophospholipid in which two fatty acids are linked to a glycerol moiety by ester bonds in carbons 1 and 2 (blue). The third carbon of glycerol is esterified to phosphorylcholine (red). Phosphatidylcholine is hydrolyzed by PLD2 to form phosphatidic acid and choline in the presence of water. VU0155072 is a small molecule PLD2-selective inhibitor

filled with ILVs (Ghossoub et al. 2014). This model is in the line with the observations of Laulagnier et al. (2004b) that stimulation of RBL-2H3 cells with ionomycin boosted the release of exosomes in a PLD2-dependent manner. Ionomycin is an ionophore that induces the hydrolysis of PI(4,5)P2 and hence IP3-triggered release of calcium into the cytoplasm. PI(4,5)P2 hydrolysis would impair the recycling pathway and indirectly favor the formation of ILVs. Moreover, high levels of intra-cytosolic calcium could facilitate the fusion events necessary for the secretion of ILVs as exosomes (Hay 2007). Interestingly, syntenin also directly interacts with PA. While ARNO is thought to be the preferred ARF6 GEF for the outward budding, one still needs to clarify which stimulator of ARF6 would support the recycling pathway. Clearly, syntenin-ALIX interaction and ESCRT are necessary for the exosomal pathway. As ESCRT was recently shown to stimulate both inward (away from the cytosol, with formation of ILVs inside the MVB) and outward (toward the cytosol) budding (McCullough et al. 2015), it would be interesting to explore the roles of ALIX and ESCRT in the syntenin recycling pathway.

3.2.1 Key Role for Phosphatidic Acid Production in Exosome Biogenesis?

PA (the product of PLD) represents the simplest phospholipid (Fig. 5). Despite its simple structure and relatively low abundance (1–4% of total phospholipids (Voelker 1991, Welti et al. 2002)), PA is important for membrane dynamics, i.e., fission and fusion events (Kooijman et al. 2003). The function of PA is likely attributable to its ability to induce negative membrane curvature because of its "small head" (forming a cone that might favor endosomal intraluminal budding) (Vitale et al. 2001). Moreover, PA can also directly interact with many different proteins (Kooijman et al. 2003, 2005; Stace and Ktistakis 2006; Huang et al. 2011; Wang et al. 2017b). However, there isn't a consensus amino acid sequence that defines a PA binding site. PA enables an electrostatic/hydrogen bond switch (Kooijman et al. 2007) when engaging with protein ligands wherein the negative charge of the PA headgroup is increased from -1 to -2 and is stabilized upon formation of hydrogen bonds with lysine and arginine residues of the interacting protein (Kooijman and Testerink 2010).

For instance, PA is implicated in regulated exocytosis in multiple cell lines (Vitale et al. 2001). It supports the secretion of von Willebrand factor from endothelial cells (Disse et al. 2009) and insulin from pancreatic β cells (Waselle et al. 2005). In RBL-2H3 cells, PA controls the trafficking of glycoconjugates from the Golgi to the plasma membrane (Marchini-Alves et al. 2015). Whether PA might be essential for outward budding in endosomes and MVB formation has not been directly investigated. PA is barely detectable in exosomes (Laulagnier et al. 2004b; Brouwers et al. 2013; Llorente et al. 2013). This is also true for exosomes produced by MCF-7 cells where ARF6-PLD2 clearly controls ILV budding and exosome secretion (Ghossoub et al. 2014).

What might explain why PA is not easily detected in exosomes? PA has important roles in cell signaling, and its level is tightly regulated inside cells by multiple phospholipases. Extending this thought, Subra and coworkers observed that intact exosomes derived from RBL-2H3 cells have phosphatidate phosphatase 1 (PAP1) activity (Subra et al. 2010). Upon the incubation of BODIPY-PA with extracellular vesicles enriched in exosomes, 60% of the PA was hydrolyzed into diglycerides within 15 min.

Yet, PA might be key at stages of the process other than budding through its biophysical properties and/or direct interactions with effector proteins involved in the process of ILV budding. It could also control the transport and plasma membrane docking of ILV-filled MVBs. Because of its negative curvature, PA production could stimulate the initiation of the ILV budding. Noteworthy, lipid-binding data suggest that syntenin can directly interact with PA (Ghossoub et al. 2014). Irrespective of the curvature, syntenin interaction with PA could concentrate the syntenin/syndecan/CD63/ALIX complexes at the nascent bud, with ALIX-ESCRT further stimulating the budding process. PA could also support ILV budding independently of ESCRT. Indeed, nSMase2 has also been proposed to interact with PA (Marchesini et al. 2003; Wu et al. 2011), and this binding activity could support nSMase2 targeting to MVBs (Wu et al. 2011). Interestingly, PA can interact with SRC in various manners: through its SH4 domain, via a unique lipid-binding region (ULRB), and also via its SH3 domains. Such interactions stimulate SRC activation by favoring the open conformation (Stith 2015). In turn, SRC can activate PLD2 in MCF-7 cells by phosphorylating tyrosine 511 (Henkels et al. 2010). Such positive feedback loop could support sustained ILV production and would be consistent with the recently established role of SRC in exosome biogenesis (Imjeti et al. 2017). Whether the production of PA is required to initiate the feedback loop is unclear, because a scenario wherein PLD2 functions as a scaffold upon SRC activation has been proposed. SRC could bind to PLD2 by interacting with its PH domain and/or via SH2-PX interactions (Banno et al. 2005). Interestingly, there is evidence that RAS mediates the activation of PLD that is induced by SRC in vivo (Jiang et al. 1995), but whether RAS might function in exosome biogenesis and cargo-loading by acting on the PLD2-PA axis is unexplored. Possibly after PLD2 action, flipping of PA from the endosomal membrane facing the cytosol to the luminal membrane could help complete the ILV bud. In support of this hypothesis, lipids such as PA can spontaneously move from one leaflet to the other within seconds or minutes (Pomorski et al. 2004).

Annexins, a family of Ca^{2+}-regulated phospholipid-binding proteins that can interact with PA (Lizarbe et al. 2013), could facilitate ILV fission. Annexins have been proposed to mediate or regulate membrane fusion by inducing membrane curvature (Boye et al. 2017), have been identified in extracellular vesicles enriched in exosomes (Dang et al. 2017), and localize at MVBs (Jackle et al. 1994). The conversion of PC to PA mediated by PLD2 might lower the Ca^{2+} requirements for membrane fusion in the presence of annexins (Blackwood et al. 1997). Signaling proteins such as ribosomal S6 kinases (S6K) are activated by PA and thereby support actin polymerization (Lehman et al. 2007). Such actin polymerization, when taking place at the MVB outer membrane, could support the procession of MVBs to the plasma membrane. Noteworthy, PA also binds to the tyrosine kinase Fer and enhances its ability to phosphorylate cortactin, a protein that promotes actin polymerization (Itoh et al. 2009). Recently, cortactin has been described to act as a positive regulator of exosome secretion (Gangoda and Mathivanan 2016; Sinha et al. 2016). Thus, PA production on the limiting membrane of MVBs could facilitate exosome release through several mechanisms.

3.2.2 PLD Inhibitors

PLD activity can be diverted (not inhibited) by supplying primary alcohols such as ethanol or 1-butanol, as is taken advantage of for in vitro and in vivo assays. PLD has the ability to transfer the phosphatidyl moiety of the phospholipid to primary alcohol rather than to water, subsequently producing phosphatidyl alcohol (e.g., phosphatidylbutanol (PtdButOH)) instead of PA (Kobayashi and Kanfer 1987). Secondary and tertiary alcohols such as *sec*-butyl or *tert*-butyl, respectively, are not PLD substrates (Munnik et al. 1995). Primary alcohols have many other effects on cells though, making it challenging to use them to identify specific roles for PLD in cellular studies, much less in vivo. Halopemide, a psychotropic agent, was identified through a high-throughput screen to inhibit PLD2 and then used as a starting point to develop analogues with increased potency (Monovich et al. 2007). One such compound, 5-fluoro-2-indolyl des-chloro-halopemide (FIPI), was subsequently shown to also inhibit PLD1 (Scott et al. 2009; Su et al. 2009). Other analogues were generated that are selective for PLD1 or PLD2 (Scott et al. 2009). FIPI is a potent in vivo inhibitor of both PLD1 and PLD2 that alters cell spreading and inhibits chemotaxis (Su et al. 2009), platelet activation and thrombosis (Stegner et al. 2013), and tumor growth and metastasis (Chen et al. 2012). FIPI might interact with conserved regions in the HDK domains, underlying its ability to inhibit both PLD1 and PLD2 (Ganesan et al. 2015).

Selective PLD2 inhibition can be achieved using the small molecule halopamide analogue VU0155072 (*N*-(2-(4-oxo-1-phenyl-1,3,8-triazaspiro[4.5]decan-8-yl) ethyl)naphthalene-2-carboxamide*N*-[2-(4-oxo-1-phenyl-1,3,8 triazaspiro[4,5]dec-8-yl)ethyl]-2-naphthalenecarboxamide) (PLD1 IC50 = 510 μM versus PLD2 IC50 = 140 nM) (Scott et al. 2009). VU0155072 has been reported to decrease tumor volume and metastasis in a mouse breast cancer model (Henkels et al. 2016) and to inhibit PLD2-dependent exosome production (Ghossoub et al. 2014).

3.3 Other Lipids Involved in Exosome Biogenesis and Release

Additional lipids can impact on exosome biogenesis and release. For example, interaction between hsc-70 (HSPA8), a cytosolic molecular chaperone, and PS at the endosomal limiting membrane is important for cargo internalization into endosomes (Morozova et al. 2016).

Lysobisphosphatidic acid (LBPA) is an isomer of phosphatidylglycerol (PG), and its concentration rises from 1 to 15% of total phospholipids between early and late endosomes in BHK cells (Kobayashi et al. 1998). LBPA has not been detected elsewhere in the cell and exhibits unique pH-dependent fusogenic properties (Kobayashi et al. 1998; Matsuo et al. 2004). LBPA can induce the formation of multivesicular liposomes when their lumen is acidic and interacts with ALIX (Matsuo et al. 2004) and the chaperon protein Hsp70 (Kirkegaard et al. 2010), indicating that LBPA can participate in exosome biogenesis.

The exosomal secretion of cholesterol depends on the presence of flotillin-2, since it recruits cholesterol to MVBs and exosomes (Strauss et al. 2010). Interestingly, U18666A [3-β-(2-[diethylamino]ethoxy)-androst-5-en-17-one, monohydrochloride], an amphiphilic drug known to inhibit cholesterol transport from the lysosomal compartment to the ER for esterification and redistribution to other cellular compartments (Appelqvist et al. 2011), blocks MVBs and lipid transport by direct inhibition of the protein Niemann-Pick type C1 (NPC1) and thus mimics the lysosomal storage disease Niemann-Pick disease type C (Sokol et al. 1988). U18666A treatment has been reported to drive formation of nonfunctional MVBs in which hepatitis C virus (HCV) particles (Elgner et al. 2016) or the HIV-1 Gag polyprotein (Lindwasser and Resh 2004) accumulate, with their release blocked. However in contrast, Strauss et al. observed a stimulation of exosome release in oligodendroglial cells treated with U18666A (Strauss et al. 2010). These authors showed that free cholesterol is partially released by exosomes, and the cholesterol enrichment of exosomes is upregulated in response to the cholesterol accumulation in late endosomal compartments, helping to ameliorate the lysosomal storage of cholesterol (Strauss et al. 2010).

Although phosphoinositides represent a small percentage of total cellular phospholipids, they are involved in diverse cellular signaling processes. Many phosphoinositide kinases (PIKs) have been described, each able to transfer a phosphate to a particular position on the inositol ring of phosphatidylinositol (PI). PIKs are grouped into three general families: phosphatidylinositol 3-kinases (PI3Ks), phosphatidylinositol 4-kinases (PI4Ks), and phosphatidylinositol 5-kinases (PI5Ks). PI can be reversibly phosphorylated at three distinct positions of the inositol ring, and thus, seven different phosphoinositides can be generated. PI3Ks and PI5Ks deserve the most attention in the present context because of their relevance in membrane trafficking and protein sorting.

PI3Ks phosphorylate the 3-hydroxyl group of the inositol ring of phosphoinositides (PIs) generating four different 3-PIs species: PI(3)P, PI(3,4)P2, PI(3,5)P2, and PI(3,4,5) P2. The multiple isoforms of PI3Ks share homologous subunits in the catalytic region and are divided into three classes (Vanhaesebroeck et al. 2001). Class I (subdivided into Class IA and Class IB) which is able to phosphorylate PI, PI(4)P, and PI(4,5)P2. This class is responsible for the production of PI(3)P, PI(3,4)P2, and PI(3,4,5)P2. Moreover, Class IA can also phosphorylate PI(5)P in vitro (Fruman et al. 1998). Class II catalyzes the production of PI(3)P from PI and PI(3,4)P2 from PI(4,5)P2. Class III produces only PI(3)P from PI (Leevers et al. 1999). PI(3)P is required for endosomal transport and MVBs formation and sorting (Schu et al. 1993; Gillooly et al. 2000). Wortmannin, a fungal metabolite, and LY294002, a flavonoid-based synthetic compound, inhibit PI(3) P production and display a similar potency in vitro for the Class I, II, and III (Vanhaesebroeck et al. 2001) kinases and inhibit MVB biogenesis. Cells treated with wortmannin or LY294002 show large vacuoles with only a few ILVs (Fernandez-Borja et al. 1999).

Finally, PI5Ks act on PI and PI(3)P to produce PI(5)P and PI(3,5)P2, respectively. PI5Ks include two mammalian enzymes, type I PIP kinase and PIKfyve. PIKfyve is the principal enzyme controlling the PI-5 pathway in the cellular context (McEwen et al. 1999; Shisheva 2001). Interestingly, PYKfyve is largely associated with the membranes of late endosomes (Shisheva et al. 2001). Its product PI(3,5)P2 is enriched in late endosomes, MVBs, and lysosomes/vacuoles. PI(3,5)P2 has been shown to be important for the transport of MVBs to lysosomes (Hessvik et al. 2016). The depletion of PIKfyve by specific siRNA increases the release of exosomes from prostatic cancer PC-3 cell line, suggesting an impairment in the fusion of MVBs with lysosomes (Hessvik et al. 2016). Hayakawa and coworkers identified a pyridofuropyrimidine compound, YM201636, as potent inhibitor of PIKfyve kinase activity in vitro (IC50 of 33 nM). The IC50 of this compound for PI-3P kinases was almost 100-fold higher (IC50 3 μM), and the compound displayed no inhibitory effect on the Class II kinases (Hayakawa et al. 2006; Jefferies et al. 2008). Interestingly, VPS24, a component of ESCRT-III, binds PI(3,5)P2 (Whitley et al. 2003). VPS24 is involved in the final steps of ILV formation driving neck constriction and membrane scission (Hanson and Cashikar 2012), and thus PI(3,5)P2-VPS24 interaction might contribute to ILV budding.

4 Conclusions and Future Perspectives

Exosomes have emerged as important organelles for cell-cell communication. Their stability and presence in biofluids make them attractive as source of biomarkers. Yet, their interest for biomedicine goes beyond biomarker discovery, as they are currently also considered as potential therapeutic targets or vehicles for efficient drug delivery. These double membrane-limited extracellular vesicles carry nucleic acids, proteins, and lipids that are able to reprogram recipient cells. Exosomes appear to be enriched in certain lipids, such as ceramide, cholesterol, and sphingomyelin, among others. The composition of exosomes is modified in various diseases, and the study of their lipid profile might provide information for clinicians. However, the field still needs to define robust pre-analytical parameters (e.g., to avoid contaminants such as lipid droplets) and to develop appropriate methods of identification to make their use amenable in daily practice.

Lipids and lipid-modifying enzymes participate in the biology of exosomes, as exemplified by the involvement of PI(3,5)P2, nSMAse2, and PLD2 in the making of exosomes. Noteworthy, both nSMase2 and PLD2 generate cone-shaped lipids (ceramide and PA, respectively) that trigger negative membrane curvature. This biophysical property might facilitate vesicular budding. Clearly, not all lipid-modifying enzymes contribute to exosome biogenesis. For instance, PLD1, hydrolyzing PC to PA and closely related to PLD2, does not participate in exosome biogenesis.

The specific relationship between lipids and protein complexes important for exosome biogenesis (e.g., ESCRTs and accessory components) remains to be elucidated. The same holds for the possible impact of lipids on the exosomal sorting of specific nucleic acids. As well, the relationship between tetraspanins, the major constituents of exosomes, and lipids, remains to be explored. Similarly, the possibility that specific lipids can have important roles on the side of the recipient cells (exosome-cell contacts, fusion, and/or uptake) and contribute to specific signaling events awaits further investigations.

No doubt, there is a huge amount of work left to discover and understand how lipids and lipid-modifying enzymes impact on exosome turnover and signaling. Yet, this knowledge might contribute to paving the way for the design of specific drugs to dampen systemic diseases and open new therapeutic opportunities for patients.

Acknowledgments Work in the laboratory of PZ is supported by grants from the Institut National du Cancer (INCa, Subvention 2013-105), the French Foundation for Cancer Research (ARC Grant PJA 20161204584), the Agence Nationale de la Recherche (ANR-18-CE13-0017, Project SynTEV), the Fund for Scientific Research–Flanders (FWO Grants G.0846.15 and G0C5718N), and the Belgian Foundation Against Cancer (STK Grant 2016-104). Antonio Luis EGEA-JIMENEZ was recipient of a postdoctoral fellowship of La Ligue contre le Cancer (France). This project has received funding from the European Union's Horizon 2020 research and innovation program under the Marie Sklodowska-Curie grant agreement No 747025.

References

Abdul-Hammed M, Breiden B, Adebayo MA, Babalola JO, Schwarzmann G, Sandhoff K (2010) Role of endosomal membrane lipids and NPC2 in cholesterol transfer and membrane fusion. J Lipid Res 51(7):1747–1760

Abusamra AJ, Zhong ZH, Zheng XF, Li M, Ichim TE, Chin JL, Min WP (2005) Tumor exosomes expressing Fas ligand mediate CD8(+) T-cell apoptosis. Blood Cells Mol Dis 35(2):169–173

Aguzzit A, Lakkaraju AKK (2016) Cell biology of prions and prionoids: a status report. Trends Cell Biol 26(1):40–51

Alvarez-Erviti L, Seow YQ, Yin HF, Betts C, Lakhal S, Wood MJA (2011) Delivery of siRNA to the mouse brain by systemic injection of targeted exosomes. Nat Biotechnol 29(4):341–345

Anderson HC (1969) Vesicles associated with calcification in matrix of epiphyseal cartilage. J Cell Biol 41(1):59

Appelqvist H, Nilsson C, Garner B, Brown AJ, Kagedal K, Ollinger K (2011) Attenuation of the lysosomal death pathway by lysosomal cholesterol accumulation. Am J Pathol 178(2):629–639

Arenz C, Gartner M, Wascholowski V, Giannis A (2001a) Synthesis and biochemical investigation of scyphostatin analogues as inhibitors of neutral sphingomyelinase. Bioorg Med Chem 9 (11):2901–2904

Arenz C, Thutewohl M, Block O, Waldmann H, Altenbach HJ, Giannis A (2001b) Manumycin A and its analogues are irreversible inhibitors of neutral sphingomyelinase. Chembiochem 2 (2):141–143

Asai H, Ikezu S, Tsunoda S, Medalla M, Luebke J, Haydar T, Wolozin B, Butovsky O, Kugler S, Ikezu T (2015) Depletion of microglia and inhibition of exosome synthesis halt tau propagation. Nat Neurosci 18(11):1584–1593

Baietti MF, Zhang Z, Mortier E, Melchior A, Degeest G, Geeraerts A, Ivarsson Y, Depoortere F, Coomans C, Vermeiren E, Zimmermann P, David G (2012) Syndecan-syntenin-ALIX regulates the biogenesis of exosomes. Nat Cell Biol 14(7):677–685

Baj-Krzyworzeka M, Szatanek R, Weglarczyk K, Baran J, Urbanowicz B, Branski P, Ratajczak MZ, Zembala M (2006) Tumour-derived microvesicles carry several surface determinants and mRNA of tumour cells and transfer some of these determinants to monocytes. Cancer Immunol Immunother 55(7):808–818

Banno Y, Ohguchi K, Matsumoto N, Koda M, Ueda M, Hara A, Dikic I, Nozawa Y (2005) Implication of phospholipase D2 in oxidant-induced phosphoinositide 3-kinase signaling via Pyk2 activation in PC12 cells. J Biol Chem 280(16):16319–16324

Blackwood RA, Smolen JE, Transue A, Hessler RJ, Harsh DM, Brower RC, French S (1997) Phospholipase D activity facilitates Ca2+-induced aggregation and fusion of complex liposomes. Am J Physiol Cell Physiol 272(4):C1279–C1285

Boye TL, Maeda K, Pezeshkian W, Sonder SL, Haeger SC, Gerke V, Simonsen AC, Nylandsted J (2017) Annexin A4 and A6 induce membrane curvature and constriction during cell membrane repair. Nat Commun 8:1623

Brouwers JF, Aalberts M, Jansen JWA, van Niel G, Wauben MH, Stout TAE, Helms JB, Stoorvogel W (2013) Distinct lipid compositions of two types of human prostasomes. Proteomics 13(10–11):1660–1666
Brugger B, Glass B, Haberkant P, Leibrecht I, Wieland FT, Krausslich HG (2006) The HIV lipidome: a raft with an unusual composition. Proc Natl Acad Sci U S A 103(8):2641–2646
Chen Q, Hongu T, Sato T, Zhang Y, Ali W, Cavallo JA, van der Velden A, Tian H, Di Paolo G, Nieswandt B, Kanaho Y, Frohman MA (2012) Key roles for the lipid signaling enzyme phospholipase D1 in the tumor microenvironment during tumor angiogenesis and metastasis. Sci Signal 5(249):ra79
Clayton A, Harris CL, Court J, Mason MD, Morgan BP (2003) Antigen-presenting cell exosomes are protected from complement-mediated lysis by expression of CD55 and CD59. Eur J Immunol 33(2):522–531
Colley WC, Sung TC, Roll R, Jenco J, Hammond SM, Altshuller Y, Bar-Sagi D, Morris AJ, Frohman MA (1997) Phospholipase D2, a distinct phospholipase D isoform with novel regulatory properties that provokes cytoskeletal reorganization. Curr Biol 7(3):191–201
Corcoran CA, He Q, Ponnusamy S, Ogretmen B, Huang Y, Sheikh MS (2008) Neutral sphingomyelinase-3 is a DNA damage and nongenotoxic stress-regulated gene that is deregulated in human malignancies. Mol Cancer Res 6(5):795–807
Costa-Silva B, Aiello NM, Ocean AJ, Singh S, Zhang HY, Thakur BK, Becker A, Hoshino A, Mark MT, Molina H, Xiang J, Zhang T, Theilen TM, Garcia-Santos G, Williams C, Ararso Y, Huang YJ, Rodrigues G, Shen TL, Labori KJ, Lothe IMB, Kure EH, Hernandez J, Doussot A, Ebbesen SH, Grandgenett PM, Hollingsworth MA, Jain M, Mallya K, Batra SK, Jarnagin WR, Schwartz RE, Matei I, Peinado H, Stanger BZ, Bromberg J, Lyden D (2015) Pancreatic cancer exosomes initiate pre-metastatic niche formation in the liver. Nat Cell Biol 17(6):816
Dang VD, Jella KK, Ragheb RRT, Denslow ND, Alli AA (2017) Lipidomic and proteomic analysis of exosomes from mouse cortical collecting duct cells. FASEB J 31(12):5399–5408
Datta A, Kim H, Lal M, McGee L, Johnson A, Moustafa AA, Jones JC, Mondal D, Ferrer M, Abdel-Mageed AB (2017) Manumycin A suppresses exosome biogenesis and secretion via targeted inhibition of Ras/Raf/ERK1/2 signaling and hnRNP H1 in castration-resistant prostate cancer cells. Cancer Lett 408:73–81
Dinkins MB, Enasko J, Hernandez C, Wang GH, Kong J, Helwa I, Liu YT, Terry AV, Bieberich E (2016) Neutral sphingomyelinase-2 deficiency ameliorates Alzheimer's disease pathology and improves cognition in the 5XFAD mouse. J Neurosci 36(33):8653–8667
Disse J, Vitale N, Bader MF, Gerke V (2009) Phospholipase D1 is specifically required for regulated secretion of von Willebrand factor from endothelial cells. Blood 113(4):973–980
Divecha N, Roefs M, Halstead JR, D'Andrea S, Fernandez-Borga M, Oomen L, Saqib KM, Wakelam MJO, D'Santos C (2000) Interaction of the type I alpha PIPkinase with phospholipase D: a role for the local generation of phosphatidylinositol 4,5-bisphosphate in the regulation of PLD2 activity. EMBO J 19(20):5440–5449
Egea-Jimenez AL, Gallardo R, Garcia-Pino A, Ivarsson Y, Wawrzyniak AM, Kashyap R, Loris R, Schymkowitz J, Rousseau F, Zimmermann P (2016) Frizzled 7 and PIP2 binding by syntenin PDZ2 domain supports Frizzled 7 trafficking and signalling. Nat Commun 7:12101
Elgner F, Ren H, Medvedev R, Ploen D, Himmelsbach K, Boller K, Hildt E (2016) The intracellular cholesterol transport inhibitor U18666A inhibits the exosome-dependent release of mature hepatitis C virus. J Virol 90(24):11181–11196
Esser J, Gehrmann U, D'Alexandri FL, Hidalgo-Estevez AM, Wheelock CE, Scheynius A, Gabrielsson S, Radmark O (2010) Exosomes from human macrophages and dendritic cells contain enzymes for leukotriene biosynthesis and promote granulocyte migration. J Allergy Clin Immunol 126(5):1032–1040
Fernandez-Borja M, Wubbolts R, Calafat J, Janssen H, Divecha N, Dusseljee S, Neefjes J (1999) Multivesicular body morphogenesis requires phosphatidylinositol 3-kinase activity. Curr Biol 9 (1):55–58

Fong MY, Zhou WY, Liu L, Alontaga AY, Chandra M, Ashby J, Chow A, O'Connor STF, Li SS, Chin AR, Somlo G, Palomares M, Li Z, Tremblay JR, Tsuyada A, Sun GQ, Reid MA, Wu XW, Swiderski P, Ren XB, Shi YH, Kong M, Zhong WW, Chen Y, Wang SE (2015) Breast- cancer-secreted miR-122 reprograms glucose metabolism in premetastatic niche to promote metastasis. Nat Cell Biol 17(2):183

Frohman MA (2015) The phospholipase D superfamily as therapeutic targets. Trends Pharmacol Sci 36(3):137–144

Fruman DA, Meyers RE, Cantley LC (1998) Phosphoinositide kinases. Annu Rev Biochem 67:481–507

Ganesan R, Mahankali M, Alter G, Gomez-Cambronero J (2015) Two sites of action for PLD2 inhibitors: the enzyme catalytic center and an allosteric, phosphoinositide biding pocket. BBA-Mol Cell Biol L 1851(3):261–272

Gangoda L, Mathivanan S (2016) Cortactin enhances exosome secretion without altering cargo. J Cell Biol 214(2):129–131

George JN, Thoi LL, McManus LM, Reimann TA (1982) Isolation of human-platelet membrane microparticles from plasma and serum. Blood 60(4):834–840

Ghossoub R, Lembo F, Rubio A, Gaillard CB, Bouchet J, Vitale N, Slavik J, Machala M, Zimmermann P (2014) Syntenin-ALIX exosome biogenesis and budding into multivesicular bodies are controlled by ARF6 and PLD2. Nat Commun 5:3477

Gillooly DJ, Morrow IC, Lindsay M, Gould R, Bryant NJ, Gaullier JM, Parton RG, Stenmark H (2000) Localization of phosphatidylinositol 3-phosphate in yeast and mammalian cells. EMBO J 19(17):4577–4588

Grigorov B, Arcanger F, Roingeard P, Darlix JL, Muriaux D (2006) Assembly of infectious HIV-1 in human epithelial and T-lymphoblastic cell lines. J Mol Biol 359(4):848–862

Gulbins E, Kolesnick R (2003) Raft ceramide in molecular medicine. Oncogene 22(45):7070–7077

Guo BB, Bellingham SA, Hill AF (2015) The neutral Sphingomyelinase pathway regulates packaging of the prion protein into exosomes. J Biol Chem 290(6):3455–3467

Haney MJ, Klyachko NL, Zhaoa YL, Gupta R, Plotnikova EG, He ZJ, Patel T, Piroyan A, Sokolsky M, Kabanov AV, Batrakova EV (2015) Exosomes as drug delivery vehicles for Parkinson's disease therapy. J Control Release 207:18–30

Hannun YA, Obeid LM (2017) Sphingolipids and their metabolism in physiology and disease. Nat Rev Mol Cell Biol 19:175–191

Hanson PI, Cashikar A (2012) Multivesicular body morphogenesis. Annu Rev Cell Dev Biol 28 (28):337–362

Harding C, Heuser J, Stahl P (1983) Receptor-mediated endocytosis of transferrin and recycling of the transferrin receptor in rat reticulocytes. J Cell Biol 97(2):329–339

Hay JC (2007) Calcium: a fundamental regulator of intracellular membrane fusion? EMBO Rep 8 (3):236–240

Hayakawa M, Kaizawa H, Moritomo H, Koizumi T, Ohishi T, Okada M, Ohta M, Tsukamoto S, Parker P, Workman P, Waterfield M (2006) Synthesis and biological evaluation of 4-morpholino-2-phenylquinazolines and related derivatives as novel PI3 kinase p110 alpha inhibitors. Bioorg Med Chem 14(20):6847–6858

Henkels KM, Peng HJ, Frondorf K, Gomez-Cambronero J (2010) A comprehensive model that explains the regulation of phospholipase D2 activity by phosphorylation-dephosphorylation. Mol Cell Biol 30(9):2251–2263

Henkels KM, Muppani NR, Gomez-Cambronero J (2016) PLD-specific small-molecule inhibitors decrease tumor-associated macrophages and neutrophils infiltration in breast tumors and lung and liver metastases. PLoS One 11(11):e0166553

Henne WM, Buchkovich NJ, Emr SD (2011) The ESCRT pathway. Dev Cell 21(1):77–91

Hergenreider E, Heydt S, Treguer K, Boettger T, Horrevoets AJG, Zeiher AM, Scheffer MP, Frangakis AS, Yin XK, Mayr M, Braun T, Urbich C, Boon RA, Dimmeler S (2012) Atheroprotective communication between endothelial cells and smooth muscle cells through miRNAs. Nat Cell Biol 14(3):249

Hessvik NP, verbye A, Brech A, Torgersen ML, Jakobsen IS, Sandvig K, Llorente A (2016) PIKfyve inhibition increases exosome release and induces secretory autophagy. Cell Mol Life Sci 73(24):4717–4737

Hofmann K, Tomiuk S, Wolff G, Stoffel W (2000) Cloning and characterization of the mammalian brain-specific, Mg2+-dependent neutral sphingomyelinase. Proc Natl Acad Sci U S A 97 (11):5895–5900

Holopainen JM, Subramanian M, Kinnunen PKJ (1998) Sphingomyelinase induces lipid microdomain formation in a fluid phosphatidylcholine/sphingomyelin membrane. Biochemistry 37(50) 17562–17570

Honda A, Nogami M, Yokozeki T, Yamazaki M, Nakamura H, Watanabe H, Kawamoto K, Nakayama K, Morris AJ, Frohman MA, Kanaho Y (1999) Phosphatidylinositol 4-phosphate 5 kinase alpha is a downstream effector of the small G protein ARF6 in membrane ruffle formation. Cell 99(5):521–532

Huang H, Gao Q, Peng X, Choi SY, Sarma K, Ren H, Morris AJ, Frohman MA (2011) piRNA-associated germline nuage formation and spermatogenesis require MitoPLD profusogenic mitochondrial-surface lipid signaling. Dev Cell 20(3):376–387

Hunter MP, Ismail N, Zhang XL, Aguda BD, Lee EJ, Yu LB, Xiao T, Schafer J, Lee MLT, Schmittgen TD, Nana-Sinkam SP, Jarjoura D, Marsh CB (2008) Detection of microRNA expression in human peripheral blood microvesicles. PLoS One 3(11):e3694

Hurley JH, Boura E, Carlson L-A, Rozycki B (2010) Membrane budding. Cell 143(6):875–887

Imjeti NS, Menck K, Egea-Jimenez AL, Lecointre C, Lembo F, Bouguenina H, Badache A, Ghossoub R, David G, Roche S, Zimmermann P (2017) Syntenin mediates SRC function in exosomal cell-to-cell communication. Proc Natl Acad Sci U S A 114(47):12495–12500

Itoh T, Hasegawa J, Tsujita K, Kanaho Y, Takenawa T (2009) The tyrosine kinase Fer is a downstream target of the PLD-PA pathway that regulates cell migration. Sci Signal 2(87):ra52

Jackle S, Beisiegel U, Rinninger F, Buck F, Grigoleit A, Block A, Groger I, Greten H, Windler E (1994) Annexin-VI, a marker protein of hepatocytic endosomes. J Biol Chem 269 (2):1026–1032

Janas T, Janas MM, Sapon K (2015) Mechanisms of RNA loading into exosomes. FEBS Lett 589 (13):1391–1398

Jefferies HBJ, Cooke FT, Jat P, Boucheron C, Koizumi T, Hayakawa M, Kaizawa H, Ohishi T, Workman P, Waterfield MD, Parker PJ (2008) A selective PIKfyve inhibitor blocks PtdIns(3,5) P(2) production and disrupts endomembrane transport and retroviral budding. EMBO Rep 9 (2):164–170

Jiang H, Lu ZM, Luo JQ, Wolfman A, Foster DA (1995) Ras mediates the activation of phospholipase-D by v-Src. J Biol Chem 270(11):6006–6009

Jung SY, Suh JH, Park HJ, Jung KM, Kim MY, Na DS, Kim DK (2000) Identification of multiple forms of membrane-associated neutral sphingomyelinase in bovine brain. J Neurochem 75 (3):1004–1014

Kai K, Dittmar RL, Sen S (2017) Secretory microRNAs as biomarkers of cancer. Semin Cell Dev Biol 78:22–36

Kakazu E, Mauer AS, Yin M, Malhi H (2016) Hepatocytes release ceramide-enriched pro-inflammatory extracellular vesicles in an IRE1 alpha-dependent manner. J Lipid Res 57 (2):233–245

Kavaliauskiene S, Nymark CM, Bergan J, Simm R, Sylvanne T, Simolin H, Ekroos K, Skotland T, Sandvig K (2014) Cell density-induced changes in lipid composition and intracellular trafficking. Cell Mol Life Sci 71(6):1097–1116

Kirkegaard T, Roth AG, Petersen NHT, Mahalka AK, Olsen OD, Moilanen I, Zylicz A, Knudsen J, Sandhoff K, Arenz C, Kinnunen PKJ, Nylandsted J, Jaattela M (2010) Hsp70 stabilizes lysosomes and reverts Niemann-Pick disease-associated lysosomal pathology. Nature 463 (7280) 549–553

Kitatani K, Idkowiak-Baldys J, Hannun YA (2008) The sphingolipid salvage pathway in ceramide metabolism and signaling. Cell Signal 20(6):1010–1018

Kobayashi M, Kanfer JN (1987) Phosphatidylethanol formation via transphosphatidylation by rat brain synaptosomal phospholipase D. J Neurochem 48(5):1597–1603
Kobayashi T, Stang E, Fang KS, de Moerloose P, Parton RG, Gruenberg J (1998) A lipid associated with the antiphospholipid syndrome regulates endosome structure and function. Nature 392 (6672):193–197
Kooijman EE, Testerink C (2010) Phosphatidic acid: an electrostatic/hydrogen-bond switch? Lipid Signal Plants 16:203–222
Kooijman EE, Chupin V, de Kruijff B, Burger KNJ (2003) Modulation of membrane curvature by phosphatidic acid and lysophosphatidic acid. Traffic 4(3):162–174
Kooijman EE, Chupin V, Fuller NL, Kozlov MM, de Kruijff B, Burger KNJ, Rand PR (2005) Spontaneous curvature of phosphatidic acid and lysophosphatidic acid. Biochemistry 44 (6):2097–2102
Kooijman EE, Tieleman DP, Testerink C, Munnik T, Rijkers DTS, Burger KNJ, de Kruijff B (2007) An electrostatic/hydrogen bond switch as the basis for the specific interaction of phosphatidic acid with proteins. J Biol Chem 282(15):11356–11364
Kosaka N, Iguchi H, Yoshioka Y, Takeshita F, Matsuki Y, Ochiya T (2010) Secretory mechanisms and intercellular transfer of MicroRNAs in living cells. J Biol Chem 285(23):17442–17452
Kowal J, Tkach M, Thery C (2014) Biogenesis and secretion of exosomes. Curr Opin Cell Biol 29:116–125
Krut O, Wiegmann K, Kashkar H, Yazdanpanah B, Kronke M (2006) Novel tumor necrosis factor-responsive mammalian neutral sphingomyelinase-3 is a C-tail-anchored protein. J Biol Chem 281(19):13784–13793
Laulagnier K, Grand D, Dujardin A, Hamdi S, Vincent-Schneider H, Lankar D, Salles JP, Bonnerot C, Perret B, Record M (2004a) PLD2 is enriched on exosomes and its activity is correlated to the release of exosomes. FEBS Lett 572(1–3):11–14
Laulagnier K, Motta C, Hamdi S, Roy S, Fauvelle F, Pageaux JF, Kobayashi T, Salles JP, Perret B, Bonnerot C, Record M (2004b) Mast cell- and dendritic cell-derived exosomes display a specific lipid composition and an unusual membrane organization. Biochem J 380:161–171
Lee C, Mitsialis SA, Aslam M, Vitali SH, Vergadi E, Konstantinou G, Sdrimas K, Fernandez-Gonzalez A, Kourembanas S (2012) Exosomes mediate the cytoprotective action of mesenchymal stromal cells on hypoxia-induced pulmonary hypertension. Circulation 126(22):2601
Leevers SJ, Vanhaesebroeck B, Waterfield MD (1999) Signalling through phosphoinositide 3-kinases: the lipids take centre stage. Curr Opin Cell Biol 11(2):219–225
Lehman N, Ledford B, di Fulvio M, Frondorf K, McPhail LC, Gomez-Cambronero J (2007) Phospholipase D2-derived phosphatidic acid binds to and activates ribosomal p70 S6 kinase independently of mTOR. FASEB J 21(4):1075–1087
Li AC, Zhang TB, Zheng M, Liu YN, Chen Z (2017) Exosomal proteins as potential markers of tumor diagnosis. J Hematol Oncol 10:175
Lindwasser OW, Resh MD (2004) Human immunodeficiency virus type 1 Gag contains a dileucine-like motif that regulates association with multivesicular bodies. J Virol 78(11):6013–6023
Lizarbe MA, Barrasa JI, Olmo N, Gavilanes F, Turnay J (2013) Annexin-phospholipid interactions. Functional implications. Int J Mol Sci 14(2):2652–2683
Llorente A, van Deurs B, Sandvig K (2007) Cholesterol regulates prostasome release from secretory lysosomes in PC-3 human prostate cancer cells. Eur J Cell Biol 86(7):405–415
Llorente A, Skotland T, Sylvanne T, Kauhanen D, Rog T, Orlowski A, Vattulainen I, Ekroos K, Sandvig K (2013) Molecular lipidomics of exosomes released by PC-3 prostate cancer cells. BBA-Mol Cell Biol L 1831(7):1302–1309
Lotvall J, Hill AF, Hochberg F, Buzas EI, Di Vizio D, Gardiner C, Gho YS, Kurochkin IV, Mathivanan S, Quesenberry P, Sahoo S, Tahara H, Wauben MH, Witwer KW, Thery C (2014) Minimal experimental requirements for definition of extracellular vesicles and their functions: a position statement from the International Society for Extracellular Vesicles. J Extracell Vesicles 3:26913–26913

Luberto C, Hassler DF, Signorelli P, Okamoto Y, Sawai H, Boros E, Hazen-Martin DJ, Obeid LM, Hannun YA, Smith GK (2002) Inhibition of tumor necrosis factor-induced cell death in MCF7 by a novel inhibitor of neutral sphingomyelinase. J Biol Chem 277(43):41128–41139

Lukic A, Ji J, Idborg H, Samuelsson B, Palmberg L, Gabrielsson S, Radmark O (2016) Pulmonary epithelial cancer cells and their exosomes metabolize myeloid cell-derived leukotriene C-4 to leukotriene D-4. J Lipid Res 57(9):1659–1669

Marchesini N, Luberto C, Hannun YA (2003) Biochemical properties of mammalian neutral sphingomyelinase 2 and its role in sphingolipid metabolism. J Biol Chem 278(16):13775–13783

Marchini-Alves CMM, Lorenzi VCB, da Silva EZM, Mazucato VM, Jamur MC, Oliver C (2015) Phospholipase D2 modulates the secretory pathway in RBL-2H3 mast cells. PLoS One 10(10): e0139888

Matsuo H, Chevallier J, Mayran N, Le Blanc I, Ferguson C, Faure J, Blanc NS, Matile S, Dubochet J, Sadoul R, Parton RG, Vilbois F, Gruenberg J (2004) Role of LBPA and Alix in multivesicular liposome formation and endosome organization. Science 303(5657):531–534

McCullough J, Clippinger AK, Talledge N, Skowyra ML, Saunders MG, Naismith TV, Colf LA, Afonine P, Arthur C, Sundquist WI, Hanson PI, Frost A (2015) Structure and membrane remodeling activity of ESCRT-III helical polymers. Science 350(6267):1548–1551

McEwen RK, Dove SK, Cooke FT, Painter GF, Holmes AB, Shisheva A, Ohya Y, Parker PJ, Michell RH (1999) Complementation analysis in PtdInsP kinase-deficient yeast mutants demonstrates that Schizosaccharomyces pombe and murine Fab1p homologues are phosphatidylinositol 3-phosphate 5-kinases. J Biol Chem 274(48):33905–33912

Meehan K, Vella LJ (2016) The contribution of tumour-derived exosomes to the hallmarks of cancer. Crit Rev Clin Lab Sci 53(2):121–131

Milhas D, Clarke CJ, Idkowiak-Baldys J, Canals D, Hannun YA (2010) Anterograde and retrograde transport of neutral sphingomyelinase-2 between the Golgi and the plasma membrane. BBA-Mol Cell Biol L 1801(12):1361–1374

Mittelbrunn M, Gutiérrez-Vázquez C, Villarroya-Beltri C, González S, Sánchez-Cabo F, González M, Bernad A, Sánchez-Madrid F (2011) Unidirectional transfer of microRNA-loaded exosomes from T cells to antigen-presenting cells. Nat Commun 2:282

Monovich L, Mugrage B, Quadros E, Toscano K, Tommasi R, LaVoie S, Liu E, Du ZM, LaSala D, Boyar W, Steed P (2007) Optimization of halopemide for phospholipase D2 inhibition. Bioorg Med Chem Lett 17(8):2310–2311

Morozova K, Clement CC, Kaushik S, Stiller B, Arias E, Ahmad A, Rauch JN, Chatterjee V, Melis C, Scharf B, Gestwicki JE, Cuervo AM, Zuiderweg ERP, Santambrogio L (2016) Structural and biological interaction of hsc-70 protein with phosphatidylserine in endosomal microautophagy. J Biol Chem 291(35):18096–18106

Mu W, Rana S, Zoller M (2013) Host matrix modulation by tumor exosomes promotes motility and invasiveness. Neoplasia 15(8):875

Munnik T, Arisz SA, deVrije T, Musgrave A (1995) G protein activation stimulates phospholipase D signaling in plants. Plant Cell 7(12):2197–2210

Pan BT, Johnstone RM (1983) Fate of the transferrin receptor during maturation of sheep reticulocytes in vitro - selective externalization of the receptor. Cell 33(3):967–977

Peinado H, Aleckovic M, Lavotshkin S, Matei I, Costa-Silva B, Moreno-Bueno G, Hergueta-Redondo M, Williams C, Garcia-Santos G, Ghajar CM, Nitadori-Hoshino A, Hoffman C, Badal K, Garcia BA, Callahan MK, Yuan JD, Martins VR, Skog J, Kaplan RN, Brady MS, Wolchok JD, Chapman PB, Kang YB, Bromberg J, Lyden D (2012) Melanoma exosomes educate bone marrow progenitor cells toward a pro-metastatic phenotype through MET. Nat Med 18(6):883

Peng Q, Zhang S, Yang Q, Zhang T, Wei XQ, Jiang L, Zhang CL, Chen QM, Zhang ZR, Lin YF (2013) Preformed albumin corona, a protective coating for nanoparticles based drug delivery system. Biomaterials 34(33):8521–8530

Perry DK (2002) Serine palmitoyltransferase: role in apoptotic de novo ceramide synthesis and other stress responses. BBA-Mol Cell Biol L 1585(2–3):146–152

Phuyal S, Hessvik NP, Skotland T, Sandvig K, Llorente A (2014) Regulation of exosome release by glycosphingolipids and flotillins. FEBS J 281(9):2214–2227

Pomorski T, Holthuis JCM, Herrmann A, van Meer G (2004) Tracking down lipid flippases and their biological functions. J Cell Sci 117(6):805–813

Raiborg C, Stenmark H (2009) The ESCRT machinery in endosomal sorting of ubiquitylated membrane proteins. Nature 458(7237):445–452

Rajagopalan V, Canals D, Luberto C, Snider J, Voelkel-Johnson C, Obeid LM, Hannun YA (2015) Critical determinants of mitochondria-associated neutral sphingomyelinase (MA-nSMase) for mitochondrial localization. BBA-Gen Subjects 1850(4):628–639

Rajendran L, Bali J, Barr MM, Court FA, Kramer-Albers EM, Picou F, Raposo G, van der Vos KE, van Nie G, Wang J, Breakefield XO (2014) Emerging roles of extracellular vesicles in the nervous system. J Neurosci 34(46):15482–15489

Raposo G, Nijman HW, Stoorvogel W, Leijendekker R, Harding CV, Melief CJM, Geuze HJ (1996) B lymphocytes secrete antigen-presenting vesicles. J Exp Med 183(3):1161–1172

Roucourt B, Meeussen S, Bao J, Zimmermann P, David G (2015) Heparanase activates the syndecan-syntenin-ALIX exosome pathway. Cell Res 25(4):412–428

Ruivo CF, Adem B, Silva M, Melo SA (2017) The biology of cancer exosomes: insights and new perspectives. Cancer Res 77(23):6480–6488

Salimu J, Webber J, Gurney M, Al-Taei S, Clayton A, Tabi Z (2017) Dominant immunosuppression of dendritic cell function by prostate-cancer-derived exosomes. J Extracell Vesicles 6 (1):1368823

Saman S, Kim W, Raya M, Visnick Y, Miro S, Jackson B, McKee AC, Alvarez VE, Lee NCY, Hall GF (2012) Exosome-associated tau is secreted in tauopathy models and is selectively phosphorylated in cerebrospinal fluid in early Alzheimer disease. J Biol Chem 287 (6):3842–3849

Sawai H, Domae N, Nagan N, Hannun YA (1999) Function of the cloned putative neutral sphingomyelinase as lyso-platelet activating factor-phospholipase C. J Biol Chem 274 (53):38131–38139

Schu PV, Takegawa K, Fry MJ, Stack JH, Waterfield MD, Emr SD (1993) Phosphatidylinositol 3-kinase encoded by yeast VPS34 gene essential for protein sorting. Science 260(5104):88–91

Scott SA, Selvy PE, Buck JR, Cho HP, Criswell TL, Thomas AL, Armstrong MD, Arteaga CL, Lindsley CW, Brown HA (2009) Design of isoform-selective phospholipase D inhibitors that modulate cancer cell invasiveness. Nat Chem Biol 5(2):108–117

Shi YH, Wang W, Yang BZ, Tian HG (2017) ATF1 and RAS in exosomes are potential clinical diagnostic markers for cervical cancer. Cell Biochem Funct 35(7):477–483

Shisheva A (2001) PIKfyve: the road to PtdIns 5-P and PtdIns 3,5-P-2. Cell Biol Int 25 (12):1201–1206

Shisheva A, Rusin B, Ikonomov OC, DeMarco C, Sbrissa D (2001) Localization and insulin-regulated relocation of phosphoinositide 5-kinase PIKfyve in 3T3-L1 adipocytes. J Biol Chem 276(15):11859–11869

Singh R, Pochampally R, Watabe K, Lu ZH, Mo YY (2014) Exosome-mediated transfer of miR-10b promotes cell invasion in breast cancer. Mol Cancer 13:256

Sinha S, Hoshino D, Hong NH, Kirkbride KC, Grega-Larson NE, Seiki M, Tyska MJ, Weaver AM (2016) Cortactin promotes exosome secretion by controlling branched actin dynamics. J Cell Biol 214(2):197–213

Skog J, Wurdinger T, van Rijn S, Meijer DH, Gainche L, Sena-Esteves M, Curry WT, Carter BS, Krichevsky AM, Breakefield XO (2008) Glioblastoma microvesicles transport RNA and proteins that promote tumour growth and provide diagnostic biomarkers. Nat Cell Biol 10 (12):1470–1476

Skotland T, Sandvig K, Llorente A (2017) Lipids in exosomes: current knowledge and the way forward. Prog Lipid Res 66:30–41

Sokol J, Blanchettemackie EJ, Kruth HS, Dwyer NK, Amende LM, Butler JD, Robinson E, Patel S, Brady RO, Comly ME, Vanier MT, Pentchev PG (1988) Type-C Niemann-Pick disease – Lysosomal accumulation and defective intracellular mobilization of low-density lipoprotein cholesterol. J Biol Chem 263(7):3411–3417

Stace CL, Ktistakis NT (2006) Phosphatidic acid- and phosphatidylserine-binding proteins. Biochim Biophys Acta 1761(8):913–926

Stegner D, Thielmann I, Kraft P, Frohman MA, Stoll G, Nieswandt B (2013) Pharmacological inhibition of phospholipase D protects mice from occlusive thrombus formation and ischemic stroke--brief report. Arterioscler Thromb Vasc Biol 33(9):2212–2217

Stith BJ (2015) Phospholipase C and D regulation of Src, calcium release and membrane fusion during *Xenopus laevis* development. Dev Biol 401(2):188–205

Stoffel W (1999) Functional analysis of acid and neutral sphingomyelinases in vitro and in vivo. Chem Phys Lipids 102(1–2):107–121

Stoll LL, Spector AA (1984) Changes in serum influence the fatty-acid composition of established cell-lines. In Vitro 20(9):732–738

Strauss K, Goebel C, Runz H, Mobius W, Weiss S, Feussner I, Simons M, Schneider A (2010) Exosome secretion ameliorates lysosomal storage of cholesterol in Niemann-Pick type C disease. J Biol Chem 285(34):26279–26288

Su W, Yeku O, Olepu S, Genna A, Park JS, Ren HM, Du G, Gelb MH, Morris AJ, Frohman MA (2009) 5-Fluoro-2-indolyl des-chlorohalopemide (FIPI), a phospholipase D pharmacological inhibitor that alters cell spreading and inhibits chemotaxis. Mol Pharmacol 75(3):437–446

Subra C, Grand D, Laulagnier K, Stella A, Lambeau G, Paillasse M, De Medina P, Monsarrat B, Perret B, Silvente-Poirot S, Poirot M, Record M (2010) Exosomes account for vesicle-mediated transcellular transport of activatable phospholipases and prostaglandins. J Lipid Res 51 (8):2105–2120

Tani H, Shiokawa M, Kaname Y, Kambara H, Mori Y, Abe T, Moriishi K, Matsuura Y (2010) Involvement of ceramide in the propagation of Japanese encephalitis virus. J Virol 84 (6):2798–2807

Théry C, Amigorena S, Raposo G, Clayton A (2006) Isolation and characterization of exosomes from cell culture supernatants and biological fluids. Curr Protoc Cell Biol 30:3–22

Tomiuk S, Zumbansen M, Stoffel W (2000) Characterization and subcellular localization of murine and human magnesium-dependent neutral sphingomyelinase. J Biol Chem 275(8):5710–5717

Trajkovic K, Hsu C, Chiantia S, Rajendran L, Wenzel D, Wieland F, Schwille P, Bruegger B, Simons M (2008) Ceramide triggers budding of exosome vesicles into multivesicular endosomes. Science 319(5867):1244–1247

Trams EG, Lauter CJ, Salem N, Heine U (1981) Exfoliation of membrane ecto- enzymes in the form of micro-vesicles. Biochim Biophys Acta 645(1):63–70

Turturici G, Tinnirello R, Sconzo G, Geraci F (2014) Extracellular membrane vesicles as a mechanism of cell-to-cell communication: advantages and disadvantages. Am J Physiol Cell Physiol 306(7):C621–C633

Valadi H, Ekstrom K, Bossios A, Sjostrand M, Lee JJ, Lotvall JO (2007) Exosome-mediated transfer of mRNAs and microRNAs is a novel mechanism of genetic exchange between cells. Nat Cell Biol 9(6):654–659

van den Boorn JG, Schlee M, Coch C, Hartmann G (2011) SiRNA delivery with exosome nanoparticles. Nat Biotechnol 29(4):325–326

van Meer G, Voelker DR, Feigenson GW (2008) Membrane lipids: where they are and how they behave. Nat Rev Mol Cell Biol 9(2):112–124

van Niel G, Charrin S, Simoes S, Romao M, Rochin L, Saftig P, Marks MS, Rubinstein E, Raposo G (2011) The tetraspanin CD63 regulates ESCRT-independent and -dependent endosomal sorting during melanogenesis. Dev Cell 21(4):708–721

Vance DE, van den Bosch H (2000) Cholesterol in the year 2000. BBA-Mol Cell Biol L 1529 (1–3):1–8
Vanhaesebroeck B, Leevers SJ, Ahmadi K, Timms J, Katso R, Driscoll PC, Woscholski R, Parker PJ, Waterfield MD (2001) Synthesis and function of 3-phosphorylated inositol lipids. Annu Rev Biochem 70:535–602
Villarroya-Beltri C, Gutierrez-Vazquez C, Sanchez-Cabo F, Perez-Hernandez D, Vazquez J, Martin-Cofreces N, Martinez-Herrera DJ, Pascual-Montano A, Mittelbrunn M, Sanchez-Madrid F (2013) Sumoylated hnRNPA2B1 controls the sorting of miRNAs into exosomes through binding to specific motifs. Nat Commun 4:2980
Vitale N, Caumont AS, Chasserot-Golaz S, Du G, Wu S, Sciorra VA, Morris AJ, Frohman MA, Bader MF (2001) Phospholipase D1: a key factor for the exocytotic machinery in neuroendocrine cells. EMBO J 20(10):2424–2434
Voelker DR (1991) Organelle biogenesis and intracellular lipid transport in eukaryotes. Microbiol Rev 55(4):543–560
Wang Y, Balaji V, Kaniyappan S, Kruger L, Irsen S, Tepper K, Chandupatla R, Maetzler W, Schneider A, Mandelkow E, Mandelkow EM (2017a) The release and trans-synaptic transmission of tau via exosomes. Mol Neurodegener 12:5
Wang Z, Zhang F, He J, Wu P, Tay LWR, Cai M, Nian W, Weng Y, Qin L, Chang JT, McIntire LB, di Paolo G, Xu J, Peng J, Du G (2017b) Binding of PLD2-generated phosphatidic acid to KIF5B promotes MT1-MMP surface trafficking and lung metastasis of mouse breast cancer cells. Dev Cell 43(2):186–197
Waselle L, Gerona RRL, Vitale N, Martin TFJ, Bader MF, Regazzi R (2005) Role of phosphoinositide signaling in the control of insulin exocytosis. Mol Endocrinol 19(12):3097–3106
Welti R, Li WQ, Li MY, Sang YM, Biesiada H, Zhou HE, Rajashekar CB, Williams TD, Wang XM (2002) Profiling membrane lipids in plant stress responses - role of phospholipase D alpha in freezing-induced lipid changes in Arabidopsis. J Biol Chem 277(35):31994–32002
Whitham M, Parker BL, Friedrichsen M, Hingst JR, Hjorth M, Hughes WE, Egan CL, Cron L, Watt KI, Kuchel RP, Jayasooriah N, Estevez E, Petzold T, Suter CM, Gregorevic P, Kiens B, Richter EA, James DE, Wojtaszewski JFP, Febbraio MA (2018) Extracellular vesicles provide a means for tissue crosstalk during exercise. Cell Metab 27(1):237–251.e4
Whitley P, Reaves BJ, Hashimoto M, Riley AM, Potter BVL, Holman GD (2003) Identification of mammalian Vps24p as an effector of phosphatidylinositol 3,5-bisphosphate- dependent endosome compartmentalization. J Biol Chem 278(40):38786–38795
Wu BX, Clarke CJ, Hannun YA (2010a) Mammalian neutral sphingomyelinases: regulation and roles in cell signaling responses. Neuromolecular Med 12(4):320–330
Wu BX, Rajagopalan V, Roddy PL, Clarke CJ, Hannun YA (2010b) Identification and characterization of murine mitochondria-associated neutral sphingomyelinase (MA-nSMase), the mammalian sphingomyelin phosphodiesterase 5. J Biol Chem 285(23):17993–18002
Wu BX, Clarke CJ, Matmati N, Montefusco D, Bartke N, Hannun YA (2011) Identification of novel anionic phospholipid binding domains in neutral sphingomyelinase 2 with selective binding preference. J Biol Chem 286(25):22362–22371
Wubbolts R, Leckie RS, Veenhuizen PTM, Schwarzmann G, Mobius W, Hoernschemeyer J, Slot JW, Geuze HJ, Stoorvogel W (2003) Proteomic and biochemical analyses of human B cell-derived exosomes - potential implications for their function and multivesicular body formation. J Biol Chem 278(13):10963–10972
Xiang XY, Poliakov A, Liu C, Liu YL, Deng ZB, Wang JH, Cheng ZQ, Shah SV, Wang GJ, Zhang LM, Grizzle WE, Mobley J, Zhang HG (2009) Induction of myeloid-derived suppressor cells by tumor exosomes. Int J Cancer 124(11):2621–2633
Yang JL, Zhang XF, Chen XJ, Wang L, Yang GD (2017) Exosome mediated delivery of miR-124 promotes neurogenesis after ischemia. Mol Ther Nucl Acids 7:278–287
Yuyama K, Sun H, Mitsutake S, Igarashi Y (2012) Sphingolipid-modulated exosome secretion promotes clearance of amyloid-beta by microglia. J Biol Chem 287(14):10977–10989

Zhou WY, Fong MY, Min YF, Somlo G, Liu L, Palomares MR, Yu Y, Chow A, O'Connor STF, Chin AR, Yen Y, Wang YF, Marcusson EG, Chu PG, Wu J, Wu XW, Li AX, Li Z, Gao HL, Ren XB, Boldin MP, Lin PC, Wang SE (2014) Cancer-secreted miR-105 destroys vascular endothelial barriers to promote metastasis. Cancer Cell 25(4):501–515

Zimmermann P, Zhang Z, Degeest G, Mortier E, Leenaerts I, Coomans C, Schulz J, N'Kuli F, Courtoy PJ, David G (2005) Syndecan recycling is controlled by syntenin-PIP2 interaction and Arf6. 9:377–388. Dev Cell 9(5):721

The manufacturer's authorised representative in the EU is Springer Nature Customer Service Centre GmbH, Europaplatz 3, 69115 Heidelberg, Germany. If you have any concerns regarding our products, please contact ProductSafety@springernature.com

Printed and bound by CPI Group (UK) Ltd, Croydon, CR0 4YY
05/10/2026
02228123-0012